Environmental
Health Risk III

WITPRESS

WIT Press publishes leading books in Science and Technology.
Visit our website for new and current list of titles.
www.witpress.com

WITeLibrary

Home of the Transactions of the Wessex Institute.
Papers presented at Environmental Health Risk III are archived in the
WIT eLibrary in volume 9 of WIT Transactions on
Biomedicine and Health (ISSN 1743-3525).

The WIT eLibrary provides the international scientific community with immediate and
permanent access to individual papers presented at WIT conferences.
http://library.witpress.com

Computational Bioengineering

THIRD INTERNATIONAL CONFERENCE ON
THE IMPACT OF ENVIRONMENTAL FACTORS ON HEALTH

ENVIRONMENTAL HEALTH RISK III

CONFERENCE CHAIRMEN

C.A. Brebbia
Wessex Institute of Technology, UK

V. Popov
Wessex Institute of Technology, UK

D. Fayzieva
Academy of Sciences, Uzbekistan

INTERNATIONAL SCIENTIFIC ADVISORY COMMITTEE

D. Adang
D.M. Bonotto
F. Garzia
O. Herbarth
G. Passerini
F. Russo

SPONSORED BY:

WIT Transactions on Biomedicine and Health

Environmental Health Risk III

Editors

C.A. Brebbia
Wessex Institute of Technology, UK

V. Popov
Wessex Institute of Technology, UK

D. Fayzieva
Academy of Sciences, Uzbekistan

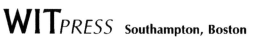

C.A. Brebbia
Wessex Institute of Technology, UK

V. Popov
Wessex Institute of Technology, UK

D. Fayzieva
Academy of Sciences, Uzbekistan

Published by

WIT Press
Ashurst Lodge, Ashurst, Southampton, SO40 7AA, UK
Tel: 44 (0) 238 029 3223; Fax: 44 (0) 238 029 2853
E-Mail: witpress@witpress.com
http://www.witpress.com

For USA, Canada and Mexico

Computational Mechanics Inc
25 Bridge Street, Billerica, MA 01821, USA
Tel: 978 667 5841; Fax: 978 667 7582
E-Mail: infousa@witpress.com
http://www.witpress.com

British Library Cataloguing-in-Publication Data

A Catalogue record for this book is available
from the British Library

ISBN: 1-84564-026-8
ISSN: 1747-4485 (print)
ISSN: 1743-3525 (on-line)

*The texts of the papers in this volume were set
individually by the authors or under their supervision.
Only minor corrections to the text may have been carried
out by the publisher.*

PREFACE

The efforts of our modern civilization to create an environment which would match human aspirations have two sides, one is the success story of constant improvements of our lifestyle and the other the increased risks to human health due to deterioration of the environment. It is questionable whether there is any part of nature that has been left unaffected due to human activities. In most cases, the closer we get to high density urban settlements, the higher the health risks due to air pollution, traffic, radiation fields, noise, and many other factors. Yet, almost all of us have to accept this way of life with the commodities that they offer and the health risks that they create.

This situation has motivated many scientists throughout the world to analyze the environmental factors that can affect our health and to calculate the levels of risk. Risks that are found to be unacceptably high require immediate action. However, it is not always straightforward to estimate all possible scenarios such as combined risks due to several factors, like for example various man-made chemicals in the environment and much more research is needed.

This book comprises the edited version of papers presented at the Third International Conference on the Impact of Environmental Factors on Health, which took place in Bologna, Italy. The conference provided a forum for the dissemination and exchange of information for the interrelation between environmental risk and health which is often complex and can involve a variety of social, occupational and lifestyle factors that emphasizes the importance of considering an interdisciplinary approach.

The book contains a series of papers dealing with some of the most recent developments in the field of Environmental Health, which are arranged in the following sessions:

- Risk analysis
- Air pollution
- Food contamination
- Occupational health
- Water quality issues
- Electromagnetic fields
- Housing and health
- Remediation
- Social and economic issues

The organizers are grateful to all the participants for having contributed to the success of the Meeting and, in particular, to the authors whose papers are published in this book. Special appreciation is due to the members of the International Scientific Advisory Committee who have helped the editors with the reviewing of abstracts and papers.

The Editors
Bologna, 2005

CONTENTS

Section 2: Air pollution

Section 5: Water quality issues

Section 6: Electromagnetic fields

Section 7: Housing and health

Section 8: Remediation

Section 9: Social and economic issues

Section 1
Risk analysis

Risk assessment for pharmaceutical products in the environment

V. Popov[1], V. Tomenko[1], C. A. Brebbia[1], A. H. Piersma[2] & M. Luijten[2]

[1]*Wessex Institute of Technology, Environmental and Fluid Mechanics, UK*
[2]*Laboratory for Toxicology, Pathology and Genetics, RIVM, The Netherlands*

Abstract

Recently, a Specific Targeted Research Project (STREP), termed F&F, supported by the European Commission under the Sixth Framework Programme Priority 5 on Food Quality and Safety (Contract No. FOOD-CT-2004-513953, http://foodandfecundity.factlink.net) on "Pharmaceutical products in the environment: Development and employment of novel methods for assessing their origin, fate and effects on human fecundity" has been established. The F&F project intends to integrate research groups from different disciplines (risk assessors managers, clinical epidemiologists, endocrinologist, biochemists, as well as experts in biochemical and chemical diagnostics) for a better understanding of the extent of the problem. Our part in the project focuses on evaluating the risk assessment of PPs in food and in the environment.

This work will pinpoint study and summarize the RA of different PPs, their origin and their influence on fecundity.

1 Risk assessment for PPs in the environment

The risk assessment part of the F&F project includes:
1. Identification of a platform of endocrine disrupting substances in the food on a regional basis within Europe;
2. Identification and assessment of other risk factors that may influence fecundity, including age, reproductive history, diet and nutrition, socio-economic status, habits and lifestyle;

3. Survey of national/regional fecundity in European populations;
4. Survey of dietary habits across the selected regions;
5. Contribution towards the development of a suite of biomarkers and high throughput screening assays, suitable for potential applications in mechanistic research and human medical and epidemiological applications;
6. Qualitative and, potentially, quantitative assessment of the risk posed to human fecundity through exposure to chemicals in food.

The main elements of the risk assessment task of the project are shown in Figure 1. It can be seen that the first step consists of Identification of potential PPs with an effect on human fecundity. Once the PPs are selected required data for Exposure Assessment as well as Dose Response curves are collected through corresponding project tasks, which is finally used for the Risk Characterization and definition of Risk Management Strategies.

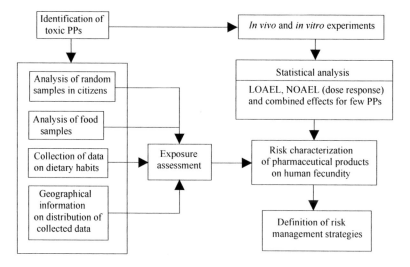

Figure 1:   Risk assessment strategy for the F&F project.

1.1 Selection of PPs

After the first six months of the project three compounds were selected that were considered relevant within the framework of F&F, though this number will be increased to twenty by the end of the project. A prioritization list of pharmaceutical products (PP) bearing a high potential of affecting human fecundity by entering the food chain has been created, based on an extensive literature search, and by considering the following issues during the selection process: (i) Does the available data indicate there is evidence that the chemical causes endocrine disrupting effects related to fecundity? (ii) Is the production volume and/or use of the PP sufficiently large to cause concern? (iii) Is the PP sufficiently persistent in the environment? (iv) Can a clear exposure route be identified by which the PP would enter the food chain?

The main problem at this stage is that there is lack of data necessary to answer the above questions for all of the PPs nowadays in use. Several chemicals have been selected for which data exists indicating positive answers to all or several of the questions (i) to (iv). In the first stage the selection process was focused on chemicals for which evidence exists for positive answer to (i). Those chemicals selected in the first stage were further investigated for additional information on the other three questions. The chemicals with more positive answers to questions (i) to (iv) and with more evidence from previous research to support those findings are of more importance to the study.

The identified compounds were ethynylestradiol, medroxyprogesterone acetate, and diethylstilbestrol.

Some of the available data on EE2 in respect to the biological effectivity, production volumes, exposures and environmental fate is given below. Similar data was gathered for the other two compounds but can be found elsewhere [1].

1.1.1 17α-Ethynylestradiol (EE2)

EE2 is used in oral contraceptives in humans. The effect of EE2 on animals has been investigated in several studies and some results are given below. These studies may give some indication of what the no observed effect concentration (NOEC) and lowest observed effect concentration (LOEC) in humans might be.

The synthetic oestrogen hormone, 17α-ethinyloestradiol can be used in human medicine to treat various gynaecological disorders and post-menopausal breast cancer. However, its largest use is in oral contraceptives, when it is usually administered in combination with a synthetic progestin. Its concentration in the contraceptive pill ranges from 20 to 50 μg, with 35 μg most commonly prescribed [2]. An annual use of 0.029 tonnes of 17α-ethinyloestradiol has been estimated in the UK [3]. By comparison, it has been estimated that 0.088 tonnes of oral contraceptives (17α-ethinyloestradiol and mestranol) are used annually in the USA [4].

Synthetic estrogens (EE2 and mestranol) are more resistant to microbial degradation than natural steroids (estradiol, estrone, estriol). The data on the physico-chemical properties of EE2 and its environmental fate indicate that the compound is relatively persistent in the aquatic environment. It is likely that adsorption of EE2 to soil is a major removal process (log Koc=3.8).

There are several routes that may lead to contamination of food or water with EE2, see Figure 2. If we neglect routes related to effects which would exist just in the vicinity of the production plant and should be negligible if the necessary precautions are in operation at the plant, then the most likely route would be through the human usage, where EE2 would either be discarded and end up in landfills or would end up in sewage through human excreta and from there would enter a sewage treatment plant (STP).

EE2 can be further transported from a landfill as effluent through the landfill effluent treatment system, and from there into the sanitary sewage or STP, or could be released into surface waters or land, depending on the level of treatment. Landfill leachate can percolate the containment system and pollute soil and groundwater, however, this route should not represent a significant treat to the environment in a well designed and maintained landfill and therefore will not considered further.

The sewage sludge from a STP, among other options like incineration for example, may be disposed into a landfill, or could be used in agriculture. From the agricultural fields the EDs compounds may be transported to surface waters, soil and groundwater by leaching, dissipation and run-off. If EE2 is transported to surface waters it may end up in the food chain by bioacumultaion in fish or as water for domestic use, and if it reaches groundwater it may further be used as tap water for human consumption. Once sewage sludge is applied to agricultural fields EE2 may end up in plants through plant uptake.

Unless direct measurements show otherwise, the risks from EE2 being present in the air due to evaporation from landfills, sewage treatment plants and agricultural fields where sewage sludge is applied, are considered to be negligible.

There is awareness of the importance of investigating the presence of EE2 in the environment, and many of the previous studies included EE2 as the main representative of the synthetic steroids.

Evidence exists of presence of EE2 in the environment. EE2 was found basically in every media where an attempt was made for its detection, i.e., raw sewage [5], STP effluent [6], rivers [7] and even groundwater [8]. The detection of EE2 is difficult since its concentrations are usually on the detection limit, but this certainly does not mean that the risk from EE2 is negligible. EE2 can cause changes in animals in very low concentrations. Chronic exposure under laboratory conditions, including studies of chronic exposure over two complete generations, to as little as 0.6 ng/l EE2 (below the limits of chemical detection for most effluents) was sufficient to sex reverse male fish (primarily zebrafish, with some work on the stickleback) and 1.5 ng/l stimulated vitellogenesis in juvenile fish (COMPREHEND 2002). Bioaccumulation can increase the EE2 concentrations by several orders of magnitude [6]. One should also not forget that EE2 concentrations in the STPs could be increased by the partial conversion of other drugs into this molecule [9]. Finally, several studies have shown that EE2 is more persistent in the environment than the natural estrogens [5,10,11].

1.2 Food to be tested

Since there is a possibility that banned growth promoting hormones may still be in use, obvious choice of food to be tested is: beef, veal, pork, poultry and fish. Food processing steps, such as cooking, smoking and fermenting, appear to have little effect on the steroid patterns.

Steroid hormones pass the blood-milk barrier. A strong correlation of the progesterone, pregnenolone, androstenedione and estrone levels with the milk fat content have been proved. The levels are higher by factor 10 to 20 in butter than in milk because of the fat content. Hartmann et al. [12] reported that the main source of natural estrogens and progesterone are dairy products (60-80%). A similar pattern can be expected for synthetic steroids, should they end up in the food of animals. Food processing does not seem to influence the amounts and ratios of the investigated hormones.

Eggs are a considerable source of hormonally active natural steroids and their precursors and therefore they should be included in the list of food to be tested for synthetic steroids, since any increase in hormone levels would naturally appear in eggs as well.

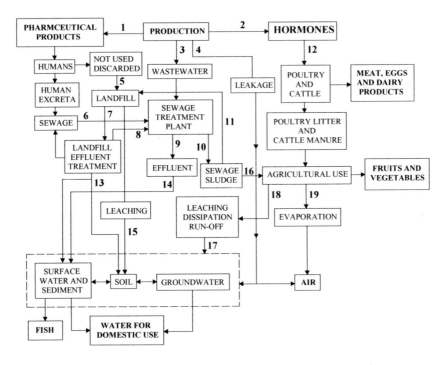

Figure 2:   Exposure routes for EE2.

The presence of 17β-estradiol and estrone in French beans *(Phaseolus vulgaris)* has been proved, with gas chromatography-mass spectrometry. It seems possible that some synthetic steroids end-up in plants through uptake from the soil, after it has been treated with sewage sludge.

Finally, baby food must be tested since children are especially vulnerable to endocrine disruptors.

1.3 Endpoints in the environment to be tested

1.3.1 Wastewater, surface water, tap water

EE2, E2 and other estrogenic compounds have regularly been detected in STPs. In several cases these compounds have been detected in surface waters as well. Finally, it is possible that they end up in the domestic water system, but the question is: in what concentrations? Water supply systems which rely mainly on rivers, like for example the water supply system of London, where 74% of the water comes from the River Thames, 15% from River Lee and 11% from groundwater, may be especially vulnerable.

1.3.2 Sewage sludge and treated soil

Sewage sludge, which is used in agriculture, will be tested in several STP for presence of selected compounds and if contaminated the crops on the treated fields with the sewage sludge will be tested and closely followed for any traces of the selected PPs.

2 Mathematical methods which will be considered for the RA

2.1 Threshold methods

It is assumed that there is a threshold of exposure below which no biologically significant effect will be produced. There is ongoing debate about whether there are true biological thresholds in the dose-response curves.

This method involves use of uncertainty factors to allow for interspecies differences and human variability – it moves the dose-response curve from the response for a group of experimental animals down to the curve for sensitive humans. Both factors are 10 giving an overall factor of 100, which has been used internationally now for 40 years.

This approach will be included in the study because uncertainty factors applied to NOAEL is the standard approach adopted by all agencies undertaking risk assessment.

2.2 Non-threshold methods

For some hazards it is considered that there may be no threshold for the mode of action, and therefore a level of exposure without significant adverse effects cannot be determined. Attempts to provide estimates of exposure associated to risks in the region of, for example, 1 in 10^6 are usually made.

This approach normally requires extrapolation of the dose-response relationship over at least four orders of magnitude. According to the extrapolation used different methods exist. Species differences can be taken into account. Though there is no clear consensus and harmonisation on the various approaches which have been used internationally, this approach is included because of the nature of the problem, which suggests that threshold for endocrine disrupting compounds may not exist.

2.3 Probabilistic risk assessment

In threshold methods the acceptable daily intake (ADI) is calculated in the following way

$$ADI = \frac{NOAEL}{UF_1 \times UF_2 \times ...}$$

where NOAEL is the No Observable Adverse Effect Level and UF_i is the ith uncertainty factors. This approach provides a single value, the uncertainty of which cannot be quantified.

In the Probabilistic Risk Assessment (PRA), the aim is to derive a range of values that are plausible, given the uncertainty in our general scientific knowledge, as well as the available data. An important advantage of the PRA is that it allows for the estimation of possible health effects given the actual exposure in the population. PRA has not received an official status yet, but is being increasingly recognized.

3 Concluding remarks

The main objective of F&F project is to determine the risks from pharmaceutical products that may end up in the food chain with an effect on human fecundity. Some studies indicate that there is some decrease in fecundity in certain areas of Europe, but it is not clear whether this is due to change in lifestyle or due to some environmental factors and/or presence of certain PPs in food.

The risk assessment (RA) part takes very important role in the F&F project since the RA is ultimately going to produce some estimate of the associated risks to human fecundity due to presence of PPs in food.

Acknowledgement

The financial support by the European Commission through the FP6 – Food Quality and Safety programme, Contract No. FOOD-CT-2004-513953, is gratefully acknowledged.

References

[1]   Luijten M, Tomenko V, Popov V, Piersma AH (2005). *A scenariospecific prioritization list of chemicals bearing a high potential of affecting human fecundity,* Deliverable number D1.1, F&F, Contract No. FOOD-CT-2004-513953.

[2]   Archand-Hoy, L.D., Nimrod, A.C. and Benson, W.H. (1998) Endocrine-modulating substances in the environment: estrogenic effects of pharmaceutical products. *International Journal of Toxicology* 17, 139-158.

[3]   Webb, S. (2000) Risk assessment for pharmaceuticals. In: Proceedings of *International Seminar on Pharmaceuticals in the Environment.* March 9th 2000, Brussels, Tecnological Institute.

[4]   Archand-Hoy, L.D., Nimrod, A.C. and Benson, W.H. (1998) Endocrine-modulating substances in the environment: estrogenic effects of pharmaceutical products. *International Journal of Toxicology* **17**, 139-158.

[5]   Ternes, T.A., M. Stumpf, J. Mueller, K. Haberer, R.D. Wilken, and M. Servos. (1999). Behavior and occurrence of estrogens in municipal sewage treatment plants – I. Investigations in Germany, Canada and Brazil. *Sci. Total Environ.* 225:81–90.

[6]   Larsson, D.G.J., Adolfsson-Erici, M., Parkkonen, J., Pettersson, M., Berg, A.H., Olsson, P.-E., Forlin, L. (1999) Ethinyloestradiol — an undesired fish contraceptive? *Aquatic Toxicology*, **45**, 91–97.

[7]   Aherne, G.W., Briggs, R. (1989) The relevance of the presence of certain synthetic steroids in the aquatic environment. *J Pharm Pharmacol* **41**, 735-736.

[8]   Hohenblum, P., Gans, O., Moche, W., Scharf, S., Lorbeer, G. (2004) Monitoring of selected estrogenic hormones and industrial chemicals in groundwaters and surface waters in Austria, *Science of the Total Environment*, **333**, 185– 193.

[9]   Kuhnz W, Heuner A, Humpel M, Seifert W, Michaelis K. (1997) In vivo conversion of norethisterone and norethisterone acetate to ethinyl etradiol in postmenopausal women. *Contraception*,**56**, 379 –385.

[10]   Ternes, T.A., Kreckel, P., Mueller, J. (1999) Behavior and occurrence of estrogens in municipal sewage treatment plants – II. Aerobic batch experiments with activated sludge. *Sci Total Environ*, **225**, 91-99.

[11]   Jurgens, M.D., Holthaus, K.I.E., Johnson, A.C., Smith, J.J.L., Hetheridge, M., Williams, R.J., 2002. The potential for estradiol and ethinylestradiol degradation in English rivers. *Environ. Toxicol. Chem.* 21 (3), 480–488.

[12]   Hartmann, S., Lacorn, M., and Steinhart, H. 1998. Natural occurrence of steroid hormones in food. Food Chemistry, 62/1, pp. 7-20.

Attending to risk in sequential sampling plans

A. J. Hamilton[1,2], V. L. Versace[1], G. Hepworth[3], F. Stagnitti[1], J. Dawson[2], P. M. Ridland[2], N. M. Endersby[2,4], N. A. Schellhorn[5], C. Mansfield[2] & P. M. Rogers[2]

[1]*School of Ecology and Environment, Deakin University, Australia*
[2]*Department of Primary Industries, Victoria, Australia*
[3]*Department of Mathematics & Statistics, The University of Melbourne, Australia*
[4]*CESAR Centre for Environmental Stress and Adaptation Research, School of Biological Sciences, Monash University, Australia*
[5]*CSIRO Entomology, Australia*

Abstract

Researchers typically tackle questions by constructing powerful, highly-replicated sampling protocols or experimental designs. Such approaches often demand large samples sizes and are usually only conducted on a once-off basis. In contrast, many industries need to continually monitor phenomena such as equipment reliability, water quality, or the abundance of a pest. In such instances, costs and time inherent in sampling preclude the use of highly-intensive methods. Ideally, one wants to collect the absolute minimum number of samples needed to make an appropriate decision. Sequential sampling, wherein the sample size is a function of the results of the sampling process itself, offers a practicable solution. But smaller sample sizes equate to less knowledge about the population, and thus an increased risk of making an incorrect management decision. There are various statistical techniques to account for and measure risk in sequential sampling plans. We illustrate these methods and assess them using examples relating to the management of arthropod pests in commercial crops, but they can be applied to any situation where sequential sampling is used.
Keywords: binomial, enumerative, risk, sampling plan, sequential sampling, Taylor's power law, Wald's sequential probability ratio test.

1   Introduction: constructing sequential sampling plans

Sequential sampling is popular in applied disciplines such as agricultural entomology as it demands the collection of the minimum number of samples necessary to make a pest management decision. Surveying crops is time-consuming and expensive, and growers cannot afford the luxury of a highly-intensive sampling programme. In sequential sampling, surveying continues until a predefined stop-rule is satisfied. That is, the ultimate sample size is determined by the results obtained as sampling progresses.

The two most commonly-used types of sequential sampling plans are the enumerative and the binomial. In the context of applied entomology, enumerative plans involve counting individual insects so as to obtain an estimate of the population's density. This estimate is then compared to an action threshold (AT). The AT represents the population density above which the grower will employ a control measure, such as pesticide application. In contrast, binomial plans only require one to record whether or not the number of insects on each sampling unit exceeds a predefined tally threshold (usually zero, hence the alternative name presence-absence sampling, Hepworth and McFarlane [1,2]). The stop-rule incorporates the AT, and upon cessation of sampling the user is informed as to whether or not action is required.

1.1 Enumerative sampling plans

As explained by Karandinos [3], the minimum sample size (n_{min}) required for a survey can be adequately approximated as

$$n_{min} = s^2 \big/ (D\,\bar{x})^2 \qquad (1)$$

where s^2 and $\bar{x}$ are the sample variance and sample mean respectively, and D is the nominal, i.e. desired, level of precision (expressed as $\sigma_{\bar{x}}/\bar{x}$, where $\sigma_{\bar{x}}$ is the standard error of the mean). Prior to sampling, however, we do not know $\bar{x}$, s^2, or $\sigma_{\bar{x}}$, so we cannot determine n_{min}. A possible solution would be to conduct a pilot survey before each sampling event so that these parameters could be estimated. This would plainly be impractical for routine sampling programmes. The problem can be resolved through the construction of a sequential sampling stop-boundary. Such a boundary is a function of the variance-mean relation of the pest (in effect, its spatial distribution) and the desired level of precision of the survey. Two stop boundaries have been proposed: Kuno [4] and Green [5].

The foundation of Kuno's [4] approach lies in the use of Iwao's [6] patchiness regression technique to characterise the variance-mean relation. Iwao modelled the relation between the sample mean ($\bar{x}$) and Lloyd's [7] mean crowding index (x^*), which is calculated as

$$x^* = \bar{x} + \big[(s^2/\bar{x}) - 1\big] \qquad (2)$$

Iwao's patchiness regression, whereby x^* is regressed against $\bar{x}$, is thus

$$x^* = \alpha + \beta\bar{x} \tag{3}$$

where the y-intercept (α) is the *index of basic contagion* and the slope (β) is the *density-contagiousness coefficient*. Finally, the minimum sample size for a prescribed level of precision can be calculated as

$$n = \left[(\alpha + 1)/\bar{x} + (\beta - 1)\right]/D^2 \tag{4}$$

Iwao and Kuno [8]. Having obtained n, Kuno's stop boundary can be calculated:

$$T_{n[\text{Kuno}]} = (\alpha + 1)/\left(D^2 - \left[(\beta - 1)/n\right]\right) \tag{5}$$

where $T_{n[\text{Kuno}]}$ is the cumulative number of individuals in samples 1 to n. Finally, a sequential stop-chart is constructed by plotting $T_{n[\text{Kuno}]}$ against n.

Green's [3] stop boundary is analogous to Kuno's, the major difference being that it uses Taylor's Power Law (TPL) Taylor [9] to model the variance-mean relation. TPL is

$$s^2 = a\bar{x}^b \tag{6}$$

where s^2 and $\bar{x}$ are as described earlier, a is a scaling factor that is dependent on sampling method and habitat, and the exponent b is a measure of spatial contagion. The parameters a and b can be estimated (i.e. $\hat{a}$ and $\hat{b}$) by regressing $\ln s^2$ against $\ln \bar{x}$:

$$\ln s^2 = \ln \hat{a} + \hat{b} \ln \bar{x} \tag{7}$$

Thus, replacing s^2 in eqn. (1) with $\hat{a}\bar{x}^{\hat{b}}$ from eqns (5) and (6) we get

$$n = \hat{a}\bar{x}^{(\hat{b}-2)}/D^2 \tag{8}$$

Green's [5] stop boundary can then be calculated as follows:

$$T_{n[\text{Green}]} = \left(\frac{D^2}{\hat{a}}\right)^{1/(\hat{b}-2)} n^{(\hat{b}-1)/(\hat{b}-2)} \tag{9}$$

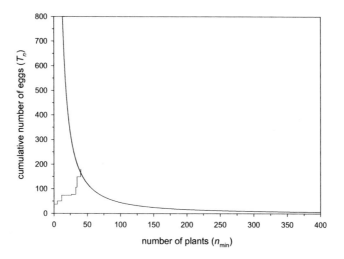

Figure 1: An enumerative sequential sampling chart for *Helicoverpa* spp. on fresh-market tomatoes (based on unpublished data of J.D. & C.M.).

Having obtained $T_{n[\text{Green}]}$ it can be plotted against $n_{\min}$ to create a sequential sampling stop chart, as shown in fig. 1. To use such a chart, or an analogous chart derived from Kuno's method, one keeps track of the number of sampling units (plants in fig. 1) and the cumulative number of individuals (eggs in fig. 1) found. Sampling ceases when the line defining this relationship intersects the stop boundary. In fig. 1. the stepped-line is a hypothetical example to demonstrate how such a chart is used. In this particular scenario, 40 plants were surveyed and a total of 180 eggs were recorded before sampling ceased.

1.2 Binomial plans

The most commonly used binomial sampling plan is Wald's [10] sequential probability ratio test (SPRT), and this is the only binomial plan considered here. The SPRT comprises lower and upper stop boundaries, and sampling continues as long as one is between the two boundaries. If the upper boundary is crossed, sampling ceases and the plan recommends implementing control. Conversely, if the lower boundary is intersected, sampling stops and no control is taken. The y-intercepts for the lower and upper stop boundaries, h_0 and h_1 respectively, are calculated as follows:

$$h_0 = \frac{\ln\left[(1-\beta)/\alpha\right]}{\ln\left[\dfrac{\theta_1(1-\theta_0)}{\theta_0(1-\theta_1)}\right]} \qquad \text{and} \qquad h_1 = \frac{\ln\left[\beta/(1-\alpha)\right]}{\ln\left[\dfrac{\theta_1(1-\theta_0)}{\theta_0(1-\theta_1)}\right]} \qquad (10), (11)$$

where θ_0 and θ_1 respectively represent the lower and upper bounds about the AT. In other words, θ_0 is the threshold below which control is not required and θ_1 is the threshold above which control would be instigated. The common slope, λ, for the two lines is given as

$$\lambda = \frac{\ln\left[(1-\theta_0)/(1-\theta_1)\right]}{\ln\left[\dfrac{\theta_1(1-\theta_0)}{\theta_0(1-\theta_1)}\right]} \tag{12}$$

2 Setting the riskiness of a plan

2.1 Enumerative plans

Risk is accounted for in sequential sampling in a variety of ways. First, consider the enumerative plan. As seen in eqns (4, 5, 8, & 9), Kuno's and Green's plans require precision to be specified. In both these instances we chose to describe it in terms of the ratio of the sample standard error to the sample mean. Note that high D-values correspond to low levels of precision, and *vice versa*. The choice of the nominal precision level is arbitrary. Many have considered a D-value of 0.2 to 0.3 to be practicable and reasonable for pest sampling in routine monitoring programs, Hamilton and Hepworth [11]. A D-value of 0.25 enables detection of either a halving or a doubling of the sample mean.

2.2 Binomial plans

Risk is attended to in binomial plans by setting the type I and II error rates (α and β respectively) and the lower and upper bounds about the AT (θ_0 and θ_1 respectively). The probability that a plan will suggest implementing control when it is not required (i.e. when $\theta \le$ AT) is represented by α, and β is the probability that no control is recommended when it is in fact needed (i.e. when $\theta >$ AT). The choice of error rates is subjective, although 0.1 has often been used for both α and β, Binns [12], Burkness *et al.* [13]. Others have argued that in a pest control context β error is more serious (from the perspective of the primary producer at least), and thus should be set at a more conservative level than α, Hamilton *et al.* [14], Mo and Baker [15]. Increases in either α or β will see a concomitant increase in the probability of either an action or no action decision and a decrease in the likelihood of a no decision outcome.

Risk is accounted for in a more indirect way in binomial plans by setting the width of the *region of indifference*, i.e. the distance between θ_0 and θ_1. This region about the AT (i.e. the width of the AT band) effectively represents the emphasis or importance one wishes to place on the exact value of the AT. The derivation of ATs is often highly subjective and it may therefore be reasonable to apply some latitude. Within the region of indifference we are not too concerned as to whether or not the crop is treated. As with the error rates, setting θ_0 and θ_1 is a somewhat subjective task. Where the sampling unit is a plant, it may be reasonable to set the region as 5% plants infested either side of AT [15].

3 Assessing the achieved riskiness of a plan

3.1 Enumerative plans

As described earlier, enumerative sequential sampling plans require precision to be set. It cannot be assumed, however, that this nominal precision level will actually be realised upon implementation of the plan. A useful way of assessing the achieved precision of a sampling plan is to statistically re-sample data-sets, Narajo and Hutchinson [16], Binns *et al.* [17]. We applied this approach to a $D = 0.3$ sampling plan for eggs of *Helicoverpa* spp. in fresh-market tomatoes (1,000 re-sampling iterations). The achieved levels of precision varied substantially (fig. 3). The mean achieved D across all data-sets (i.e. mean of all means of 1,000 iterations) was 0.32 (SD 0.14), with the minimum and maximum being 0.22 (SD 0.27) and 0.46 (SD 0.21) respectively. In general, the plan failed to satisfy the nominal precision at densities of less than 0.2 eggs/plant, whereas it often over-performed at higher densities. In this example the nominal and actual precision levels were close, on average. But this may not always be the case, and validation of precision is a prudent step that should be undertaken in the development of a sampling plan.

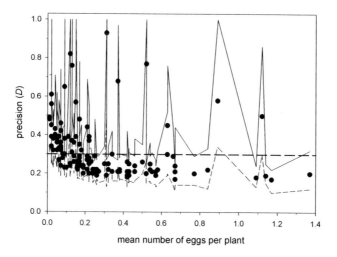

Figure 2: The mean (dots), minimum (light dashed line), and maximum (solid line) levels of precision (*D*) achieved over 1,000 re-sampling iterations when implementing a sampling plan for *Helicoverpa* on fresh-market tomatoes. The heavy dashed line denotes the nominal level of precision (*D* = 0.3). Based on unpublished data of J.D. & C.M.

3.2 Binomial plans

The performance of binomial plans is typically assessed through the construction of operating characteristic (OC) and average sample number (ASN) curves. The OC function describes the probability that the plan will *not* recommend control, and the ASN function calculates the mean number of samples required to satisfy the sequential sampling stop rule. The OC of a perfect plan would be a stepwise function, as one would go from being 100% certain of the need to take action when above the AT (even if only by an infinitesimally small amount) to being 100% certain that no action is required when the level of infestation is at or below the AT. Thus, the steepness of the OC curve indicates the relative riskiness of the plan, where a steep slope implies a high-precision (and thus low risk) plan. Hamilton *et al.* [14] used the slope parameter of a four-parameter sigmoidal model (fitted to OC data generated by re-sampling—see below) as the criterion for comparing the relative precision of plans. The OC function can also be used to assess the level of conservativeness of a plan. If the OC is < 0.5 at the AT then the plan is conservative, since at the AT it is more likely to recommend treatment than no treatment. Conversely, it is anti-conservative if the OC > 0.5 at the AT. The ASN curve is also useful from a risk management perspective in that it enables one to assess the likelihood of having to collect large sample sizes, which is often an important logistical consideration.

The OC function ($L(\theta)$) can be calculated according to Wald's [10] theoretical equations, where:

$$L(\theta) = \frac{\left[(1-\beta)/\alpha\right]^{h(\theta)} - 1}{\left[(1-\beta)/\alpha\right]^{h(\theta)} - \left[\beta/(1-\alpha)\right]^{h(\theta)}}$$

(13)

where α and β are the type I and II error rates, respectively, θ is a random variable of the population, which in the case of the binomial distribution (i.e. the distribution we are concerned with here) will represent the proportion of plants infested, and $h(\theta)$ is the non-zero solution for

$$\int_{-\infty}^{\infty} \left[\frac{f(x,\theta_1)}{f(x,\theta_2)}\right]^{h(\theta)} f(x,\theta)\,dx = 1 \qquad \text{or} \qquad \sum_x \left[\frac{f(x,\theta_1)}{f(x,\theta_2)}\right]^{h(\theta)} f(x,\theta) = 1$$

(14), (15)

when x is continuous (eqn 14) or discrete (eqn 15). Fowler and Lynch [18] provide a useful iterative procedure for computing OC values whereby dummy-values are set for $h(\theta)$. They also explain how to attend to the special case where $h(\theta) = 0$ (for OC and ASN curves). The ASN function, $E_\theta(n)$, is calculated as follows:

$$E_\theta(n) = \frac{\left[\beta/(1-\alpha)L(\theta)\right] + (1-\beta)/\alpha\left[1 - L(\theta)\right]}{\theta.\ln\left[\frac{\theta_1(1-\theta_0)}{\theta_0(1-\theta_1)}\right] + \ln\left[\frac{1-\theta_1}{1-\theta_0}\right]}$$

(16)

Construction of OC and ASN curves using Wald's algorithms is tedious, and it assumes that the population can be adequately described by a statistical distribution and that the sampling process can also be explained by a theoretical distribution. An alternative approach, developed by Naranjo and Hutchison [16], is to simulate sampling by re-sampling data-sets. In this instance, the OC is more specifically defined as the proportion of re-sampling iterations for which the proportion of plants infested did not exceed the lower of the two sequential stop lines. Similarly, the ASN represents the average number of samples (over all re-sampling iterations) that were collected before the stop-rule terminated sampling. Wald's OC and ASN algorithms are approximations as they do not account for overshooting of the decision boundaries. Re-sampling circumvents this problem, and it can accommodate for a minimum sample size that must be collected each time—there are at present no published adjustments to Wald's equations that do this. A potentially significant pragmatic constraint of the re-sampling method is that two independent data-sets are required, one to construct and one to validate the plan. Also, the number and spread of data-points is important, so as to enable the fit of a sensible model.

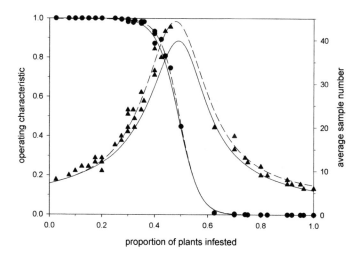

Figure 3: OC and ASN curves caluclated using Wald's algorithms (solid lines) and re-sampling (dashed). The specifications of the plan are: $\alpha = 0.1$, $\beta = 0.05$, $\theta_0 = 0.4$ and $\theta_1 = 0.6$. Dots and triangles represent the operating characteristic and mean sample size values respectively, calculated over 1,000 iterations, for data-sets of *P. xylostella* counts in broccoli fields (see [14]).

We determined OC and ASN curves for a binomial sampling plan for *P. xylostella* in broccoli crops (fig. 3). Theoretical and re-sampling approaches were used. The re-sampling-derived OC and ASN curves were obtained by fitting four-parameter sigmoidal and five-parameter Lorentzian models, respectively, to the resampled data using SigmaPlot [19]. The models respectively explained > 99.9% and 97.3% of the variance). The OC curves derived via theory and re-sampling were highly similar. Both implied a slightly conservative plan. There was a marked disparity between the ASN curves though, particularly around the AT (ASN at AT = 39.4 and 43.4), although such differences are unlikely to be of practical significance in this situation.

4 Conclusion

Sequential sampling offers a practical alternative to traditional high-power designs, and has particular applications in situations where phenomena are monitored on a routine basis and finances or time are limiting. The premise of sequential sampling is that the minimum possible number of samples should be collected each time a population is surveyed. As sample size decreases, however, confidence in our estimates of population parameters decreases, which plainly leads to an increase in the risk of making an inappropriate management decision. Therefore, the level of risk one is prepared to take needs to be stated and incorporated into the sampling plan, which then needs to be validated to determine how well it performed with respect to the risk level we specified. Risk is attended to enumerative plans through the concept of precision, and this can be assessed via re-sampling methods. For binomial plans, risk is incorporated through type I and II error rates and the upper and lower bounds of the AT. The performance of the plan can then be assessed through the construction of OC and ASN curves, which can be calculated theoretically or empirically.

References

[1]   Hepworth, G. & McFarlane, J. R., Variance of the estimated population density from a presence-absence threshold sample. Journal of Economic Entomology, 85(6), pp. 2240–2245, 1992a.

[2]   Hepworth, G. & McFarlane, J. R., A systematic presence-absence sampling method applied to twospotted mite, Tetranychus utricae Koch (Acari: Tetranychidae) on strawberries in Victoria, Australia. Journal of Economic Entomology, 85(6), pp. 2234–2239, 1992b.

[3]   Karandinos, M.G., Optimal sample size and comments on some published formulae. Bulletin of the Entomological Society of America, 22(3), pp. 417-421, 1976.

[4]   Kuno, E., A new method of sequential sampling to obtain population estimates with a fixed level of precision. Researches in Population Ecology, 11: pp. 127–136, 1969.

[5]   Green RH., On fixed precision level sequential sampling. Researches in Population Ecology, 12, pp. 249–251, 1970.

[6]   Iwao, S., A new regression method for analyzing the aggregation pattern of animal populations. Researches in Population Ecology, 10, pp. 1–20, 1968.

[7]   Lloyd, M., Mean Crowding. Journal of Animal Ecology, 36(1), pp. 1–30, 1967.

[8]   Iwao, S. & Kuno, E., Use of regression of mean crowding on mean density for estimating sample size and the transformation of data for the analysis of variance. Researches in Population Ecology, 10, pp. 210–214, 1968.

[9]   Taylor, L.R., Aggregation, variance and the mean. Nature, 189(4766), pp. 732–735, 1961.

[10]   Wald, A., Sequential analysis, John Wiley and Sons: Dover, NY, 1947.

[11]   Hamilton, A.J. & Hepworth, G., Accounting for cluster sampling in constructing enumerative sequential sampling plans. Journal of Economic Entomology, 97(3), pp. 1132–1136, 2004.

[12]   Binns, M. R. Sequential sampling for classifying pest status (Chapter 8). CRC Handbook of Sampling Methods for Arthropods in Agriculture, eds. L.P. Pedigo & G.D. Buntin,CRC Press: Boca Raton, pp.137-174, 1994.

[13]   Burkness, E. C., Venette, R. C., O'Rourke, P. K., & Hutchinson, W. D., Binomial sequential sampling for management of aster Leafhopper (Homoptera: Cicadellidae) and Aster Yellows phytoplasma in Carrot: impact of Tally Threshold on the accuracy of treatment decisions. Environmental Entomology, 28(5), pp. 851-857, 1999.

[14]   Hamilton, A.J., Schellhorn, N.A., Ridland, P.M., Endersby, N.E. & Ward, S.A., A dynamic binomial sequential sampling plan for diamondback moth, Plutella xylostella. Journal of Economic Entomology, 97(1), pp. 127–135, 2004.

[15]   Mo, J. & Baker, G., Evaluation of sequential presence-absence sampling plans for diamondback moth (Plutellidae: Lepidoptera) in cruciferous crops in Australia. Journal of Economic Entomology, 97(3), pp. 1118–1125, 2004.

[16]   Naranjo, S. E. & Hutchinson, W. D., Validation of arthropod sampling plans using a resampling approach: software and analysis. American Entomologist, Spring, pp. 48-57, 1997.

[17]   Binns, M.R., Nyrop, J.P. & van Der Werf, W., Resampling to evaluate the properties of sampling plans (Chapter 9). Sampling and monitoring in crop protection, CABI Publishing: Oxon and New York, pp. 205–226, 2000.

[18]   Fowler, G. W., & Lynch A. M., Sampling plans in insect pest management based on Wald's sequential probability ratio test. Environmental Entomology, 16(2), pp. 345–354, 1987.

[19]   SigmaPlot 2002 for Windows Version 8.02a, Systat Software, Inc.

Brownfield redevelopment, integrating sustainability and risk management

K. Pediaditi, W. Wehrmeyer & J. Chenoweth
Center of Environmental Strategy, University of Surrey, U.K.

Abstract

Different definitions of risk too easily lead to differences in the type and level of risk accepted by varying stakeholders involved in the remediation process and redevelopment of contaminated sites as a whole. This can be rooted in the way risk information is interpreted and evaluated: technical risk definitions are largely evidential and based on engineering or technical contents, whereas social risk definitions are typically experiential and based on shared understanding and interpretation of information, including history and events. Brownfield redevelopments are characterised as high risk projects, due to potential onsite contamination, with some developers effectively redlining such sites. Yet, the Sustainable Urban Brownfield Regeneration Integrated Management (SUBRIM) Consortium identified that although contamination may be present on a site it may not always be the primary concern of the community affected by the redevelopment. It is argued here that risk is perceived by the public in a much more holistic, social way, which bears similar characteristics to the concept of sustainable development. The paper presents the results of a survey of perceived risks and impacts of a proposed development in Greater Manchester, UK, and draws conclusions for the need for risk communication and integration of the concepts of sustainability and risk, specifically with regards to brownfield regeneration projects.
Keywords: risk, sustainability, public, contamination.

1 Introduction

In 2004, brownfield redevelopment became a core objective to achieve sustainable communities [1] which is subsequently reflected in a number of strategic guidance and policy documents. In fact, the UK government has set a target that 60% of new homes should be built on previously developed land [2].

The rationale is that brownfield redevelopment offers the opportunity to create a more spatially integrated, mixed use urban environment but also to introduce resource efficient, high quality buildings [3]. Most importantly, Brownfield Redevelopment Projects (BRP) reduce the pressure to develop Greenfield sites.

However, POST [4] suggests that a significant proportion of developers effectively 'red-line' brownfield sites and prefer to develop on Greenfields as they perceive BRP to involve additional or at least increased risk. This comes from the potential for contamination and the risks this poses to the success and feasibility of the project [5]. In addition, BRPs have to deal with more, and more complex, issues and stakeholders, which itself causes uncertainty, in turn caused by a lack of environmental and redevelopment information on the type, location and significance of contamination [6]. Equally, environmental or health risks from contamination are subject to regulatory and planning procedures under Part IIA. Such procedures essentially require the assessment and management of risk and deal exclusively with technical, science-based risk. However risk is defined and perceived in many different ways and it is argued here that these different definitions of risk easily lead to differences in risk perception and acceptance by different stakeholders involved in the BRP and therefore the acceptability of the BRP as a whole (Section 2).

When deciding to start a BRP, a number of factors need to be considered, including human and ecological risks, technical feasibility, stakeholders, costs and benefits as well as more recently sustainability. However, [7] shows that these factors are interlinked and interdependent. This paper explores the interdependency of risk and sustainability (Section 3) and discussed their integrated consideration and management. It does so by reporting on a survey, questioning residents adjacent to a BRP on the risks they felt they were facing from the proposed BRP (Section 5 and 6). The extent to which contamination and its risks was seen as significant by the public is examined. Conclusions are drawn for future BRPs, including the need for a holistic integration of sustainability and risk management.

2   Defining risk

There are four broad ways in which people define risk, the first two are broadly evidential, the last two are largely experiential in their heuristic method.

2.1 Technical definition

Risk can be defined as the statistical probability for an event occurring, multiplied by the magnitude / scope of the event, often multiplied by some form of social response:

$$Risk = [\Pr obability * Magnitude * Outcry]$$

Technical risk underlies most engineering-based approaches to remediation, including site sampling, and thus the complex decision-making process to remediate, and subsequently regenerate the site. This is particularly relevant under the UK approach to restoring sites according to "suitability for use" [5], where the level of remediation and the future land use are evaluated interdependently. It is labeled here as "evidential" because it uses empirically-derived values as the basis for risk assessment and management. Because of its perceived objectivity and its technical background, it is also favoured by regulatory agencies, Local Authorities (LAs) and lawyers.

2.2 Economic definition

Here, risk is defined by means of an economic interpretation of the likely damage attributed to a statistical probability of an event, most notably in the calculation of damage under the Polluter Pays Principle [8]. Economic risk assessment of contaminated land typically includes issues of liability relating to:

- The clean-up costs themselves
- Liability for the remediation
- Loss of earning through project delay or reduced prices
- Future liability for residual contamination
- Legal recourse for specific aspects of the regeneration process

As with the technical definition, the economic definition of risk is essentially evidential because the assessment of risk depends on the data gathered on costs, and benefits, to the polluter.

2.3 Psychological definition

Psychologically, risk is subjectively based on personal backgrounds, culture circumstances, and institutional factors [9]. Risk is not expressed as a technically-derived number (a probability assessment), but is a qualitative and typically holistic, evaluation of something being "risky", "dangerous", "threatening" or "hazardous". Therefore it is essentially experiential.

Although there is a relationship between the technical assessment of risk and its psychological perception, they are not proportional in all cases. Equally, a psychological evaluation of low risk is not necessarily accepting it. This is because the empirical and experiential origins of risk are paradigmatically and ontologically distinct and are not immediately comparable, let alone tradable. Yet technically derived low estimates of risk are often seen as sufficient to define a risk as "residual" or "background", implying approval for accepting risk as "inevitable" or "normal" [10].

Previous and on-going research has identified some issues influencing psychologically-defined risk estimates which also affect risk acceptance of individuals or groups [10]. These are summarised in [7, pg 28] as:

- *the degree to which the institutions assessing and managing the risk are trusted by the various stakeholders (i.e. involving issues of fairness openness and participation in decision making);*
- *the degree of dread felt by people in relation to the hazards present;*
- *the degree to which people feel familiar with the risks involved;*
- *the degree to which people feel in control of the risks to which they are exposed;*

- *the degree to which the risks are known (including assumptions about contamination);*
- *the degree to which alternative options have been explored (and the use of the Precautionary Principle) [4, pg 3].*

2.4 Sociological and cultural definition

Here, risk is defined through social and cultural factors, which provide a sense-making framework of the situation [9]. This assumes the ability to develop a shared interpretation and understanding of hierarchical, egalitarian, individualistic, fatalistic and autonomous cultural patterns [12]. Beck [13] argues that we, as a society, through our individual activities and tacit as well as open acceptance of risk, define collectively the levels of risk we deem acceptable.

Currently, when dealing with potentially contaminated sites developers are required to focus on dealing with technical risks. It is also these technical risks and their regulatory or land use implications which deter some developers from BRPs.

3 Sustainability and risk: two sides of the same coin?

Grays and Wiedemann [14] argue that risk and sustainability could each benefit from more intensive recognition of their interdependence. The review of the most popular definition of sustainable development - *"development which meets the needs of the present without compromising the ability of future generations to meets their own needs"* [15: 43] – shows two important elements relating to risk: Firstly, sustainability is concerned with the future and decisions which affect it, yet the future is unknown so that such decisions involve uncertainty and thus risk with regard to unknown implications of current decisions. For instance, the Precautionary Principle states that *"where there are threats of serious or irreversible damage, lack of full scientific certainty shall not be used as a reason for postponing cost-effective measures to prevent environmental degradation"* [8: Principle 15]. However, in the sustainability literature risk is not directly expressed as an element of sustainable development.

Secondly, sustainable development and risk are ambiguous and mean different things to different people. Inherent to such understanding of both terms are personal values and perceptions – the psychological and cultural definitions of risk. These values shape what is to be sustained. Equally with risk, as the value attributed to a resource shapes what and how it is to be protected. Decision making with regard to sustainability and risk are based on human values and involves trade offs between risks and benefits.

Finally, a practical examination of BRPs and their relation to sustainability and risk show an important interrelation: Currently, a developer of such a site is unlikely to consider the sustainability of the project unless it is demonstrated that failure to do so involves (technically or economically defined) risks. A survey of a local community adjacent to a contaminated BRP in Greater Manchester evaluates below whether developers are right to worry about contamination risk and its public's perception or whether their concerns are in fact misplaced.

4 Case study background and survey methodology

1200 residents were surveyed living adjacent to a contaminated brownfield site of 18ha in the Greater Manchester area. The site borders an active landfill site, and consists of derelict paper mill, ancillary lodges (ponds) and some recreational facilities. A desk study of the site history and potential sources of contamination identified potential contaminants as metals and metalloids, acids, alkalis, inorganic chemicals, organic chemicals (e.g. PCB, PAH, fuel oils) and asbestos. Proposals have been made to develop some industrial units, a high school and 800 residential units, with the remediation survey currently ongoing.

The survey aimed to identify perceived impacts residents felt would occur as a result of the development and consisted of questions on different impact categories coded on a score from -5 to + 5 as to whether they felt a significant positive or negative impact would occur, followed by a the option for a qualitative justification or explanation of their scoring. Open questions asked to write three main concerns regarding the proposal as well as aspirations for the site. Respondents were also asked to prioritise given social, economic and environmental objectives, considering the locality's needs. This offered an evaluation of respondents' key values and sustainability priorities. Finally, respondents were asked about the perceived importance of different types of risks from the BRP to study the role which technically defined and risk of contamination plays in gaining public acceptance of the overall proposals.

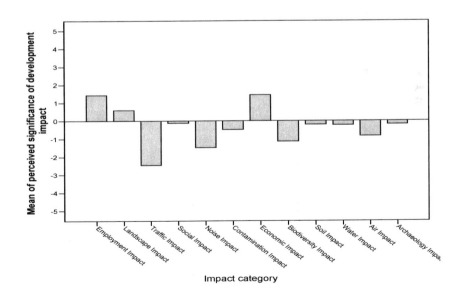

Figure 1:   Perceptions of the BRP on different issues.

5 Results

A 11.75% response rate was achieved, typical of this type of survey. Regarding the perceived significance of the proposal's impact on different issues or topics (fig 1), residents believed the proposals would have slight positive significant impact with regard to the economy, employment and the landscape. This was justified by stating that new residents would strengthen the town economy, and that employment would be generated during the construction phase. Residents identified traffic as the most significant negative impact and gave negative scores to noise and air quality which they attributed to the traffic. Biodiversity also was perceived to be affected negatively which many residents justified as occurring as a result of loss of the lodges and park/ recreational facilities.

Table 1:   Priorities of sustainability objectives

	N	Mean	Std. Deviation
Provide a safe environment for people to work and live in	139	3.25	2.607
Minimise pollution and remediate existing contamination	139	3.63	2.654
Protect the landscape	139	4.24	2.911
Protect biodiversity and the natural environment	139	4.25	3.213
Provide adequate local service to serve the development	139	4.83	2.745
Promote the local economy	139	5.34	3.191
Integrate development within the locality	139	5.53	3.119
Provide employment opportunities	139	5.71	3.948
Protect heritage and historic buildings	139	6.37	3.608
Provide accessibility for all	139	6.81	3.515
Provide housing to meet needs	139	6.83	3.444
Minimise the use of resources	139	7.04	3.878
Provide transport infrastructure to meet business needs	139	7.94	4.221
Support local business diversity	139	8.40	4.086
Enable businesses to be efficient and competitive	139	9.55	4.667

Regarding the perceived priorities of sustainability objectives according to local needs (Table 1), although a social objective (provision of a safe environment), ranked first, many environmental objectives ranked highly such as the minimisation of pollution and the remediation of contaminated land, the protection of the landscape and biodiversity. Economic objectives in general were not a priority. This can be justified when looking at the context of the site, which mainly consists of social housing and many derelict buildings with limited open green areas and limited landscape amenities.

When questioned on the extent they faced different types of risks, environmental risks ranked the highest (Figure 2). However, all types of risks were of some concern mainly in the slightly (2) to moderately zone (3) with economic risks scoring the lowest followed by human heath and safety risks.

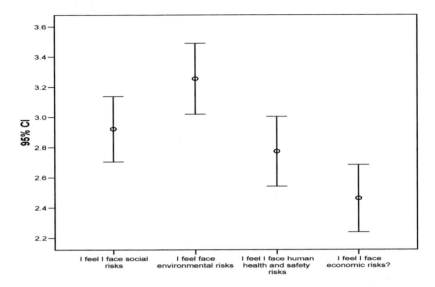

Figure 2:   Perception of different types of risks faced.

6   Discussion

Although the remediation of contaminated land and reduction of pollution was ranked as the second most important sustainability objective for the site (Table 1) residents did not seem to perceive a significant negative impact from contamination (fig 1). Although overall a slightly negative impact score was achieved, the responses span between positive and negative, unlike traffic for example where all responses were negative. Respondents who saw the proposal as having a positive impact on pollution and contamination justified it with reference to the remediation works carried out at the time of survey. However, where respondents saw a negative impact they were not referring to the ground contamination but to traffic pollution being generated by HGV movements on the site during remediation, as well as concerns of littering once the proposed school is operative. Interestingly, respondents overall only felt slightly concerned by potential health and safety risks associated with the BRP (fig 2) with social and environmental risks ranking higher, although many respondents will be sending their children to the school on the site, which is known to be contaminated. Equally, when asked about their three greatest concerns, the site's contamination was never mentioned. The above results show how the public perceives and evaluates risk using the psychological and socio-cultural definition of risk which, as argued, is not directly correlated to the technical definition of risk. Likewise, it is useful to explore the factors which may have played a role in developing the above perceptions and relate it to risk perception literature.

Familiarity is considered to play an important role in influencing risk perception. As many of the residents surveyed potentially worked on the Paper Mill prior to its closure in 2002, respondents may be shaped by an experiential approach to risk perception and familiarity with the site may not have felt human health risks related to the contamination as being of particular concern and thus the "dread factor" was reduced [7]. However it is these human health and safety risks which mainly deter developers from developing of brownfield sites and it is these types of risks which are addressed through current planning and regulatory processes, thus failing to address the socio-cultural and psychological definitions of risk by the public which are more experiential.

Interestingly in this case study, environmental risks were considered to be of the greatest concern and had a significant difference in relation to human health risks and economic risks (Fig 2). This result is also supported through the perceived impact results (Fig 1) and the qualitative responses, where traffic was identified as most important as well as the loss of biodiversity (Fig 1). Here the experiential nature of risk perception is once again dominated as the area is known for its traffic and congestion problems therefore residents have the familiarity of the risk issue, which they associate with negative experiences. As traffic has been an ongoing phenomenon, a lack of confidence and trusting the Local Authority managing (or not) the issue has been fostered in the community. Furthermore, the loss of biodiversity which is also included in the environmental risk category and the perceived risk once again can be related to factors such as the lack of trust but also that of control [7] as the lodges had recently been drained when the survey was conducted.

Therefore, the public considers different types of risk using mainly psychological and socio-cultural definitions of risk. The levels of these experiential perceptions of risk were based on factors such as familiarity, trust perceived control as well as previous experience of the perceived risks, which is in line with much of the literature [7, 9]. It is also demonstrated the different definitions of risk are not mutually exclusive, but do co-exist (Fig 2). Roth [17] also argues that lay people assess risk in a more holistic way which takes into account social environmental and economic impacts of risk related decisions, rather than narrowly focusing on the technical aspect of risks relating to health impacts. This is more in line with the concept of sustainable development, as it allows a balancing or a trade-off between different aspects of risk and it sees risk not in a reductionist, compartmentalised manner. This was illustrated through the results where residents were able to weigh the environmental risks up against the perceived economic benefits of the BRP, such as strengthening of the local economy and increased employment and thus expressed only slight concern with regard to economic risks. However, risk decision-making, as currently undertaken in the UK, and beyond, is one-dimensional considering predominantly the technical aspect of risk, as defined by experts, thus failing to take a multidimensional holistic assessment, which also integrates lay people's perceptions of risk which do not necessarily focus on the issue of contamination either.

However, to suggest that, therefore, technical risk assessments (including site surveys and their resulting remediation strategies etc) can be replaced by public consultation would be irresponsible. The need for expert information on technically defined risk regarding contamination is not disputed, but the exclusive consideration of technically defined risks in BRP decision making is, as important issues affecting the overall sustainability and potential public acceptability of the BRP may omitted through this approach.

When considering remediating a site, technical risks will be assessed and, based on the results, a risk management plan potentially incorporating a remediation strategy will be implemented. However, due to the nature of the technical risk assessment the social, environmental and economic direct and indirect risks will not have been considered when designing the risk management strategy. This omission can have serious repercussions, as even technically perfect remediation strategies have to be subsumed under their socio-economic, regulatory and public policy context. In this case study it was demonstrated that respondents where not so much concerned by the actual contamination on the site but rather with the traffic being generated for its remediation. Thus it is demonstrated that the narrowly focus approach to risk consideration purely on technically defined risk with contamination levels has resulted in jeopardising the sustainability as well as the public acceptability of the project. It is thus proposed by [16] that with regard to risk management decision-making, sustainability should be part of the factors in the equation, rather than basing decisions purely on technical elements of risk. This would then also provide the intellectual basis for integrating risk-based information under the planning mantra of sustainable development.

7 Conclusion

From this case study it can be concluded that a BRP in fact is no different to a Greenfield development especially with regard to public risk perception and acceptability as in both cases a large range of issues and potential risks need to be considered. Here, the public appears more concerned with environmental risks relating to traffic and biodiversity which are equally applicable to Greenfield projects, if not more. Therefore, developers should not necessarily be scared or put off by risks with regard to BRP because with regard to public perception they do not have to be different to a Greenfield project. If anything, developers should obtain the confidence to involve local people as they can weigh the risks against the benefits such as increased employment, improved landscape etc, against the potential human health risks, a task not possible through the technical definition of risk and related processes. In addition, the study shows that the public can and do weigh different dimensions of risk and different sustainable development dimensions in a complex trade-off, which it is sometimes suggested the public cannot or would not do. Furthermore, it was demonstrated that through the use of the concept of sustainable development, many different aspects and risks can be addressed in a way which the public can relate to. In conclusion, an inclusive approach involving both experts and the public in risk assessment and which ensures the inclusion and consideration of all definitions of risk through the utilisation of the concept of sustainable development is proposed.

References

[1] ODPM, *Consultation paper on Planning Policy Statement1: Creating Sustainable communities*, London, 2004.
[2] DETR, *A better quality of life: A strategy for sustainable development in the UK*, Cm 4345, The Stationary Office, London, 1999.
[3] DETR, *Planning for sustainable development: Towards Better Practice*, DETR, HMSO, London, 1998.
[4] POST, *A brown and pleasant land- Household growth and brownfield sites*, Parliamentary Office of Science and Technology, London, 1998.
[5] Syms, P., *Contaminated Land, The practice and economics of redevelopment,* Blackwell Science, Oxford, 1997.
[6] Wylie, J., & Sheehy, N., Contaminated Land & Risk Communication: Developing communication guidelines using a Mental Models approach, *Land Contamination & Reclamation,* **7(4)**, pp 285-289, 1999.
[7] Pediaditi K., Wehrmeyer W. & Chenoweth, J., Risk, its role in Brownfield redevelopment project decision making and conceptual commonalities to sustainability, *CES Working Paper*, 02/2005, ISSN 1464-8083, 2005.
[8] UNCED, 1992, *Rio Declaration on Environment and Development*, www.unep.org/Documents/Default.asp?DocumentID=78&ArticleID=116 3
[9] Renn, O, Three Decades of Risk Research: Accomplishments and new Challenges, *Journal of Risk Research*, **1**, pp. 49-71, 1998.
[10] Roth, E., Morgan, G., Fischhoff, B., Lave, L, Bostom, A. What do we know about making Risk Comparisons? *Risk Analysis*, 10(3), pp.375-387, 1990
[11] Slovic, P, Informing and educating the public about risk, *Risk Analysis,* **6**, pp. 403-415, 1986.
[12] Thompson, M., Ellis, R., Wildavsky, A., *Cultural Theory.* Westview Press, Boulder, Colorado, 1990.
[13] Beck, U., *Risk Society*, Sage, London, 1992
[14] Grays R.C.R, & Wiedemann, P.M., Risk Management and sustainable development: mutual lessons from the approaches to the use of indicators, *Journal of risk research*, Vol 2, No 3, pp201-218, 1999.
[15] WCED, *Our Common Future*. Oxford, Oxford University Press, 1987.
[16] Vegter, J.J., Sustainable contaminated land management: a risk-based land management approach, *Land contamination and reclamation*, 9(1), pp 95-100, 2001.

Risk in anthropic environments: methodologies for risk evaluation and exposition reduction

F. Russo & A. Vitetta
Department of Computer Science, Mathematics,
Electronics and Transportation, University of Reggio Calabria, Italy

Abstract

The simulation of an anthropic environments system in emergency conditions requires the study of two strictly connected models: risk analysis and evacuation design. To reduce the exposure component of the risk, evacuation measures have to be implemented. When an event happens in a system or is forecasted in the short term, the evacuation measures have to be applied and in some cases have to be designed in real time. This paper is developed with the following main objectives: the formalization of the risk problem; the definition of the probability (or the frequency) that the event occurs, the vulnerability and the exposition with particular reference to a transportation system; the specification of evacuation measures for the reduction of exposition and risk.
Keywords: risk analysis, evacuation, simulation, network design.

1   Introduction

This paper proposes methods for the simulation and design of a transportation system under conditions of safety and/or security. Safety and security problems are connected with events that generate emergency conditions, such as the 9/11 attack, Atocha station, and the Asian tsunami. Methods for planning a transportation system in an urban area when exogenous events affecting the system occur and/or in emergency conditions, have received little attention from transportation and risk researchers as well as research institutions and journals. Emergency conditions related to safety and/or security problems in a transportation system can be activated by exogenous events (power failure, radiation leak, etc.) or by endogenous events to the transportation system (dangerous emissions, etc.). The dangers for the population could be immediate (such as the emission or the discharge of hazardous goods from a truck, earthquake, bomb attack, etc.) or delayed (such as flooding, tsunami, lava flow, power station failure, hurricane, toxic or radioactive cloud, tsunami, etc.).

The developments of decision support systems for emergency conditions have not received much attention in the literature. Only specific aspects are treated concerning large-scale emergencies when a nuclear event occurs [1], in urban systems when general hazards occur [2, 3] and in buildings during fires [4, 5].

In general, there is no systematic analysis of the general risk theory applied in the transportation system and very often the vulnerability and exposure in the transportation system are considered as similar variables, or in other cases the exposure variables are treated as vulnerability variables.

When an event occurs in a system or is bound to happen in the short term, evacuation measures must be applied and in some cases have to be designed in real time. Models and algorithms specified and calibrated in ordinary conditions [6, 7, 8, 9] cannot be directly applied in emergency conditions.

The emergency plan, in general, is defined considering two elements: each person knows exactly what to do (information); each person follows instructions exactly (coordination and organization). The assumptions are that the emergency plan is well coordinated and organized and the information is optimal. But who guarantees that: The available choice set for the authorities and operational forces is good, where the choice set is defined in terms of information, coordination and organization? The choice made is the best? The assumptions are true?

In real conditions very often to verify the quality of an evacuation strategy a real simulation on the real system is tested. This approach is very close to real conditions but is costly in terms of money, organization and people involved. During real experimentation if some of the scenario configurations have to be modified, a new real evacuation has to be organized. In real conditions also some new users could be present in the system and a priori experimentation is impossible.

Transportation risk analysis consists in developing a quantitative estimate of risk based on engineering assessments and possible mathematical techniques for combining estimates of incidents, consequences and frequencies [10]. In this paper, transportation risk analysis is proposed through a simulation approach with quantitative models where real conditions are reproducible on a computer. Computer simulation is cheaper than real simulation in terms of cost and time, and different strategies and scenarios can be tested. Real simulation may be useful to calibrate some parameters. For new users some hypotheses can be made; stochastic models may help in this direction.

This paper is developed with the following main objectives: (a) to formalize the risk problem with clear diversification in the definition of the vulnerability and exposure in a transportation system; thus the paper gives improvements in consolidated quantitative risk analysis models, especially transportation risk analysis models; (b) to specify a system of models for evacuation simulation and design.

In relation to the proposed objectives in this paper: (a) a general framework is reported with specific methods and models (section 2) for analyzing urban transportation system performances in emergency conditions when exogenous phenomena occur and for the specification of the risk function; (b) the evacuation problem could be studied in the standard simulation context of a "what if" approach or in the more recent optimization "what to" approach (section 3).

Some conclusions and indications for research developments are reported in section 4.

2 Risk function

Risk can be defined as a cardinal measure of potential economic loss, human injury, or environmental damage in terms of both incident probability and the magnitude of the loss, injury, or damage [10].

Risk has to be assessed in all its components (probability, vulnerability and exposure) and a numeric value has to be obtained. This value can be considered a cardinal measure of the safety and security level. An increase in the risk level is equivalent to a reduction in safety and security. A general formulation for risk assessment in all its components has to be developed. Two types of risks can be defined: individual risk and societal risk. Individual risk is associated with a particular person or at a particular location; societal risk is associated with an activity to a particular population. In [10] risk assessment is proposed by means of quantitative analysis defining:

- for individual risk
  A) the individual risk level that gives the risk level for a person at a particular location;
  B) the average individual risk that gives the average risk to all the population;
  C) the maximum individual risk that illustrates the highest risk to any one individual of a population;
- for societal risk
  D) the societal risk level that gives the total risk level associated with an activity to a particular population.

Moreover, in [10] risk assessment is proposed by means of geographic (map) analysis:

- for individual risk
  E) the individual risk contour that illustrates the geographical distribution of individual risk;
- for societal risk
  F) the societal risk curve that illustrates the curve of the probability and the consequences of the total risk associated with an activity to a particular population.

Risk above a certain level (in one or more indicators) is considered intolerable and not justified and some measures have to be introduced to prevent the risk exceeding pre-defined risk level, named intolerable risk. The risk limit is not defined by scientific calculation but by observation of what society at present tolerates [11]. The change in intolerable risk during the years combined with recent events shows how the risk limit for society changes in time.

Individual intolerable risk is defined as a maximum level that the individual accepts for the individual risk level indexes. Over these values there is an alarm level and below these values an acceptable level. The definition of individual intolerable risk can be extended to societal intolerable risk but there are some conceptual difficulties in defining this limit. This is due to the complexity of societal intolerable risk as there is difficulty allowing different types of events with the same level.

Starting from the definition of risk by which it depends on the probability (or the frequency) that the event occurs and on the magnitude of the loss, injury, or damage, in a simplified version *societal risk* R can be defined as:

$$R = P M \qquad (1)$$

where
- P is the *probability* that an emergency event occurs;
- M is the *magnitude* defined as a cardinal measure of the consequences for a particular population.

Eq. (1) can be also written in the form:

$$R = P V N \qquad (2)$$

where
- M is defined as $M = V N$
- V is *vulnerability*;
- N is *exposure*.

In the literature there is no clear distinction between vulnerability and exposure, especially in transportation systems. Hence in this paper we state the definition straightaway and propose a mathematical formulation.

The *vulnerability* of the system can be defined as the resistance of the infrastructures (material and immaterial) when the emergency occurs. Vulnerability is thus related only to the resistance of the infrastructures when the emergency occurs and there is no dependence on demand. Vulnerability is a supply characteristic. Examples of vulnerability are: the degree of resistance of a bridge when an emergency occurs; the period of time during which a data network and servers function properly before a crash. Vulnerability could also be connected to buildings that collapse on road surfaces or to traffic lights at junctions that are out of order due to the event.

The *exposure* of the system can be defined as the equivalent homogeneous weighted value of people, goods and infrastructures affected during and after the event. Exposure is a demand and demand/supply interaction characteristic. An example of exposure is the number of users in the system area that could die if not evacuated when an emergency occurs. To use the same example as above, exposure is also the value of the bridge and/or the buildings that collapse on the road surface and also the number of people on the bridge or inside the buildings and again that can be evacuated.

Considering eq. (1) two types of measure for risk reduction may be defined (Fig. 1):

- *prevention*, which consists in reducing the level of P;
- *protection*, which consists in reducing the level of M.

Currently, the reduction of P is possible only for some kinds of events which occur in relation to human activities (power failure, radiation leak, hazardous freight, etc.) and is the main objective of safety planners.

The magnitude (M = V N) can be reduced with two classes of measure (Fig. 1):

- *resistance*, which consists in reducing the level of V;
- *evacuation*, which consists in reducing the level of N.

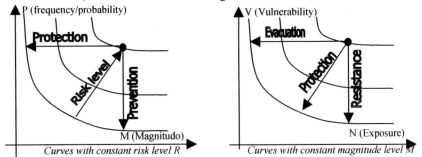

Figure 1:   Possible measures for societal risk reduction.

In this paper a generalized formulation is proposed for societal risk assessment that goes beyond the traditional formulation where vulnerability and exposure are considered constant throughout the area studied. Having defined an emergency event E (for example a radiation leakage in a nuclear power station) in an area T (land around the power station), event E may occur in T with an intensity level in the range L_E (for example the intensity of radiation emissions between two prefixed values), in the time slice Δ (for example in the next 2 years).

For each event a probability density function $p(x,y,z)$ can be defined where x, y and z are respectively the variables for the intensity level in the range L_E, the area T and the time slice Δ. The function p is a probability function and can be defined as:

$$\int_{x\in L_E} \int_{y\in T} \int_{z\in\Delta} p(x,y,z) \, dz \, dy \, dx = P \qquad (3)$$

with the constraint $P \in [0, 1]$. P is the probability level that at least an event E may occur in T, with an intensity level in the range L_E, in the time slice Δ.

The function p is a probability density function and the value p(x,y,z) dz dy dx is the probability that the event E happens with intensity level between x and x + dx in the surface area dy around point y in the time slice between z and z + dz.

If the probability function p assumes a value p in L_E, T and Δ, the relation between p and P is:

$$p \left(\int_{x \in L_E} dx \right) \left(\int_{y \in T} dy \right) \left(\int_{z \in \Delta} dz \right) = P \qquad (4)$$

The function can be obtained from the frequency that the event occurs if there are the available data. In this case different probability density functions can be tested with the Kolmogorov-Smirnov test in order to find the best distribution.

The level of magnitude that produces an event E with intensity level x at point y of T is $M(x, y)$ given by the product of:

$$M(x, y) = V(x, y) \, N(x, y) \qquad (5)$$

where
- vulnerability $V(x, y)$ is the capacity of infrastructures (building, road, bridge, ….) at point y of T not to withstand event E with intensity level x;
- exposure $N(x, y)$ is the equivalent homogeneous weighted value of people, goods and infrastructures at point y of T affected during and after the event occurring with intensity level x in the range L_E.

With the given definitions and notations, assessments can be made with a set of indexes:
- for individual risk
  A) the individual risk level, $R^i_{L_E,T,\Delta}(y)$, for event E, at point y of area T, with intensity level in the range L_E, in a time slice Δ, can be defined as:

$$R^i_{L_E,T,\Delta}(y) = \int_{x \in L_E} \int_{z \in \Delta} M(x,y) \, p(x,y,z) \, dz \, dx$$

  B) the average individual risk level, $R^a_{L_E,T,\Delta}(y)$, for event E, in area T, with intensity level in the range L_E, in a time slice Δ, can be defined as:

$$R^a_{L_E,T,\Delta} = \int_{x \in L_E} \int_{y \in T} \int_{z \in \Delta} M(x,y) \, p(x,y,z) \, dz \, dy \, dx \, / \left(\int_{y \in T} dy \right)$$

  C) the maximum individual risk level $R^m_{L_E,T,\Delta}(y)$, for event E, in area T, with intensity level in the range L_E, in a time slice Δ, can be defined as:

$$R^m_{L_E,T,\Delta} = \max_{y \in T} R^i_{L_E,T,\Delta}(y) = \max_{y \in T} \left(\int_{x \in L_E} \int_{z \in \Delta} M(x,y) \, p(x,y,z) \, dz \, dx \right)$$

- for societal risk
  D) the general cardinal measure of societal risk for event E in T, with intensity level in the range L_E, in a time slice Δ, can be defined as:

$$R_{L_E,T,\Delta} = \int_{y \in T} R^i_{L_E,T,\Delta}(y) \, dy = \int_{x \in L_E} \int_{y \in T} \int_{z \in \Delta} M(x,y) \, p(x,y,z) \, dz \, dy \, dx$$

Considering eq. (5) societal risk can be expressed as:

$$R_{L_E,T,\Delta} = \int_{x \in L_E} \int_{y \in T} \int_{z \in \Delta} V(x,y) \, N(x, y) \, p(x,y,z) \, dz \, dy \, dx \qquad (6)$$

Eq. (2), considered for risk assessment, is a particular case of eq. (6) under several restrictive hypotheses.

In the hypothesis of
- constant vulnerability $V(x, y)$ with respect to T and in the range L_E and equal to V;
- constant exposure $N(x, y)$ in T and in the range L_E and equal to N;

societal risk assumes the simple form:

$$R_{L_E,T,\Delta} = V \ N \int_{x \in L_E} \int_{y \in T} \int_{z \in \Delta} p(x,y,z) \ dz \ dy \ dx \qquad (7)$$

Considering eq. (3), the risk reported in (7) is equal to:

$$R_{L_E,T,\Delta} = P \ V \ N \qquad (8)$$

Eq. (8) is equal to eq. (2) but they are equivalent only in the particular hypothesis described.

3   Risk exposure in a transportation system

To be consistent with the main objectives defined, in this paper we consider that the risk has to be evaluated and reduced when an event happens or is bound to happen in the short term and an evacuation plan has to be generated (also in real time). Hence the risk is formulated taking the following into account:
- an event happens with a predefined intensity level and in a homogeneous area with respect to the event;
- vulnerability $V(x, y)$ is constant.

An analysis of the effect of frequency or probability and vulnerability on the risk function may be found in papers belonging to other research areas. For frequency or probability, examples of events and theories are: for earthquakes, geotechnical and geologic theory; for chemical effects, chemistry theory; for terrorist attacks, policing and security theories. For vulnerability some examples of structures and theories are: for building vulnerability, construction theory; for vehicles, mechanical theory.

Exposure in the past was not considered a problem, nor was evacuation studied with a quantitative approach. Nowadays, exposure reduction with evacuation design has to be developed in transportation science.

Starting from the position given, a general formulation for designing transportation systems can be developed. The aim is to minimize the risk function R as it is defined in eq. (6). It is supposed that for each event E, with intensity level in the range L_E, in an area T:
- the vulnerability function V cannot be modified and is given equal to V (constant values in L_E and T);
- the exposure function N is constant with respect to x in the range L_E and equal to the function $N^*(y)$;
- the probability function p cannot be modified and is given and equal to the constant value p in L_E, T and Δ.

Considering these hypotheses, societal risk R reported in eq. (6), given eq. (4) is:

$$R_{L_E,T,\Delta} = Vp(\int_{x \in L_E} dx)(\int_{z \in \Delta} dz)\int_{y \in T} N^*(y) \ dy = V \ P \ (\int_{y \in T} N^*(y) \ dy) \ / \ (\int_{y \in T} dy) \quad (9)$$

with the hypothesis that the function $N^*(y)$ allows the triple integral to separated into three single integral.

For $N^*(y)$, in relation to the optimization problem considered, different specific exposure functions can be defined as objective functions to identify evacuation measures in transportation systems. The area system and the transportation supply relative to area T can be discretized in a finite number of homogeneous areas with respect to exposure represented by:

- links representing sections of road and relative area activities and buildings giving onto them (if a road is not homogeneous in terms of exposure the sections are represented with different links in series);
- nodes representing the junctions between links, the fictitious points (r) where the origin of the user journey towards the assembly centres is assumed to be concentrated, the assembly centres (s) (safe points).

It is thus possible to represent transportation supply by a graph consisting of an ordinate pair of sets, a set of elements called nodes (i or j) and a set of pairs of nodes (i,j) called arcs or links that are homogeneous with respect to the evacuation. To each link may be associated:

- a link flow f_{ij} (**f** being the link flow vector) which represents the average number of users using the link in the time unit; the flow vector can only assume values belonging to its feasibility set denoted by S_f;
- a link cost scalar function $c_{ij}(\mathbf{f})$ (**c** being the link cost vector) which allows us to calculate the average transport cost of each link corresponding to a link flow vector.

We may associate to each loop-less path k of the graph connecting the fictitious points to the assembly centres:

- a path flow h_k (**h** being the flow path vector) which represents the average number of users who, in the time unit, use path k from their origin (in a fictitious point) to their destination (in an assembly center);
- a path cost g_k (**g** being the cost path vector) which represents the average cost of users who, in the time unit, use path k from their origin (in a fictitious point) to their destination (in an assembly center).

The path cost g_k is the sum of the link cost $c_{ij}(\mathbf{f})$ that belong ($\in$) to path k: $g_k = \Sigma_{ij \in k} \, c_{ij}(f)$. Considering the binary index $\delta_{ij,k}$ that is 1 if link ij belongs to path k and 0 otherwise, the path cost g_k can be also written as the sum of the cost $c_{ij}(\mathbf{f})$ of links ij that belong to path k:

$$g_k = \Sigma_{ij} \, \delta_{ij,k} \, c_{ij}(\mathbf{f}) \tag{10}$$

The link flow f_{ij} is the sum of the path flow gk that contains ($\supset$) the link ij: $f_{ij} = \Sigma_{k \supset ij} \, h_k$. Considering the binary index $\delta_{ij,k}$ the link flow f_{ij} can be also written as the sum of the flow h_k of paths h that contain the link ij:

$$f_{ij} = \Sigma_k \, \delta_{ij,k} \, h_k \tag{11}$$

In this context the integral reported in eq. (9) to assess the risk can be transformed in a sum relative to the homogeneous elements (nodes and links). The exposure $N^*(y)$ in T can be evaluated separately for each homogeneous zone r as the sum of the cost for all users to reach the safe points s, departing from r and considering all the paths ($\Rightarrow$) that connect r and s:

$$N^*(r) = \Sigma_s \Sigma_{k \Rightarrow rs} \, g_k \, h_k \tag{12}$$

Global exposure evaluated in T reported in eq. (9) ($\int_{y \in T} N^*(y)$ dy) can be expressed as the sum of $N^*(r)$ in all the homogeneous zones r:

$$\int_{y \in T} N^*(y) \, dy = \Sigma_r \, N^*(r) = \Sigma_r \, \Sigma_s \, \Sigma_{k \Rightarrow rs} \, g_k \, h_k$$

Considering the paths k that connect all the origins r to all the destinations s is equivalent to considering all the path k. The previous equation can be written as:

$$\int_{y \in T} N^*(y) \, dy = \Sigma_k \, g_k \, h_k$$

Considering the relation between path costs and link costs, eq. (10), and path flows and link flows, eq. (11), global exposure can also be written as:

$$\int_{y \in T} N^*(y) \, dy = \Sigma_{ij} \, c_{ij}(\mathbf{f}) \, f_{ij} = \mathbf{c}^T \, \mathbf{f}$$

Societal risk reported in eq. (9) finally is:

$$R_{L_E,T,\Delta} = V \, P \, (\mathbf{c}^T \, \mathbf{f}) \, / \, (\int_{y \in T} dy) \tag{13}$$

Other risk exposure can be considered, such as evacuation time or the time at which the last vehicle exits from the network.

In a transportation system and with the previous hypotheses (constant values of the function V, p and the function N constant in L_E), the minimization of the risk function R is expressed as the minimization of the exposure function $N^*(y)$ with the integral throughout area T. The optimization problem consists in obtaining the flows $\mathbf{f}^*$ (arg min) that minimize the risk function (13):

$$\mathbf{f}^* = arg \, min_{f \in Sf} \, R_{L_E,T,\Delta} = arg \, min_{f \in Sf} \, V \, P \, (\mathbf{c}^T \, \mathbf{f}) \, (\int_{y \in T} dy) \tag{14}$$

From a transport point of view, the terms V and P are supposed constant as other research areas study the problem to reduce them. The $\int_{y \in T} dy$ is the size of T and is constant. The optimization problem (14) is equivalent to the following:

$$\mathbf{f}^* = arg \, min_{f \in Sf} \, R_{L_E,T,\Delta} = arg \, min_{f \in Sf} \, \mathbf{c}^T \, \mathbf{f} \tag{15}$$

Risk $R_{L_E,T,\Delta}$ can be valued considering the optimal flow $\mathbf{f}^*$ in eq. (13).

The problem reported in eq. (15) is a formulation in terms of design (or "what to") approach where an objective function (in this context $\mathbf{c}^T \, \mathbf{f}$ represents the sum of the cost for all users to reach the safe points) is minimised. At the minimum for the objective function, the path and link flows and costs are obtained. The flow and the costs are carried out with an optimum set of path choice by the users. This optimal path must be followed by users minimize global exposure.

The conditions for the existence and uniqueness of the solution for the eq. (15) are relative to the cost function that has to be continuous, differentiable and monotone and are demonstrated in [9].

In the problem, vulnerability may not be constant. The problem can be solved with different levels of vulnerability and different optimal solutions can be obtained. This is possible for example if the risk and the optimal system configuration have to be defined in real time after an event happens on the system. In this context the infrastructural configuration is defined in real time and the new optimal configuration can be generated.

4 Conclusions

In this paper a general model for risk evaluation in transportation systems is proposed and vulnerability and exposure are explained. Methods for evacuation are proposed for designing evacuation in a road urban network system in emergency conditions. Research for the analysis and modelling of transportation systems in emergency conditions requires further studies. In emergency conditions there is the need to develop new methods and rearrange standard procedures such as: network vulnerability analysis in terms of the "safety coefficient" of the supply system in relation to events with different levels of danger and different probabilities of fulfilment; specification and calibration of link cost functions to use in system simulation in over-saturation conditions in the periods analysed; specification and calibration of demand models for the different choice levels for users and for the public decision-maker. In this paper it is evident that the definition of the best scenario emerges only from the simulation of pre-defined scenarios, taking into account supply, demand and their interaction. The management of emergency conditions and evacuation of an urban area must necessarily be supported by quantitative analyses.

References

[1]   R. Goldblatt, R., "Development of Evacuation Time Estimates for the Davis Nuclear Power Station", (Tech. Rep. 329 KLD, 1993).
[2]   F. Russo, Vitetta A., "The road network design problem to improve the safety during exogenous flow perturbations", *Proceedings of the 29th ISATA Conference* (Florence, 1996).
[3]   R. Goldblat, "Evacuation planning. Human factor and traffic engineering perspectives". *Proceedings of the European Transport Conference* (Strasbourg, 2004).
[4]   University of Maryland, Fire and Rescue Institute - http://www.mfri.org.
[5]   M. Di Gangi, A. Luongo, R. Polidoro, "Una procedura di carico dinamico per la valutazione dei piani di evacuazione", *Proceedings of 2° seminario scientifico su Metodi e Tecnologie dell'Ingegneria dei Trasporti, Università di Reggio Calabria*, (Franco Angeli, Milan, 2000).
[6]   M. Ben Akiva, S. Lerman, *Discrete choice analysis: theory and application to travel demand* (MIT Press, Cambridge, MA, 1985).
[7]   Y. Sheffi, *Urban transportation networks* (Prentice Hall, Englewood Cliff, NJ, 1985).
[8]   K. Train K., *Discrete choice methods with simulation* (Mit Press Cambridge, Massachusetts, 2003).
[9]   E. Cascetta, *Transportation systems engineering: theory and methods* (Kluwer, Academic Press, 2001).
[10] CCPS, *Guidelines for chemical transportation risk analysis* (American Institute of Chemical Engineers, New York, 1995).
[11] Health and Safety Commission, Major hazard aspects of the transport of dangerous substances. Report and appendices (HMSO, London, 1991).

Biomonitoring in environmental medicine – results of LARS

U. Rolle-Kampczyk[1], U. Diez[2], M. Rehwagen[1], M. Richter[1], M. Borte[2] & O. Herbarth[1]
[1]Centre for Environmental Research Leipzig-Halle,
Department of Human Exposure Research and Epidemiology, Germany
[2]Hospital Sankt Georg Leipzig,
Children's Hospital and Outpatient Ambulance, Germany

Abstract

The Leipziger allergy risk study (LARS) investigated, during a period of five years, the influence of a typical indoor contaminant burden on the development of allergies and upper respiratory tract infections in children with an allergy-risk. During the third year of life, biomonitoring with the focus on passive smoking was carried out. Therefore, typical tobacco smoke related indoor volatile organic compounds (VOC) as well as excretion of certain VOC metabolites in urine were measured. The data analyses are based on parent-completed questionnaires, exposure measurements and medical examination. Generally, residences with a high burden of passive smoking showed higher benzene concentrations than non-smoking ones. Significant differences between the excretion of VOC metabolites could be found between passive smoking and unburdened children. Obstructive bronchitis was observed more frequently in the children being exposed to increased concentrations of benzene as well as toluene, m,p-xylene and styrene. In addition, occurrence of atopic symptoms like eczema was found to be associated with the excretion of the VOC metabolite of toluene   S-benzyl-mercapturic acid (SBMA). Therefore, evaluation of external exposure should be supplemented with the evaluation of internal exposure.
Keywords: biomonitoring, passive smoking, allergy risk children, VOC, metabolites.

WIT Transactions on Biomedicine and Health, Vol 9, © 2005 WIT Press
www.witpress.com, ISSN 1743-3525 (on-line)

1 Introduction

Little is known about the influence of the environment on the occurrence of allergies in the first years of life, but allergic diseases are increasing all over the world [1, 2].

The LARS study is a prospective cohort study investigating the influence of chemical indoor exposure on the occurrence of atopic symptoms and upper respiratory tract infections in children during their first years of life.

Chemical indoor exposure is defined as the burden of volatile organic compounds (VOC) in the children's residences.

Indoor VOC concentrations are influenced by certain factors such as renovation, furniture and passive smoking. Evidence is mounting that VOCs have different effects on human health such as development of atopic diseases [3–5]. This study wanted to clarify the role of passive smoking on the development of atopic diseases by assessment of the internal dose of tobacco smoke related VOC eliminated in urine. The influence of passive smoking on the children's health has been described by various authors [6–12].

Tobacco-smoke related VOCs in indoor air were analysed by different research groups. The International Agency for Research on Cancer (IARC) defined benzene as one component related to smoke exposure [13]. Other authors reported toluene, xylenes, styrene and ethylbenzene as relevant as well [3, 14, 15]. The biomonitoring had the aim to objectify the external exposure and to look for exposure associated health effects. Because, only a contaminant in the body can cause effects. Therefore, the internal exposure was analyzed by measuring metabolites of the contaminants in urine [14–17]. The measurement of specific metabolites is important, because so it is possible to avoid an overload by endogenous metabolic processes. S-phenylmercapturic acid (SPMA) and S-benzylmecapturic acid (SBMA) were measured as specific metabolites for the exposure to benzene and toluene [18–28]. Measurement of cotinine, a biomarker for nicotine, was used to objectify the questionnaire data of concerning the burden of the children's passive smoking.

2 Material and methods

2.1 Study population

For the original "LARS-Study" (Leipzig's Allergy Risk Study) 475 premature infants and newborns with parental risk for allergic disease were recruited from a total of 3540 live births in the city of Leipzig, born between March 1995 and March 1996.

The allergic risk factors were defined as (a) cord blood IgE >0.9 kU/l , (b) children with double-positive allergy history, [c] children with a birth weight of 1500–2500g. Infants of the same study population with these risk factors but without indoor burden (assessed by indoor measurements and questionnaire responses) served as control subjects. This is case-control study within the prospective cohort study.

At the end of the infants' third year of life, the study plans called for a clinical examination, indoor VOC measurements, biomonitoring and completion of a detailed questionnaire on the children's illnesses and disease symptoms (e.g., wheezing, obstructive bronchitis and eczema), parental lifestyle factors (e.g., smoking, renovation of residence, area of residence, pets etc.). Only 192 3-year-olds were entered into biomonitoring as they fulfilled all 4 conditions of participation: written informed parental consent, a completed questionnaire especially concerning the part on smoking, a consent to perform indoor measurements and a urine sample. Parents who did not give their consent were not followed further.

2.2 VOC measurement

Samples for the analyses of the indoor VOC burden were collected in the children's bedrooms using OVM 3500 passive collectors (3M, Neuss, Germany) for a period of four weeks.

VOCs were quantitatively analysed by capillary gas chromatography with FID and ECD. A gas chromatograph type Autosystem by Perkin Elmer was used (capillary columns PVMS/5, SB 11 and DMS; 50 m, ID=0.32, slice thickness 1 μm; carrier gas nitrogen, 14.5 psi, injection volume 2 μl, split 1:10; temperature program: 40°C, 2°C/min--150°C). To check the correctness, all analyses were measured with two different polar columns and using the method of the internal standard (internal standard = cyclododecan).

2.3 Urine analysis

The mercapturic acids were analyzed after chromatographical separation with a RP 18 column (15 cm) and ionisation with the Turbo-Ionspray-source (TIS) on LC/MS/MS device API 300 by PE SCIEX, using tandem-mass spectrometry in negative mode.

Cotinine was analyzed after extraction with dichloromethan from urine and chromatographic short separation with a RP 18 column (5cm) using chemical ionization under atmospheric pressure (APCI) also on LC/MS/MS device in positive mode.

Analysis of creatinine as a measure for individual urinary dilution was used for standardization of the metabolite concentrations, therefore, referring to 1g of creatinine. For the measurements, the HPLC Gold by Beckmann (with Diodenarray-detector, column: RP18, 4.6 mm ID, 5 μm, 15 cm column of Knauer) was used.

2.4 Statistical analysis

Statistical analyses were performed applying the work package STATISTICA for Windows (version 5.1, 1997 edition, Statsoft Inc., Tulsa OK, USA). The Kolmogorov-Smirnov test revealed non-normal distribution of data. The Mann-Whitney U-test was used to analyze differences between data concerning VOC burden and excretion of metabolites and questionnaire data concerning passive smoking and health complaints. In addition, odds ratios (OR) based on the maximum likelihood method with a 95% confidence interval (CI) were calculated. As a reference data set was not available, evaluation was carried out by comparing the results with percentile data based on our own measurements. Concentrations exceeding the 75%, 80%, 90% or 95% percentile were defined as threshold values for certain compounds.

3 Results

Only 192 3-year-olds were entered into biomonitoring as they fulfilled all conditions of participation. 27% of the parents confirmed to smoke in the home. Trend analysis revealed a higher benzene concentration in residences where either or both parents smoked as presented in figure 1.

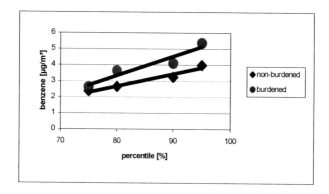

Figure 1: Concentrations of benzene in indoor air of children with and without burden of passive smoking. Measured concentrations in both groups are presented on the y-axis and assigned to the 75%, 80%, 90% and 95% percentile presented on the x-axis.

In contrast, significant differences could be found for the excretion of the specific metabolites SPMA, SBMA and cotinine as shown in table 1.

Table 1: Association between burden of passive smoking and excretion of metabolites.

Metabolite	p	non-burdened children mean value [μg/g creatinine]	burdened children mean value [μg/g creatinine]
SPMA	0.044	2.44	3.32
SBMA	0.043	37.97	44.4
Cotinine	0.002	4.43	9.08

Than was tested which health effects are associated with passive smoking related VOC. The Mann-Whitney-U-test showed significant associations to the occurrence of eczema and obstructive bronchitis like demonstrated in table 2.

Toluene concentration exceeding the 75% percentile of the in indoor air (>19.83 µg/m³) was significantly associated with the occurrence of eczema during the third year of life in burdened children (OR=13, CI: 1.63-103.12, p=0.008).

Table 2:   Associations between single VOCs and occurrence of symptoms in participants under burden of passive smoking.

Symptom	VOC	p	mean value [µg/m³] non-burdened children	Mean value [µg/m³] burdened children
Eczema	Toluene	0.03	15.12	29.34
Bronchitis	Toluene	0.018	14.79	25.98
	Benzene	0.013	1.76	3.11

Further association between certain VOC and bronchitis could be found for styrene concentrations above the 75% percentile (>1.17 µg/m³) revealed an OR of 6.4 (CI: 1.01-40.53, p=0.04), and m,p-xylene concentrations above the 80% percentile (>11.1 µg/m³) revealed an OR of 10 (CI: 1.045-161.7, p=0.02).

Moreover, associations between excretion of metabolites and the occurrence of certain illnesses were observed. OR calculation showed that the occurrence of eczema in burdened children was significantly related to an increased excretion of the toluene metabolite SBMA in urine above the 80% percentile and are shown in table 3.

Table 3:   Association between burden with passive smoking and the occurrence of eczema.

SBMA percentile [%] and (concentration [µg/g creatinine])	p	Odds ratio (OR) and confidence interval (CI)
> 80 (> 30.14)	0.019	9 1.24-65.1
> 90 (> 69.58)	0.03	16 1.07-239.1
> 95 (> 385.16)	0.03	16 1.00-2.39

No significant relationship could be found between concentrations of single VOCs in the air of the children's rooms and excretion of the metabolites.

Thus, we looked for another relationship between indoor VOC burden and the elimination of metabolites. We could find that, despite the lack of metabolic relationship, measured benzene concentrations were associated with excretion of the nicotine metabolite cotinine (table 4). This emphasize the relationship of the indoor benzene burden to passive smoking. So, it was possible to reflect from a body burden to an exogenous exposure source.

Table 4:   Association between single VOC burden and urinary cotinine excretion without considering passive smoking.

	Cotinine 95%
Benzene 75%	p=0.013, OR=11.6, CI: 1.21-110.39
Benzene 80%	p=0.003, OR=17.27, CI: 1.79-165.98
Benzene 90%	p=0.004, OR=18, CI: 2.6-124.45
Benzene 95%	p=0.0002, OR=57, CI: 6.66-487.1
Styrene 80%	p=0.004, OR=7.27,CI: 1.11-47.28

Abbreviations: OR=Odds ratio, CI=Confidence interval, n=122.

To improve the interpretation of the association between cotinine excretion and benzene, SPMA, the benzene metabolite was further metabolised. A significant relationship to passive smoking was found when SPMA excretion exceeded the 75% and 80% percentile and cotinine excretion exceeded the 75% and 80% percentile (table 5).

Table 5:   Associations between burden of passive smoking with cotinine and SPMA.

Metabolite in urine	Burden with passive smoking	Metabolite in urine	Burden with passive smoking
Cotinine >75% percentile (10.17 [µg/g] creatinine)	p=0.0006, OR=4.42 CI: 1.85-10.53	SPMA >75% percentile (4.44 [µg/g] creatinine)	p=0.03, OR=2.46 CI: 1.09-5.54
Cotinine >80% percentile (13.99 [µg/g] creatinine)	p=0.0002, OR: 5.38 CI: 2.16-13.36	SPMA > 80% percentile (4.89 [µg/g] creatinine)	p=0.025, OR=2.79 CI: 1.17-6.64

Abbreviations: OR=Odds-Ratio, CI=Confidence interval.

4 Discussion

The data analysis showed that apart from benzene no increased VOC concentrations could be found in the residences under burden of passive smoking.

A reasonable explanation could be that measurements were conducted in the children's bedrooms where active smoking is usually avoided. The measured significant higher concentrations of the metabolites SPMA, SBMA and cotinine in urine of passive smoke burdened children may due to exposure while staying in common rooms of the residence.

Assignment of single VOCs to certain symptoms and illnesses revealed a significant association between the toluene burden and the occurrence of eczema. Significant associations of obstructive bronchitis were found with benzene and toluene as well as for styrene and m,p-xylene when in higher concentrations, caused possibly by resulting from the irritating mucosal effects of these substances at those concentrations. These findings correspond to results of previous investigations revealing associations between passive smoking and the occurrence of certain symptoms in 1-year old children [6, 14].

Furthermore, the excretion of SBMA as a specific toluene metabolite was related to passive smoking and occurrence of eczema. The burden of passive smoking may contribute to atopic sensitization by increasing the IgE synthesis [10]. The MAS study revealed a relationship between pre- and postnatal burden of passive smoking and sensitization to food allergens [10, 11]. Already collected data will be further analyzed to help explain these aspects.

Additional, an association between the burden of passive smoking and the related exposure to benzene and toluene was indirectly analyzed by measuring urinary excretion of metabolites. Therefore, evaluation of external exposure should be supplemented with the evaluation of internal exposure to clarify possible associations with certain health effects.

Our findings indicate that children under risk of atopy do react sensitively to chemical substances such as passive smoking. They further show that these children have an increased risk to obstructive bronchitis and eczema.

References

[1]   ISAAC: Worldwide variation in prevalence of symptoms of asthma, allergic rhinoconjunctivitis, and atopic eczema: ISAAC. *The Lancet*, 351, pp. 1225, 1998.

[2]   Schäfer, T., Ring, J., Epidemiology of allergic diseases. *Allergy*, 52 (38), pp. 14-22, 1997.

[3]   Wallace, L., Pellizzari, E., Hartwell, T.D., Perritt, R., Ziegenfuß, R., Exposure to benzene and other volatile compounds from active and passive smoking. *Arch Environ Health*, 42 (5), pp. 272-279, 1987.

[4]   Wieslander, G., Norbäck, D., Björnsson, E., Janson, C., Boman, G., Asthma in the indoor environment: The significance of emission of formaldehyde and volatile organic compounds from new painted indoor surfaces. *Int Arch Env Health*, 69, pp. 115-124, 1997.

[5]   Norbäck, D., Björnsson, E., Janson, C., Widström, J., Boman, G., Asthmatic symptoms and volatile compounds formaldehyde and CO_2. *Occ Env Med*, 52, pp. 388-395, 1995.

[6]   Tager, I.B., Hanrahan, J.P., Tosteson, T.D., Castile, R.G., Brown, R.W., Weiss, S.T., Speizer, F.E., Lung function pre- and postnatal smoke

exposure and wheezing in the first year of life. *Am Rev Respir Dis,* 147, pp. 811-817, 1993.

[7]   Etzel, R.A., Indoor air pollution and childhood asthma: effective environmental interventions. *Environ Healt. Pers.,* 103 (6), pp. 55-58, 1995.

[8]   Skolnick, E.T., Vonvolakis, M.A., Buck, A., Mannino, M.A., Sun, L.S., Exposure to Environmental Tobacco Smoke and the Risk of Adverse Respiratory Events in Children Receiving General Anesthesia. *Anethesiology* 88, pp. 1141-1142, 1998.

[9]   Knight, J.M., Eliopoulos, C., Klein, J., Greenwald, M., Koren, G., Pharmacokinetic Predisposition to Nicotine from Environmental Tobacco Smoke: A Risk Factor for Pediatric Asthma. *J Asthm,* 35 (1), pp. 113-117, 1998.

[10] Wahn, U., Environmental factors facilitating allergic sensitization and atopic manifestation in early childhood. *Nutrition Research,* 18, pp. 1363-1371, 1998.

[11] Kulig, M., Luck, W., Lau, S., Niggemann, B., Bergmann, R., Klettke, U. et al., Effect of pre and postnatal tobacco smoke exposure on specific sensitization to food and inhalant allergens during the first 3 years of life. Multicenter Allergy Study Group, Germany. *Allergy,* 54 (3), pp. 220-228, 1999.

[12] Joad, J.P., Smoking and pediatric respiratory health. *Clin Chest Med,* 21(1), pp. 37-46, 2000.

[13] IARC Working Group: Tobacco smoking 38, pp. 1-421, 1985.

[14] Diez, U., Kroeßner, T., Rehwagen, M., Richter, M., Wetzig, H., Schulz, R., et al., Effects of indoor painting and smoking on airway symptoms in atopy risk children in the first year of life results of the LARS-study. *Int J Hyg Environ Health,* 203, pp. 23-28, 2000.

[15] Hajimiragha, H., Ewers, U., Brockhaus, A., Boettger, A., Levels of benzene and other volatile aromatic compounds in the blood of non-smokers and smokers. *Int Arch Occup Environ Health,* 61, pp. 513-518, 1989.

[16] Rolle-Kampczyk, U., Herbarth, O., Rehwagen, M., Noninvasive diagnostic methods in environmental medicine - Biomonitoring of specific exposure dependent Metabolites. *J Env Med,* 1, pp. 65-70, 1999.

[17] Ong, C.N., Lee, L.B., Determination of benzene and its metabolites application in biological monitoring of environmental and occupational exposure to benzene. *J Chromatogr B,* 660, pp. 1-22, 1994.

[18] Greim, H., Csanady, G., Filser, J.G., Schwarz, L., Wolff, Th., Werner, S., Biomarkers as Tools in Human Health Risk Assessment. *Clin Chem,* 12, pp. 1804-1808, 1995.

[19] Ikeda, M., Exposure to complex mixtures: implications for biological monitoring. *Toxicol Lett,* 77, pp. 85-91, 1995.

[20] Lowry, L.K., Role of biomarkers of exposure in the assessment of health risks. *Toxicol Lett,* 77, pp. 31-38, 1995.

[21] Van Sittert, N.J., Booggaard, P.J., Beulink, G.D.J., Application of the urinary S-phenylmercapturic acid test as a biomarker for low levels of exposure to benzene in industry. *Br J Ind Med*, 50, pp. 460-469, 1993.

[22] Takahashi, S., Matsubara, K., Hasegawa, M., Akane, A., Shiono, H., Detection and measurement of S-benzyl-N-acetylcysteine in urine of toluene sniffers using capillary gaschromatography. *Arch Toxicol*, 67, pp. 647-650, 1993.

[23] Takahashi, S., Kagawa, M., Shiwaku, K., Matsubara, K., Determination of S-benzyl-N-acetyl-L-cysteine by Gas Chromatograhy/Mass Spectrometry as a new marker of toluene Exposure. *J Anal Toxicol*, 18, pp. 78-80, 1994.

[24] Angerer, J., Schildbach, M., Krämer, A., S-p-toluylmercapturic acid in the urine of workers exposed to toluene: a new biomarker for toluene exposure. *Arch Toxicol*, 72, pp. 119-123, 1998.

[25] Boogaard, P.J., van Sittert, N.J., Biological monitoring of exposure to benzene: a comparison between S-phenylmercapturic acid, trans, trans-muconic acid, and phenol. Occup Environ Med, 52, pp. 611-620, 1995.

[26] Einig, D., Dunemann, L., Dehnen, W., Sensitive gas chromatographic method for determination of mercapturic acids in human urine. *J Chromatogr B*, 687, pp. 379-385, 1996.

[27] Norström, A., Andersson, B., Aringer, L., Levin, J.O., Löf, A., Näslund, P., Wallen, M., Determination of specific mercapturic acids in human urine after experimental exposure to toluene or o-xylene. *IARC SciPubl*, 89, pp. 232-234, 1988.

[28] Rolle-Kampczyk, U., Rehwagen, M., Herbarth, O., Is the Internal Burden in Human Beings reflected by Air Pollution Measurements? *Air Pollution*, 7, pp. 447-455, 1999.

Measures of network vulnerability indicators for risk evaluation and exposure reduction

M. Di Gangi & A. Luongo
Dip.to di Architettura Pianificazione ed Infrastrutture di Trasporto, Università degli Studi della Basilicata, Potenza, Italy

Abstract

Reliability of transportation systems can be affected by events both exogenous to the system (i.e. earthquakes, floods, terrorism attack, etc.) and endogenous to the system (i.e. dangerous freight, etc.). Hazardous events can introduce disconnections in transportation systems whose effects can be relevant both in the short term (difficulties in evacuation procedures and aids to population) and in the long term (effects in local services and local economies). For these main reasons, in particular considering nonurban situations, to guarantee an acceptable level of accessibility among urban centers an analysis of network vulnerability is relevant. In this paper, after an introduction concerning the concept of network vulnerability, it is proposed an enhanced method, based on consolidated procedures generally adopted in the analysis of transport networks, to explore a transport network in order to put in evidence weakness in some of the links by computing quantitative indicators. The proposed methodology can be adopted, once defined a risk scenario, both to select where to plan necessary adjustments on transport system and to define adequate operations for evacuation and to come to the aid of population, in order to reduce exposure. An explicative application to a real system is also shown to put in evidence capabilities of the proposed indicators.
Keywords: network vulnerability, risk analysis.

1 Introduction

A large amount of studies concerning vulnerability of single structures can be found in literature, whilst more rarely such studies concern vulnerability of either transportation or territorial systems.

Aims of a vulnerability reduction policy are to favour emergency management in order to guarantee timely aids to victims and an orderly and gradual evacuation of population, taking care in avoiding congestion phenomena on links.

As a matter of fact interventions to reduce vulnerability of a transportation system allow not only to enhance the capacity to evacuate a certain area if a hazardous event occurs but also to reduce those accessibility problems that can occur in certain settlements

Reliability of a system can be defined as the capability to work properly, within a certain period of time and in the predicted conditions. This, for transportation system, can be represented, in normal conditions, as the possibility to connect each other the several origins and destinations of displacements and, in emergency conditions, as the guarantee that links are able to bear stresses and flows due to evacuation avoiding congested situations.

In this paper, after a short description of methodological framework, it is presented an analytical procedure to evaluate quantitative measures that can be used both to compute the degree of reliability of connections of the several origin-destination pairs and to quantify the potential exposure due to the vulnerability of the network. Furthermore the results of some applications to real cases are also reported.

2   Methodological framework

An increase in the interest in road network reliability by scientific community can be observed since 1990s. In particular, after the seismic event of Kobe in 1995, a significant interest has been concentrated in those aspects concerning reliability of transportation network.

Several definitions and classifications of reliability have been proposed in literature [1]. A first classification of the studies conducted on transportation network reliability can be done between those methodologies considering only supply system and those ones that take into account also interaction between demand and supply.

Within the first case it is possible to distinguish two aspects: in the first one, concerning connectivity reliability [2, 3], analytical procedures are proposed to individuate reliability of connections; moreover D'Este and Taylor [4] suggest some indicators to evaluate weakness points of a network. The second one take into account capacity reliability [5, 6] defined as the probability that a network, whose state may be normal or degraded, is able to satisfy a certain level of demand that is can accept a fixed traffic volume. This probability is defined by Chen et al. [5] as the probability that residual capacity of a network results, once fixed the capacity loss due to degradation, greater than or equal to the required demand.

In the latter case reliability of travel times has been considered, defined as the probability that a journey between an origin-destination pair is concluded within a definite time interval [2]. To evaluate travel time reliability several measure methodologies have been proposed [7, 8].

Starting from the concept of network weakness proposed by D'Este and Taylor [4], this work develops the concept of robustness of connections proposed by the author [9], taking advantage of the properties of an assignment model recently proposed by Russo and Vitetta [10], and allows the definitions quantitative measures usable both to evaluate a degree of reliability of connections among the several origin-destination pairs and to quantify the level of potential exposure due to the network vulnerability.

A particular evidence should be put on the concept of network vulnerability connected to the consequences of the lapse of performance of one (or more) of the links that make it up, in terms of impact on the whole territorial system served.

3   The proposed approach

Starting from the application of the concept of vulnerability to the existing connection of a generic origin-destination (in the following o/d) pair, it is possible to develop the analysis to the access from a particular site to the network and, finally, to analyses that can involve the whole network.

A first definition of point (or node) vulnerability can be given as [4]: *"a node is vulnerable if loss (or substantial degradation) of a small number of links significantly diminishes the accessibility of the node, as measured by a standard index of accessibility"*.

By means of this definition, vulnerability can be defined in terms of the quality of accessibility from a given node to the remaining part of the network.

One of the aims of the proposed vulnerability analysis is to estimate those points constituting a weakness for the network where possible interruptions and/or damages can cause unpredictable effects on the performances of the whole network and, consequently, give some indications on actions to carry out to strengthen the level of connection.

An outline of dependencies among the several operative tasks in which the proposed approach can be divided is shown in Figure 1. As it can be seen, a first analysis can be conducted exclusively on the supply model of the considered transportation system leaving aside the demand.

Subsequently, starting from results on the reliability analysis of the supply system and introducing evaluations on the involved demand, passing through the definition of a risk scenario, it is possible to analyse the exposure of the considered network.

In the following activities to be developed in order to conduct the described analyses are described; they can be summarised as follows:

- definition of the type of the analysis;
- individuation of suitable variables (indicators) able to quantify the level;
- measure of values assumed by considered indicators.

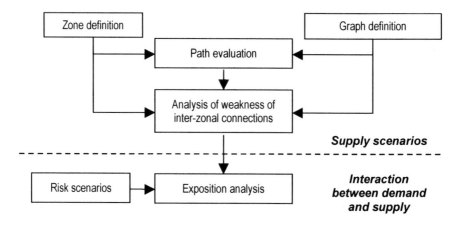

Figure 1: Dependencies among the several operative tasks of the proposed procedure.

3.1 Deterministic measures

A first approach for the analysis of weakness of connections can be based on the evaluation of connectivity in terms of existence and characteristics of alternative paths connecting the considered zones.

Let N be the set of nodes, L the set of links and $G(N, L)$ the graph representing the considered transportation system. Let the generic o/d pair od connected by a number N^k_{od} of paths that make up the set K_{od}; let a_k be the number of links that compose the generic path $k \in K_{od}$. Let define an incidence link-path matrix Δ, whose generic element δ_{ij}^k is equal to 1 if link ij belongs to path k and 0 otherwise, and an incidence link-o/d pair matrix Γ whose generic element γ_{ij}^{od} is equal to 1 if link ij belongs at least to one of the paths connecting the pair od, otherwise it is equal to 0.

Following these definitions, once fixed an o/d pair od, $n^K_{od} = \Sigma_{k \in Kr} a_k$ represents the total number of links belonging to the paths connecting the considered pair and $n^G_{od} = \Sigma_{i \in N} \gamma_{ij}^{od}$ represents the number of links of the graph crossed by the paths connecting the considered pair.

It can be introduced, as synthetic measure, a *Weakness Index* (WI_{od}) of the connections defined as follows:

$$WI_{od} = \frac{\dfrac{n^K_{od}}{n^G_{od}} - 1}{N^k_{od} - 1} \qquad \text{if } N^k_{od} > 1$$

$$WI_{od} = 1 \qquad \text{if } N^k_{od} = 1$$

This indicator, whose values are between 0 and 1, is related to each o/d pair and give information on the overlapping among the paths connecting the considered pair. A value $WI_{od} = 0$ means that to each link belonging to a path corresponds a unique infrastructural section that is different paths are absolutely not overlapped each other. Otherwise, a value $WI_{od} = 1$ implies that all the paths are exactly overlapped and coincide to one path.

So, the closer to zero is the value of this indicator the more different are the paths and the more the connectivity of the considered o/d pair improves; that is weakness due to events that could cause impassability of some road section reduces. To compute such indicator it is necessary to evaluate a set of paths connecting the considered o/d pairs; path evaluation can be conducted by means of a k-path algorithm taking into account of network characteristics.

3.2 Stochastic measures

In the approach that follows, the computation of paths is performed introducing probabilistic path choice models and, in particular, C-Logit formulation proposed by Cascetta et al. [11]. In such approach path choice is based on the mathematical framework of a multinomial Logit model with a modification in systematic utility given by:

$$V^*_k = V_k - CF_k$$

where CF_k,, defined as commonality factor of path k, takes into account of the overlapping of path k with all the other paths belonging to the set K_{od} connecting the o/d pair od.

In particular, considering the D-C-Logit model developed by Russo and Vitetta [10], for each link ij crossed by effective paths connecting the o/d pair od it is possible to evaluate link choice probability as:

$$p_{ij,od} = w_{ij,od} / \Sigma_{m \in B(j)} w_{mj,od}$$

where $w_{ij,od}$ represents the link weight, depending on the considered pair od and $B(j)$ represents the set of the initial nodes of those links entering node j (the backward star of node j).

In order to determine such weight, the link multiplicity $N_{ij,od}$ of link ij respect pair od is defined, it indicates the number of paths crossing link ij that connect o/d pair od.

Starting from the definition of multiplicity for each link, it is possible to evaluate the total number of paths N^k_{od} connecting pair od as:

$$N^k_{od} = \Sigma_{m \in B(d)} N_{md,od}$$

where $B(d)$ represents the set of the initial nodes of those links entering destination node d.

The total number of links building up the set of paths connecting the o/d pair (n^K_{od}) is computed by cumulating, for all the links belonging to the paths, the values of multiplicity $N_{ij,od}$ of link ij respect o/d pair od:

$$n^K_{od} = \Sigma_{ij} N_{ij,od} \quad \forall ij : p_{ij,od} \neq 0$$

Furthermore the number n^G_{od} of links of the graph involved by paths connecting the same o/d pair is given by the cardinality of the set of links belonging to paths:

$$n^G_{od} = ||\{ ij : p_{ij,od} \neq 0 \}||$$

Weakness Index (WI_{od}) can be then computed and it is possible to define, for each link and each o/d pair, another indicator taking into account not only the number of paths connecting the considered o/d pair crossing the link but also the link choice probability referred to each path connecting the considered o/d pair. This yields to a *Weighted Weakness Index* ($WWI_{ij,od}$) where the ratio between multiplicity $N_{ij,od}$ of link ij concerning o/d pair od and the total number of paths N^k_{od} connecting pair od is weighted with the link choice probability $p(ij/j)$ as follows:

$$WWI_{ij,od} = \frac{N_{ij,od} \; p_{ij,od}}{N^k_{od}}$$

If for each o/d pair $max_{ij} \{WWI_{ij,od}\}$ is evaluated, it is possible to consider as more at risk (referring to the considered o/d pair) the link for which such value occurs. In order to obtain a synthetic link indicator referred to the whole set of o/d pairs, a *Link Weakness Index* (LWI_{ij}) is built up similarly to the previous one by considering for each link the values of all the o/d pairs:

$$LWI_{ij} = \frac{\Sigma_{od} N_{ij,od} \; p_{ij,od}}{\Sigma_{od} N^k_{od}}$$

This indicator allows one to put in evidence all those infrastructural sections more interested by the considered o/d pairs and can be used to define a hierarchy among the sections to find out those ones whose working conditions and effectiveness are essential to preserve network connectivity.

Using the parameters above defined and considering not only the vulnerability among connections but also the potential exposure of the network, it is necessary to take into account the level of demand existing among the several o/d pairs. So, a first approach indicator of potential exposure for each link can be introduced by weighting previously defined *Link Weakness Index* ($LWI_{ij,od}$) values with the demand flow d_{od} interesting each o/d pair, obtaining a *Link Exposure Index* (LEI_{ij}):

$$LEI_{ij} = \frac{\Sigma_{od} \; WWI_{ij,od} \cdot d_{od}}{\Sigma_{od} \; d_{od}}$$

Also this indicator can be used in ranking links, on the basis of the level of the potential exposure associated to each one of them, to define priority rules for those operations aimed to the protection and safeguard of the network.

4   Applicative example

The aim of the example here shown is to individuate the connectivity level existing within the territory of the province of Potenza (Fig. 2), located in South Italy that, for its particular nature, is subjected to natural hazards such as landslides and earthquakes.

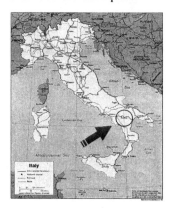 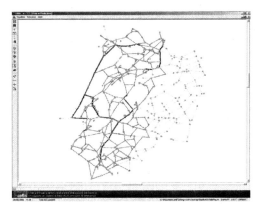

Figure 2:   Location of the province of Potenza and graph of the provincial road network.

The considered area has been divided into 100 zones, coinciding with the territory of municipalities, and the definition of the road network has been conducted by considering the main road sections up to the provincial level. Link travel time has been evaluated by assuming an average speed for each link depending on both physical and functional characteristics of the road section that it represents. Main characteristics of the graph of the road network are summarised in Tab. 1.

Table 1:   Main characteristics of the graph of the road network.

Number Of zones	Number of nodes	Number of links	Number of O/D pairs
100	397	1156	9900

In the following are reported the main results obtained by applying the proposed procedure to the above described network. The aim of this example is only to show one of the possible use of the proposed indicators. For this reason all those particular comments on the results obtained, such as identifiyng the section of the network corresponding to the links of the graph, are not reported.

4.1.1   Computation of indexes

The proposed set of indicators has been evaluated on the provincial road network. First of all, the number n^K_{od} of paths for each O/D pair has been deducted and classified.

Table 2: Distribution of the number of paths for each O/D pair.

n^K_{od}	1	2 - 5	6 - 10	11 - 20	21 – 50	51 - 100	> 100	
O/D	2904	5062	1202	454	213	51	14	9900
Pairs	29.3%	51.1%	12.1%	4.6%	2.2%	0.5%	0.1%	100.0%

As it can be seen from values shown in Tab. 2, more that the 90% of O/D pairs result connected by a number of paths less than 10 and about the 29% of the O/D pairs have only one path connecting them.

Then results obtained in terms of *Weakness Index* for the considered O/D pairs have been classified and summarised in Tab. 3. As it can be seen, the same O/D pairs connected by only one path show a value for this measure equal to 1, that is present the highest level of weakness.

Table 3: Distribution of the *Weakness Index* for each O/D pair.

WI	=0	0 -.1	.1 -.2	.2 -.3	.3 -.4	.4 -.5	.5 -.6	.6 -.7	.7 -.8	.8 -.9	.9 - 1	=1
n. of	22	12	101	578	890	995	1213	1621	1124	440	0	2904
pairs	0.2%	0.1%	1.0%	5.8%	9.0%	10.1%	12.3%	16.4%	11.4%	4.4%	0.0%	29.3%

From the shown indicators, together with the WWI indicator, considerations on weakness (or robustness) of connectivity among the several O/D pairs can be made.

From the operational point of view, it is also important to define not only what kind of interventions must be done to reduce weaknes but, especially in a context either of limited resources or of priorities, it is really important to individuate where such interventions should be conducted. Hence, one of the main purposes can be to identify those links whose "weight", in terms of guaranteed connectivity, is more relevant.

Information on the role assumed by each link of the network in assuring connectivity among the O/D pairs can be obtained by the above defined *Link Weakness Index* (LWI_{ij}). As a matter of fact all those links of the graph, corresponding to infrastructural sections, that are more interested by the considered O/D pairs can be put in evidence. Referring to the test network here introduced, it is possible to obtain a classification of links, as shown in Tab. 4.

In particular, it is also possible to go more in depth and explicitly identify those links whose contribution to the weakness of the whole network is more relevant, rearranging the set of links in a ordered list those critical links whose level of service must be protected in order to guarantee connectivity among O/D pairs, as shown in Fig. 3.

Table 4: Distribution of the *Link Weakness Index* for each link of the network.

LWI	=0	0 -.03	.03 -.06	.06 -.09	.09 -.12	.12 -.15	.15 -.25
n. of	284	764	56	24	8	16	4
links	24.5 %	66.1 %	4.8 %	2.1 %	0.7 %	1.4 %	0.4 %

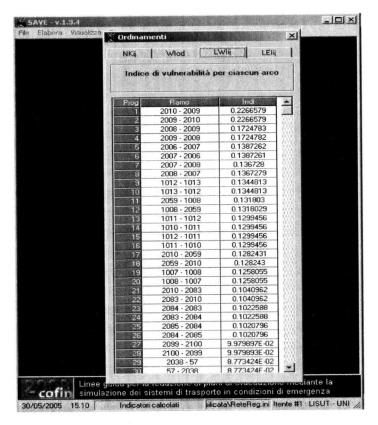

Figure 3: Example of the output of the ranking procedure among the link of the road network.

Similarly, it is possible to obtain an ordered list of links in terms *Link Exposure Index* (LEI_{ij}), once the level of demand for each O/D pair is introduced.

5 Some considerations

The method proposed in this work, based on consolidated procedures generally adopted in the analysis of transport networks, exploring a transport network can put in evidence network weakness by means of the computation of the defined quantitative indicators.

As briefly shown in the example, it is given a possible way, once defined a risk scenario in terms of supply system and demand, to identify those critical sections of the transport system where necessary adjustments must be planned to guarantee level of service of the network. This is very important expecially in those cases where a good functionality of the network is critical, as those events of evacuation or coming to aid of population, in order to reduce exposure.

 WIT Transactions on Biomedicine and Health, Vol 9, © 2005 WIT Press
www.witpress.com, ISSN 1743-3525 (on-line)

References

[1]   Berdica, K. An introduction to road vulnerability - what has been done, is done and should be done. *Transport Policy*, vol. **9**, no. 2, 117-127, 2002

[2]   Bell, M. G. H., Iida, Y. Transportation network analysis. John Wiley & Sons, Chichester, 1997

[3]   Iida, Y. Basic concepts and future direction of road network reliability analysis. J. Adv. Transpn., 33(2), 125-134, 1999

[4]   D'Este, G. M., Taylor, M. A. P. Network vulnerability: an approach to reliability analysis at the level of national strategic transport networks. In The Network Reliability of Transport, (M. G. H. Bell & Y. Iida, eds.) pp. 23-44, Pergamon, 2003

[5]   Chen, A., Yang, H., Lo, H. K., Tang, W. H. A capacity related reliability for transportation networks. J. Adv. Transpn., 33(2), 183-200, 1999

[6]   Yang, H., Lo, H. K., Tang, W. H. Travel time versus capacity reliability of a road network. In Reliability of Transport Network, (M. G. H. Bell & C. Cassir, eds.), Research Studies Press, Baldock, 2000

[7]   Asakura, Y., Kashiwadani, M. Road network reliability caused by daily fluctuation of traffic flows. Proc. 19th PTRC Summer Annual Meeting, University of Sussex, Brighton, July, 73-84, 1991.

[8]   Inouye, H. An evaluation of the reliability of travel time in road networks based on stochastic user equilibrium. In The Network Reliability of Transport, (M. G. H. Bell & Y. Iida, eds.) pp. 79-91, Pergamon, 2003

[9]   Di Gangi, M., Luongo A.S. Definizione della vulnerabilità di un sistema di trasporto in condizioni di emergenza: indicatori quantitativi per l'analisi sperimentale. Presented at VII annual seminar "Metodi e tecnologie dell'ingegneria dei trasporti", Reggio Calabria, 2-3 Dec.2004

[10]   Russo, F., Vitetta, A. An assignment model with modified Logit , which obviates enumeration and overlapping problems. Transportation 30 177-201, 2003

[11]   Cascetta, E., Nuzzolo, A., Russo, F., Vitetta A. A modified logit route choice model overcoming path overlapping problems, specification and some calibration results for interurban networks. In Transportation and Traffic Theory (J.B. Lesort editor), Pergamon, 1997

Methemoglobin and hemolytic anemia as potential markers for drug side-effects

H. Singh & E. T. Purnell
Department of Natural Sciences and Mathematics,
College of Sciences and Technology, Savannah State University,
Savannah, USA

Abstract

Methemoglobinemia and hemolytic anemia are the most prominent side-effects of a wide variety of arylamine drugs including agricultural and industrial chemicals. Symptoms of this hemotoxicity include headache, fatigue, dizziness respiratory and cardiac arrest, and possibly death. Parent compounds are usually converted to their toxic metabolites (N-hydroxylamine) and react with oxyhemoglobin with the consequent reduction of molecular oxygen to active oxygen species leading to hemotoxic damage. We are investigating the role of redox cycling and an alternative hypothesis; viz., that a "hydroxylamine-centered" radical formed during an arylhydroxylamine-oxyhemoglobin reaction causes hemotoxic damage. We examined the time-course methemoglobin potential and hemolytic anemia potential of four laboratory synthesized halogenated phenylhydroxylamines based on their decreasing electronegativity: phenylhydroxylamine (PHA), p-fluoro-, p-bromo-, and p-iodo-PHA. Methemoglobin (MetHb) was determined spectrophotometrically and erythrocyte hemolysis was studied by collecting whole blood from male Sprague-Dawley rats, labeling the cells with radioactive chromium-51 and by infusing the labeled erythrocytes via tail vein in isologous rats. The time course of blood radioactivity was followed by serial sampling of blood from the orbital sinus for 14 days. Results showed dose- and time-dependent changes in the induction of methemoglobin by aniline-derivatives. The MetHb levels peaked to more than 70 percent within 10 minutes at 60 µM and remained elevated for 240 minutes in certain treatments. All tested agents produced dose-dependent reductions in the labeled red blood cells indicating the loss of blood cells from circulation. The dose- and time-dependent methemoglobin and hemolytic anemia responses suggest these hydroxylamines as potential active metabolites and biomarkers that may mediate aniline-induced hemotoxicity. The minimum dose required to induce these effects varies with the test agent based on their electronegativity potential.
Keywords: aniline, methemoglobin, hemolytic anemia, hemoglobin biomarkers, halogenated phenylhyroxylamines.

1 Introduction

Biological markers are usually endpoints in events leading from exposures to toxic damage. Such markers are potentially useful for risk assessments by linking exposures to given amounts of a chemical with the induction of specific health effects. Strategies for the use of biomarkers in the prediction of risk for disease should include mechanistic research to determine the earliest steps leading to disease. Studies should be done to determine which of the DNA and hemoglobin adducts formed by a chemical may lead to neoplasia based on chemical and physical properties of a toxicant. Once the mechanism of disease is known, pharmacodynamic models of the disease process may help in using biomarkers to predict risk and develop safer drugs. In general, DNA and hemoglobin adducts formed by a chemical exposure are likely to lead to a toxic injury based on structural properties. Therefore, it is desirable to understand the relationship between exposures and the probability of disease development in relation to structure and physical properties of a chemical (Henderson [1]).

In this study, we present mechanistic data on the relationship between the chemical structure and its two potential blood biomarkers, methemoglobin and blood hemolysis as toxic side-effects accompanied after treatment with industrial chemical aniline and its derivatives. Studies in rats with aniline and dapsone have led to the identification of N-hydroxy metabolites as the potentials hemotoxic mediators for certain chemicals especially arylamine compounds (Harrison and Jollow [2, 3] Grossman et al. [4]). There is little information, however, regarding the potential hemotoxicity from exposure to halogenated arylamine derivatives, particularly industrial and agricultural chemicals such as aniline.

Methemoglobin (MetHb) is formed in erythrocytes even under normal conditions but reducing mechanisms present in the normal cell maintain most of the hemoglobin in a functioning state. The normal reducing mechanism utilizes NADH (reduced nicotine adenine dinucleotide) methemoglobin reductase and NADPH that provide electrons and protons for the enzymatic reduction of methemoglobin. In most cases, the methemoglobinemia is an acquired condition and results from the action of certain drugs, chemical agents and food. Certain nitro- and amino-derivatives of the aromatic compounds like aniline, nitrobenzene, nitrotoluene, phenylhydromine, and sulfonamides have been known to cause methemoglobinemia (Kiese [5]).

A number of toxic metabolites that produce methemoglobin are also responsible for inducing hemolytic activity. Compounds of industrial interest (aniline), agricultural chemicals (Propanil) and drugs (dapsone, phenacetin, primaquine) have been shown as methemoglobinemic and hemolytic agents. The objective of this study was to examine the methemoglobinemic and hemolytic capacities of structurally related halogenated arylhydroxylamines with decreasing electronegativity such as N-hydroxy derivatives of aniline phenylhydroxylamine: p-fluoro-, p-bromo-, and p-iodo-phenylhydroxylamines.

Aniline (benzeamine, phenylamine, MW 93.12) is an oily liquid, colorless but darkens upon exposure to light and air. This chemical is used as a solvent in manufacturing dyes, medicinal products, resins, perfumes and shoe polish.

The present study attempts to understand the mechanisms underlying arylamine-induced methemoglobinemia and hemolytic anemia biomarkers with respect to structure/activity requirements of aniline derivative-analogs.

2 Materials and methods

2.1 Synthesis of arylhydroxylamines

Various halogenated hydroxylamines were synthesized from the corresponding nitroanilines by zinc dust/NH_4CI reduction or by catalytic reduction with hydrogen (Harrison and Jollow [2], Grossman and Jollow [4]). Both techniques have been used routinely for the preparation of arylhydroxylamines in the literature. The following synthesized arylhydroxylamines were crystallized purified and stored at -80^0C: phenylhydroxylamine (PHA), 4-fluoro-, 4-bromo-, and 4-iodo-phenylhydroxylamines. Structures of these analogs were confirmed by MS, NMR and HPLC.

2.2 Blood collection

Whole blood was collected from male, Sprague-Dawley rats, weighing 100-150 gms via aortic puncture. Seven to 10 ml of whole blood was collected into heparinized syringes and placed in 50 ml conical tubes. The blood was washed at 37^0 C with PBSG at pH 7.4 then centrifuged at 10,000 rpm for 5 minutes in a desktop Eppendorf Centrifuge 5403. The supernatant was aspirated into a vacuum flask. The resulting RBCs were washed twice more with the final wash lasting for 7 minutes to better pellet the cells. The final pellet was diluted with the phosphate buffered saline solution with glucose (PBSG) to yield a 40% hematocrit.

2.3 Methemoglobin assay

The halogenated phenylhydroxylamines were prepared in acetone to yield concentrations from 30-300 µM. Ten µl of the test agent versus the vehicle (acetone) was added to the PBSG. Two ml samples in scintillation vials for incubations were placed in a 37-degree shaker bath and methemoglobin levels were measured at various time points ending at 180-240 minutes. Fifteen ml plastic tubes, one for each sample, were placed on ice. Five ml of ice-cold hemolysis buffer (0.277% Potassium Phosphate, 0.289% Sodium Phosphate, and 0.05% Triton x100) was placed in each tube. Then 75 µl of the 40% hematocrit blood was pipetted into 5ml of the hemolysis buffer and vortexed. For each sample, 4 cuvettes were arranged. To cuvettes 2 and 4, 20 µl of 10% KCN was added. To cuvettes 3 and 4, 20 µl of 20% K3Fe (CN) $_6$ was added. One ml of the hemolyzed blood sample was pipetted into each of the 4 cuvettes. The absorbance was measured at 635 nm on an UltroSpec 2000 UV/Visible Spectrophotometer. Incubations in the presence and absence of the various chemical agents described above were performed in triplicate. Methemoglobin levels relative to total hemoglobin were measured by a modification of the spectrophotometric technique of Evelyn and Malloy [6].

2.4 Measurement of the hemolytic response

Rat erythrocytes were collected, washed three times with PBSG, labeled with radioactive sodium chromate (0.1 m ^{51}Cr/1.0 ml of packed cells), incubated for 15 minutes at 37^0 C on shaker bath, washed once again with PBSG, adjusted hematocrit to 40%, treated cells with specified doses, incubated again for two hours at 37^0 C before injecting into rats (0.5 ml/animal). The initial blood sample 75-μl (T_0) was taken from the orbital sinus within 30 minutes after the infusion of tagged erythrocytes in rats. Control incubations received acetone as a vehicle. The treated erythrocytes were administered via tail vein to isologous rats as previously described elsewhere (International Committee for Standardization in Hematology [7], Harrison and Jollow [2]). Serial blood samples (75 μl) from each rat were then collected into heparinized capillary tubes at designated intervals for 14 days. At the end of experiment, all of the samples were counted in a well-type γ-counter, with the counts per minute above background for each sample expressed as a percentage of the T_0 sample. Data were expressed in terms of % decrease in values relative to the radioactive ^{51}Cr values of the red cells in that animal at time zero (T_0) in the control.

2.5 Animals

Male Sprague Dawley rats weighing 100-150 gms were used for this study. The usage of rats falls into two categories: (1) RBC donors, (2) hemotoxicity assays. For RBC donation, the animals were placed under ether anesthesia and blood was obtained by cardiac puncture. For the hemotoxicity studies, the animals received radiolabelled Cr- 51 tagged red blood cells iv via tail vein under light ether anesthesia. Serial blood samples were taken subsequently from the orbital sinus. At the end of all experiments, the animals were placed under ether anesthesia and sacrificed by decapitation.

3 Results

3.1 Methemoglobin

Figure 1 shows dose dependent changes in the induction of methemoglobin following exposure to various halogenated phenylhydroxylamines. The MetHb induction peaked to 35% at 50 μM, 56% at 100 μM and to 67 % at 150 μM within 10 minutes before declining after treatment with *para*-fluoro-PHA. At the end of 240 minutes the, MetHb level was 5 to 42 % depending on the dose compared to 2 % in control. Similarly, para-bromo-PHA produced dose dependent MetHb that peaked to almost 78 % within 20 minutes at 120 μM before declining. The MetHb remained eight to thirteen-fold elevated (40 to 65 %) compared to 5 % in control at 240 minutes post-treatment. With *para*-iodo-PHA, the MetHb level peaked to 75 % at the 90 μM dose before started declining. At the end of 240 minutes, the percent MetHb stayed elevated from 20 to 35 % depending on the dose and this represented 3 to 7 fold increase in MetHb compared to control. The data presented showed the highest peak with *para* -bromo-PHA followed by *para* iodo-PHA, *para* -fluoro-PHA and PHA. With PHA, the MetHb peaked within 60 minutes before declining. However, with *para* -bromo- PHA and *para* -iodo-PHA, the percent MetHb remained elevated by 7-8 fold at the end of 240 minutes.

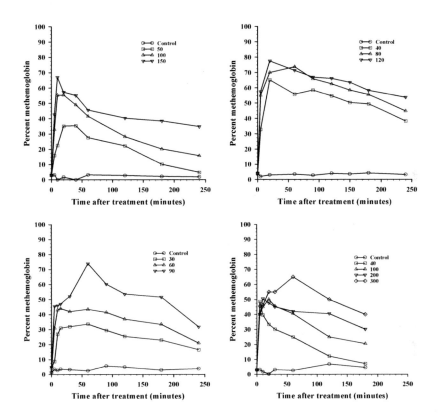

Figure 1:   Time course of percent methemoglobin formation with para-fluoro-, para-bromo-, para-iodo-phenylhydroxylamine and PHA (dose in µM).

3.2 Hemolytic anemia

The three aniline hydroxylamines tested produced dose dependent reduction in the labeled red blood cells indicating the loss of blood cells from circulation (Figure 2 a-c). The most pronounced reduction was observed at doses from 175 to 250 µM. The dose of 100 µM appeared to be the threshold level and the dose of 325 µM did not show much further reduction in the radioactivity than that observed at 250 µM. Results showed that *para* -iodo-PHA was two times more toxic than para-fluoro-PHA in the induction of hemolytic anemia after treatment with 175 µM. All the three tested halogenated phenylhydroxylamines appeared to be potential biomarkers in the induction of hemolytic anemia in this study.

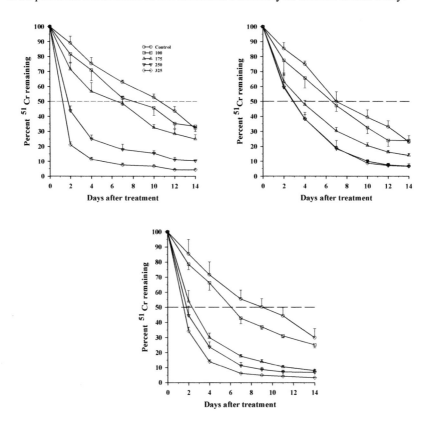

Figure 2:   Percent ^{51}Cr remaining in erythrocytes after treatment with *para*-fluoro-, *para*-bromo-, and *para*-iodo-PHA (dose in µM).

The hemolytic effect of *para*-bromo- and *para*-iodo-PHA as shown in Figure 2 was almost similar. At 100 µM, there was little effect on the reduction of tagged cells from circulation with either phenylhydoxylamine compared to respective controls but the level of tagged cells dramatically reduced in circulation as the dose increased to 250 µM or above. It appeared that the maximum drastic effect peaked at 250 µM with either phenylhydroxylamine, thereby, reducing the circulation of tagged cells to less than 10 percent compared to approximately 30 percent in control.

The T_{50} (50% removal from circulation) values for PHA at 150 and 250 µM were approximately 4.0 days and 8.5 and 1.75 days with para-fluoro-PHA, respectively, compared to 8.5 days in control.

4 Discussion and conclusion

The current study showed that induction MetHb and blood hemolysis varied with dose, time and the electronegativity of halogenated phenylhydroxyamines tested. The *para* -fluoro-PHA produced the most rapid response by elevating the MetHb level from 2-5 percent in control to almost 70 percent within 10 minutes before declining. Whereas the MetHb steadily declined with time in all cases except with *para* -bromo-PHA that still showed 40-65 percent MetHb at the end of 240 minutes experimental period compared to less than 5 percent in control.

Aniline induced a dose-dependent methemoglobinemia in rats after intraperitoneal injection, but did not cause methemoglobin formation when it was present in erythrocyte suspensions in concentrations associated with *in vivo* methemoglobinemia. This finding is consistent with previous reports in the literature and with the conclusion that methemoglobinemia after aniline is me-diated by one or more toxic metabolites formed during the hepatic clearance of aniline (Kiese [5]).   Although phenylhydroxylamine, nitrosobenzene, or further breakdown products of aniline metabolism have not been demonstrated in urine (von Jagow et al. [8]) but Kiese [9] has shown that nitrosobenzene is present in blood after aniline administration.   Production of nitrosobenzene and/or phenylhydroxylamine from aniline has also been observed in microsomal systems (Kiese [5]) and in the isolated perfused rat liver (Eyer et al. [10]).

The time course of methemoglobinemia in rats given aniline halogenated hydroxylamines is much different from that observed after treatment of the rats with the other phenylhydroxylamines. In general, halogenated aniline-induced a much extended duration of methemoglobinemia for a given peak level than did PHA as was observed in the present study. Whereas the metabolites produced parallel increases in peak and total methemoglobinemia with increasing dose, higher doses of aniline analogs were associated with a disproportionate increase in the duration and level of methemoglobinemia. This was confirmed in the present study.

Among the halogenated anilines the p-substituted compounds have been found to be most active in cats (McLean et al. [11]) and dogs (Kiese [12]). In dogs the high yield of ferrihemoglobin by 4-chloroaniline is due to the slow elimination of the parent amine and its N-hydroxy metabolite. According to Kiese and Renner [13], 4-Chlorophenylhydroxylamine and 4-chloronitrosobenzene accumulate to high concentrations, up to 2×10^{-4} M and probably produce most of the ferrihemoglobin. Ferrihemoglobin formation by halogen-anilines has also been observed in humans (Williams and Challis [14], Hughes and Treon [15], Faivre et al. [16]).

All three aniline hydroxylamines tested produced dose-dependent reduction in the labeled red blood cells indicating the loss of blood cells from circulation. The most pronounced reduction was observed at doses from 175 to 250 μM. The dose of 100 μM appeared to be the threshold level and the dose of 325 μM did not show much further reduction in the radioactivity than that observed at 250 μM. Results showed that *para* -iodo-PHA was two times more toxic than *para* -fluoro-PHA in the induction of hemolytic anemia in rats. These three phenylhydroxylamines tested appeared to be active metabolites that mediate aniline-induced hemolytic anemia. The study showed the following hemotoxic potencies of the hydroxylamines tested: p-iodo-PHA > p-bromo-PHA> p-fluoro-PHA >PHA>. Overall, aniline-derivatives produced a dose-dependent reduction in the circulation of tagged red cells as indicated by the radioactivity count.

It is generally known that hemolytic arylamines require metabolism to N-hydroxylamine's in order to produce toxic effects on red blood cells. The reactive N-hydroxy metabolites subsequently react with oxyhemoglobin to produce reactive oxygen species and sulfur-center free radical of hemoglobin resulting in formation of adducts with a variety of membrane associated proteins altering cytoskeletal structure and function. These membrane alterations result in the premature removal of damaged cells from the circulation by the spleen. This study was an attempt to compare the hemotoxicity of a variety of laboratory-synthesized arylhydroxylamine analogs of aniline selected based upon their differences in electronegativity. The aryl hydroxylamines selected for examination vary in electron donation/withdrawal in the para position and hence were expected to vary the stability of the generated hydronitoxide radical that might act as an intermediary in inducing hemotoxic damage.

All phenylhydroxylamines in the present studies act as probable mediators of aniline-induced hemolytic anemia in rats; however, the interactions between phenylhydroxylamine and erythrocyte components which result ultimately in splenic sequestration of erythrocytes are poorly understood. It is known that phenylhydroxylamine is metabolized within erythrocytes and is a highly potent methemoglobin-forming agent in erythrocytes (Kiese, [5]). In as much as phenylhydroxylamine itself is a reducing agent, phenylhydroxylamine mediated hemoglobin oxidation is proposed to occur via a "coupled oxidation" with oxyhemoglobin in the erythrocyte, forming methemoglobin, nitrosobenzene and partially reduced oxygen species (e.g., peroxide and/or superoxide; Kiese [5]). Nitrosobenzene thus formed may be bound to deoxyhemoglobin or may be reduced to phenyl hydroxylamine by an NADPH dependent diaphorase, leading to the formation of a redox cycle producing many equivalents of methemoglobin for each equivalent of phenylhydroxylamine. The cycle is depleted eventually by side reactions involving phenylhydroxylamine or nitrosobenzene, or by reduction of phenylhydroxylamine to aniline within erythrocytes (Eyer [17], Kiese [5], Murayama [18]). Side reactions which may occur within erythrocytes include binding of phenylhydroxylamine to erythrocytic protein (Kiese and Traeger [19] and binding of both nitrosobenzene and phenylhydroxylamine to sulfhydryl groups in glutathione or protein (Boyland et al. [20], Eyer [17]. The findings presented here support that several aniline metabolites of known structure mediate the hemolytic effect of aniline or any aniline-related compounds. Although it has been proposed previously that N-hydroxydapsone might mediate the hemolytic effects of dapsone (Glader and Conrad [21]), N-hydroxy metabolites have not otherwise been considered as mediators of the hemolytic effects of aniline, primaquine or other hemolytic drugs. Further experiments are required to determine whether aniline-induced hemolytic anemia is an appropriate model for hemolytic anemia induced by primaquine and other drugs which are aniline derivatives. Our data indicate that N-hydroxyl metabolites should be considered as possible mediators of chemical -induced hemolytic anemia, and thus are potential biomarkers for assessing chemical toxicity.

Acknowledgements

The authors thank Dr. David Jollow and Dr. David McMillan for the guidance and supervision of this study, Dr. John E. Otis for assistance in the synthesis of aniline analogs, Ms. Jennifer Schulte for the technical assistance and Dr. Sivapatham Paramasivam for the assistance in graphic presentation of data.

References

[1]   Henderson, R.H., Biomarkers: The Genome & the Individual, Charleston, SC, pp. 11, 1997.

[2]   Harrison, J.H., Jr., Jollow, D.J., Role of aniline metabolites in aniline-induce hemolytic anemia. J Pharmacol Exp Ther 238:1045-1054, 1986.

[3]   Harrison, J.H., Jr., Jollow, D.J., (Contribution of aniline metabolites to aniline-induced methemoglobinemia. Mol Pharmacol 32:423-431, 1987.

[4]   Grossman, S.J., and Jollow, D.J., Role of Dapsone Hydroxylamine in Dapsone-Induced Hemolytic Anemia. The Journal of Pharmacology and Experimental Therapeutics 244(1): 118-125, 1987.

[5]   Kiese, M., Methemoglobinemia: a comprehensive treatise. CEC Press, Cleveland, 1974.

[6]   Evelyn, KA, Mallory, HT. Microdetermination of oxyhemoglobin, methemoglobin, and sulfhemoglobin in a single sample of blood. J Biol Chem 126:655-662, 1938.

[7]   International Committee for Standardization in Hematology: Recommended methods for radioisotope red cell survival studies. Blood 38:378-386, 1971.

[8]   von Jagow R, Kiese M, Renner G. Urinary excretion of N-hydroxy derivatives of some aromatic amines by rabbits, guinea pigs, and dogs. Biochem Pharmacol 15:1899-1910, 1966.

[9]   Kiese, M., The biochemical production of ferrihemoglobin-forming derivatives from aromatic amines, and mechanisms of ferrihemoglobinemia formation. Pharmacol Rev 18:1091-1161, 1966.

[10]   Eyer, P., Kampffmeyer H., Maister, H., Rösch-Oehme Biotransformation of nitrosobenzene, phenylhydroxylamine, and aniline in the isolated perfused rat liver. Xenobiotica 10:499-516, 1980.

[11]   McLean, S., Starmer, G.A., Thomas, J., Methemoglobin formation by aromatic amines. J Pharm Pharmacol 21, 441, 1969.

[12]   Kiese M. Oxydation von aniline zu nitrosobenzol in hunde. Nauyn Schmiedebergs Arch Pharmacol 235:360-364, 1969.

[13]   Kiese, M., Renner, G., the isolation of p-chloronitrosobenzene from the blood of dogs injected with p-chloroaniline. Naunyn-Schmiedebergs Arch Exp Pathol Pharmakol 246, 163, 1963.

[14]   Williams JR, Challis FE Methylene blue as an antidote for aniline dye poisoning. Case report with confimatory experimental study. J Clin Med 19, 166, (1933).
[15]   Hughes, J.P., Treon, J.F., erythrocytic inclusion bodies in the blood of chemical workers. Arch Ind Hyg Occup Med 10, 192, 1954.
[16]   Faivre, M., Armand, J., Everux, JC., Duverneuil, G., Colin, C., Méthémoglobinémie toxique par des dérivés de paniline: parachloroaniline et paratoluidine (deux cas). Arch Mal Prof Méd trav 32, 575, 1971.
[17]   Eyer, P., Reactions of nitrosobenzene with reduced glutathione. Chem.- Biol. Interact. 24:227-239, 1979.
[18]   Murayama M. The combining power of normal human hemoglobin for nitrosobenzene. J Biol Chem 235: 1024-1028, 1960.
[19]   Kiese M, Traeger K. The fate if phenylhydroxylamine in human red cells. Naunyn-Schmiedeberg's Arch Pharmacol 292:59-66, 1976.
[20]   Boyland, E, Mansi, D., and Nery, R. The reaction of phenylhydroxylamine and 2-naphthylhydroxylamine with thiols. J. Chem. Soc. Part I: 606-611,1962.
[21]   Glader, B.E., and Conrad, M.E. Hemolysis by diphenylsulfones: Comparative effect of DDS and hydroxylamine-DDS. J. Lab. Clin. Med. 81:267-272, 1973.

Quantitative microbial risk assessment modelling for the use of reclaimed water in irrigated horticulture

A. J. Hamilton[1], F. Stagnitti[1], A.-M. Boland[2] & R. Premier[2]
[1]School of Ecology and Environment, Deakin University, Australia
[2]Department of Primary Industries Victoria, Australia

Abstract

Reuse of treated sewage effluent for the irrigation of horticultural crops is being propounded and practiced as a means of alleviating pressure on freshwater resources. Concerns have been raised, however, as to the risk to human health, primarily disease, associated with this practice. Quantitative Microbial Risk Assessment (QMRA) is a useful tool for estimating this risk. We describe how QMRA works and the current state of knowledge of the components of QMRA models for the horticultural reuse scenario.
Keywords: food-safety, horticulture, pathogen, quantitative microbial risk assessment, reclaimed water, recycled water, vegetable.

1 Introduction

Increasing human population sizes are placing significant strain on the World's freshwater resources. Rivers are becoming polluted, extraction for agricultural use is substantially reducing flows, and competition for freshwater is intensifying. Moreover, with the growth of large cities, there is a concomitant escalation in sewage output, and thus a likely increase in detrimental effects associated with discharge of effluent to receiving waters. One means of alleviating such stresses is to reuse wastewater for horticultural irrigation (Hamilton *et al.* [1]). But this practice has been approached with a degree of trepidation, owing primarily to concerns about risks to human health via contamination of food with pathogenic microorganisms [1]. In theory at least, such risks can be mitigated through combinations of low- and high-technology engineering solutions. At the recent *Integrated Concepts in Recycled Water* conference (Wollongong, February 2005), Professor Don Bursill made this pertinent observation: "You can turn anything wet into drinking water if you filter it through enough money".

But this is also where risks can enter a system: it is usually not economically feasible to employ almost fail-safe treatment. Little wastewater in the developing world undergoes treatment of any kind, and even in affluent countries the cost of treatment is a key criterion determining the likely success or failure of a reuse scheme (Robinson [2]). Thus, we need methods to determine the risk that different recycled water irrigation scenarios pose to human health, so that safe and economically realistic schemes can be developed.

Recent years have seen a general movement towards the use of QMRA for determining health risks. The brief for the revised World Health Organisation (WHO) guidelines for agricultural reuse (due for release in 2005) was to use QMRA (Blumenthal et al. [3]). Australia is also currently revising its national guidelines for recycled water use, and these will include QMRA (Cunliffe et al. [4]). The purpose of this review is to outline how QMRA works, and to progress ideas on how it can best be applied to horticultural reuse scenarios. Knowledge gaps relating to such QMRA models are identified and subsequent recommendations for strategic research are made.

2   What is Quantitative Microbial Risk Assessment (QMRA)?

Quantitative Risk Assessment (QRA) modelling is a formal process for calculating probabilities of risk associated with defined scenarios. It was originally developed to determine risks to humans of environmental exposure to various hazards, especially chemicals (NRC [5]). Recent times have seen the emergence of a specific form of QRA, namely, QMRA. QMRA comprises four distinct steps: (i) hazard identification, (ii) exposure assessment, (iii) dose-response analysis, and (iv) risk characterisation (Haas et al. [6]).

The first QMRAs for reclaimed water irrigation of food crops were simplistic models where the various parameters—such as the concentration of viruses in the irrigation water or the amount of food consumed—were represented as point-estimates (Asano and Sakaji [7], Asano et al. [8], Rose et al. [9], Shuval et al. [10]). More recent models have used probability distributions to define parameters (Tanaka et al. [11], van Ginneken and Oron [12], Petterson et al. [13]). This is an important step forward, as it means that a more accurate estimate of risk can be calculated, since variability and uncertainty are accounted for. QMRA is applied to a conceptual model such as the one we present below for the irrigation of horticultural crops with treated wastewater, fig. 1.

3   Hazard identification

In the context of QMRA, hazard identification primarily involves determining the microbiological agent(s) likely to be of potential significance with respect to human health. There have been many reported cases of human pathogen

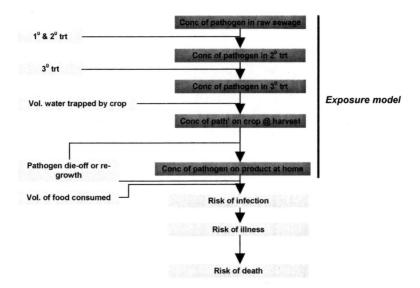

Figure 1:   Conceptual model of risk pathway associated with consumption of horticultural crops irrigated with wastewater.

contamination of crops irrigated with reclaimed water (summarised by Fegen et al. [14]. But establishing a cause-effect relationship between contaminated produce and disease outbreaks has proved rather difficult. One of the more convincing cases is the 1970 cholera outbreak in Jerusalem (Shuval et al. [15], Fattal et al. [16]). Illicit irrigation of vegetables with reclaimed water and subsequent purchase by around 100,000–200,000 people was followed by about 200 cases of cholera. The cause-effect connection was strengthened by the fact that the risk analysis model of Shuval et al. [10], when applied to this irrigation scenario, proved to be a good predictor of the magnitude of the epidemic. There is also reasonable evidence to suggest that outbreaks of cholera and typhoid fever in Chile in the late 1970s to early 1980s could be attributed to contaminated food from wastewater-irrigated horticulture (Shuval [17]).

Recent QMRA models have primarily been concerned with risk of disease from enteric viruses [11, 12, 13]. The rationales for using viruses are that they (i) are generally highly persistent in the environment, (ii) have low-dose infectivity, and (iii) are relatively difficult to remove/inactivate in wastewater treatment systems. Asano et al. [8] have argued that the difficulty of routine monitoring for enteric viruses is another reason for developing QMRAs that address this group. A wide variety of enteric viruses are found in wastewaters (Irving [18]). The most commonly problematic from a human health perspective are enteroviruses, rotaviruses, hepatitis A virus, and Norwalk or Norwalk-like viruses.

4 Exposure assessment

The objective of exposure assessment is to determine the quantity of pathogenic organisms consumed by a person eating or drinking the product of interest. This can be achieved relatively easily for drinking water scenarios by determining the concentration of pathogens in the water and the amount of water typically consumed by an individual (Haas *et al.* [19]). But the situation is somewhat more complex when considering horticultural irrigation. In addition to information on the concentration of pathogens in the raw wastewater and the amount of food consumed, factors such as treatment efficiency, irrigation method, and pathogen die-off need to be accounted for.

4.1 Pathogen concentration in wastewater

Asano *et al.* [8] collated the largest database in the USA for enteric virus concentrations in treated wastewater. It comprises 424 secondary-treated effluent samples and 814 tertiary-treated samples. The concentration of pathogens such as enteric viruses in tertiary-treated effluent is a function of the concentration in the secondary-effluent and the efficiency of the tertiary-treatment process. Possibly the most comprehensive study of a tertiary-treatment plant's pathogen removal efficiency is that of Rose *et al.* [9], table 1. Parkinson and Roddick [20] reviewed the literature on the pathogen removal efficiencies of fourteen different wastewater treatment technologies, and categorised them into broad efficiency classes.

Table 1: Pathogen removal efficiencies (as %, with log removals in parentheses) of different tertiary treatment processes. After Rose *et al.* [9].

Pathogen	Biological/ clarification	Filtration	Chlorination	Storage (16–24 hr)	Complete treatment
Enteroviruses	98.0 (1.71)	84.0 (1.71)	96.5 (1.45)	90.91 (1.04)	99.999 (5.01)
Giardia	93.0 (1.19)	99.0 (2.00)	78.0 (0.65)	49.5 (0.30)	99.993 (4.14)
Cryptosporidium	92.8 (1.14)	97.9 (1.68)	61.1 (0.41)	8.5 (0.04)	99.95 (3.27)
Helminths	>75.0	no data	no data	no data	<99.6

4.2 Volume of water on crop and attachment of pathogens to crop

A critical step in the development of horticultural reuse QMRAs is the determination of the volume of water caught by plants. The concentration of pathogens on the plant at harvest is plainly a function of this. Surprisingly, there is a dearth of information on the process. Glass-house experiments simulating spray-irrigation of cucumber and lettuce revealed that on average 0.36 and 10.8 mL of water was retained by 100 g of each product, respectively [10]. The latter point-estimate was subsequently used by Petterson *et al.* [13] in their lettuce irrigation QMRA. Aside from the theoretical limitations associated with point estimates, it should be noted that Shuval *et al.*'s estimates are based on small sample sizes: 26 and 12 for cucumber and lettuce, respectively. Moreover, it appears that each vegetable was represented by one cultivar only (the cultivars were not reported, but the lettuce was referred to as 'long leaf'). While cultivar effects are likely to be trivial for cucumbers, they may be significant for more structurally complex and diverse plants like lettuce. In an unpublished field-study we irrigated three cultivars of lettuce—Iceberg, Cos, and Romaine—and measured the amount of water trapped by 25 plants of each. Analysis of variance on $\log_{10}$-transformed data demonstrated a significant cultivar effect ($P = 0.045$, $df_{\text{total}} = 74$), and *post hoc* Least Significant Difference tests revealed a significant difference ($P < 0.05$) between Iceberg (37.3 mL) and Romaine (26.8 mL), with neither of these cultivars being significantly different from Cos (30.7 mL). Data on mass were not recorded, so it is not possible to compare these values to those of Shuval *et al.* [10]. Nonetheless, it does highlight the potential significance of cultivar variation.

4.3 Pathogen decay

Pathogens on a plant's surface, being exposed to sunlight, are susceptible to desiccation and inactivation or death by ultra-violet light. A significant positive correlation between mean hours of monthly sunshine and the rate of die-off has been demonstrated for bacteria on salad crops (Fattal *et al.* [21]). Schwartbrod [22] estimated that there would be a < 6 $\log_{10}$ reduction in virus concentration on a plant from the time of irrigation to consumption. While useful, this is a very rough estimate, and QMRAs would probably be best to use models that describe decay rates as a function of time (and possibly other factors). Moreover, it may be fruitful to break down the production and distribution chain into field and post-harvest events when addressing pathogen decay.

The decay of pathogens in the environment can be modelled using a simple first-order rate equation such as

$$f = \mu_1 / \mu_0 = e^{(-kt)} \tag{1}$$

where f is the proportion of pathogens remaining (viable) after time t (d), μ_0 and μ_1 are the respective initial and final pathogen concentrations, and the slope parameter k is the decay coefficient (d^{-1}). Asano and Sakaji [7] and Asano *et al.* [8] used this function in their deterministic models. They were concerned with a variety of risks (vegetable and golf-course irrigation, recreational waters, and groundwater recharge) and assumed a generic k for enteric viruses of 0.69 d^{-1}; a justification for this value was not given. van Ginneken and Oron [12] subsequently used this estimated k–value in their stochastic model. Experiments on the decay of *Bacteriodes fragilis* bacteriophage B40-8 on glasshouse-grown lettuce yielded an estimated k of 0.47 d^{-1} (Petterson *et al.* [23]).

In the log-linear model in eqn. (1) the probability of a pathogen being inactivated remains constant over time and is described by the parameter k.

Thus, inactivation is assumed to be a single-phase process, and the model does not accommodate multi-phase inactivation kinetics that may be appropriate where persistent sub-populations exist. Petterson et al. [23] fitted the following bi-phasic inactivation model to their bacteriophage survival data on lettuce and carrot crops:

$$\mu_1 = \mu_0 \left[ae^{-k_1 t} + (1-a)e^{-k_2 t} \right] \qquad (2)$$

where a is a mixing parameter that describes the proportionate size of the sub-population, k_1 and k_2 are the respective decay coefficients for the main and sub-populations, and t, μ_0, and μ_1 are as defined above. For both crops the bi-phasic model showed a statistically superior fit over the single-phase, thus inferring the presence of persistent sub-populations.

The k parameter(s) in eqn. (1) and eqn. (2) are not the only constants that require careful consideration when developing a QMRA model. The time, t, that the viruses are exposed to the environment could have a marked effect on the model output. Asano et al. [8] assumed that irrigation would cease two weeks before harvest, and they consequently assigned a t-value of 14 d to their model. In doing so they implicitly assumed that no virus inactivation took place after harvest. Petterson et al. [13] also used $t = 14$ d, but stated that consumption was assumed to take place this long after the last irrigation event. van Ginneken and Oron [12] adopted a novel approach whereby the elapsed time between final irrigation and consumption was optimised for their specific QMRA so as to obtain a total risk of infection of $< 10^{-4}$ (i.e. to comply with US EPA [24]). The optimal value was 20 d for spray irrigation of vegetables.

4.4 Pathogen re-growth

Viruses are not able to grow outside their hosts. Thus, considering most QMRA models for horticultural re-use have been based on viruses, pathogen re-growth has not needed to be addressed. Bacterial and fungal pathogens, on the other hand, do have the potential to re-grow on the produce. Several models that describe growth as function of time and environmental variables have been constructed (see review by López et al. [25]). Detailed re-growth models for pathogens on vegetables are generally lacking.

4.5 Quantity of food consumed

Quantification of the amount of food consumed is an important step in a QMRA model. Unfortunately, unlike drinking water scenarios, Rosebury and Burmaster [26], comprehensive data on consumption rates are difficult to obtain. In their model, Shuval et al. [10] simply used point-estimates, and assumed that Israelites consumed 100g of lettuce or cucumber d^{-1} for 150d. Petterson et al. [13] based their assumption of 100 g of lettuce per consumption event on Shuval et al.'s point-estimate. Asano et al. [8] and Tanaka et al. [11] assumed that consumers of crops irrigated with reclaimed water were exposed to an average daily dose of 10 mL of reclaimed water. van Ginneken and Oron [12] used a more realistic approach, whereby consumption behaviour of raw fruits and vegetables (combined) was described using probability distributions.

5 Dose-response models

Dose-response models describe the relationship between the mean number of microorganisms ingested and the probability of a specific outcome (usually infection) in individuals that have received that mean dose (Vose [27]). The two most commonly-used dose-response models in QMRA are the exponential and the β-Poisson. The best-fit parameters for the models are determined from trials where subjects are challenged with specific doses of a pathogen or a substitute for it.

The exponential model is:

$$P_{\text{inf}}\left(\lambda;r\right)=1-e^{(-r\lambda)},\tag{3}$$

where λ is the number of potentially infective microorganisms consumed and r is the probability that each microbe has of causing infection to a consumer (pathogen-host survival probability). The model carries the following assumptions: (i) there is a constant probability of infection across all individuals in a population, (ii) each individual microorganism has the same infective capability, and (iii) survival of a microorganism within a host is independent of the survival of any other microorganism in the same host. The exponential model has found particular application for enteric protozoan pathogens such as *Cryptosporidium parvum* and *Giardia lamblia*, which are typically found in low numbers [6].

The β-Poisson dose-response model, derived by Furumoto and Mickey [28], is an extension of the exponential. In addition to describing λ with a probability function (the Poisson), r is described with the β-probability distribution. Thus, the β-Poisson infectivity model is

$$P_{\text{inf}}\left(\lambda;\alpha,\beta\right)=1-{}_1F_1\left(\alpha,\alpha+\beta,-\lambda\right)\tag{4}$$

where α and β are fit-parameters (but also have biological meaning, [27], and ${}_1F_1()$ is the Kummer confluent hypergeometric function. This model cannot readily be fitted to dose-response data to obtain maximum likelihood estimates of its parameters. The problem is circumvented by using an approximation, [28]. If $\beta \gg 1$ and $\beta \gg \alpha$ then P_{inf} can be estimated as

$$P_{\text{inf}}=1-\left(1+\lambda/\beta\right)^{-\alpha}\tag{5}$$

This approximation of the β-Poisson has been used widely in QMRA.

The β-Poisson is a useful alternative to the exponential as it allows one to incorporate individual variability, both in the pathogen and host. This property is particularly valuable where subpopulations, such as pregnant women, immunodeficient people (e.g. AIDS sufferers), children, or the elderly, are prevalent or of particular interest. Thus, the β-Poisson is generally more appropriate than the exponential for pathogens that illicit an immune response. A β-Poisson dose-response model for rotavirus infection of humans was developed by Ward *et al.* [29], and has this been widely used for drinking water, [9, 11], and horticultural reuse QMRAs [12, 13]. Rotaviruses form a sub-group of enteric viruses. They are known for being highly infective, and are particularly common in susceptible sub-populations such as the young and the elderly. They are thus considered to represent an adequate worst-case scenario of enteric viruses. Best-fit parameters of other dose response studies were tabulated by Hass *et al.* [6].

5.1 Risk characterisation

Risk characterisation combines the exposure and dose-response models so that a risk probability can be estimated. As alluded to above, risk can be determined in one of either two ways. Point estimates of model parameters can be used and a single probability describing risk calculated. Alternatively, the model parameters can be represented by probability distributions, which can be sampled from at random many times over using computer simulation techniques such as Monte Carlo. Such stochastic models are preferred because they accommodate variation. More specifically, they can account for variability and uncertainty. Variability is the natural variation among data. It cannot be reduced through improved experimental design or measurement techniques. Uncertainty, on the other hand, represents one's ignorance about the parameter of interest. It can be reduced through more accurate and/or precise sampling. It is not always possible to separate variability and uncertainty, but simply including variation, or total uncertainty (Vose [30]), in a QMRA model gives a truer representation of risk than simple point-estimate models [6, 30].

The discussion hitherto has been concerned with determining the level of risk. An equally important agendum is defining the *acceptable* level of risk. There has been little guidance for setting suitable risk levels for reuse scenarios. To this end, QMRA models for effluent reuse have generally followed the lead of the drinking water industry. The US EPA [24] set an arbitrary acceptable risk level of one infection per 10,000 people per year (i.e. $< 10^{-4}$) for human consumption of drinking water. This has been used as the critical risk level or reference point for several wastewater reuse QMRAs [8, 9, 10, 11 15]. The appropriateness of this standard was questioned by Haas [31] who propounded a more conservative benchmark of 10^{-3}.

Recent years have seen the emergence of a new approach to setting acceptable risk standards—the disability adjusted life year (DALY) (WHO [32]). The DALY metric is calculated as the sum of years of life lost (YLL) due to premature death and the number of years lived with a disability (standardised for severity) (YLD). Thus,

$$DALY = YLL + YLD \qquad (6)$$

The exact calculation of YLL and YLD is complex and is outlined by WHO [32]. The DALY is the chosen metric of acceptable risk for the WHO's new drinking water guidelines WHO [33] and their revised recycled water guidelines that are in progress (Carr et al. [34]). It is also to be used in the revised Australian recycled water guidelines.

5.2 Conclusion

The use of reclaimed water in irrigated horticulture is a contentious issue, owing primarily to concerns about the microbiological safety of produce grown in such a manner. QMRA has much to offer the debate. It will allow objective characterisation of risks associated with different scenarios. It is already starting to have an impact as several key reuse guidelines are based on it. Nonetheless, there is still substantial scope for improved QMRA models. Data upon which the models are based are still poor for certain steps, especially (i) the volume of water trapped by a plant, (ii) pathogen decay kinetics, (iii) and produce consumption behaviour of consumers. Also, most models are restricted to one or a few scenarios. Computerised decision support tools wherein a scheme-developer could run a QMRA for a specifically-defined scenario could be developed in the future, and could prove useful for viability and safety of the scheme.

References

[1]   Hamilton, A. J., Boland, A.-M., Stevens, D., Kelly, J., Radcliffe, J., Ziehrl, A., Dillon, P. J. & Paulin, R., Position of the Australian horticultural industry with respect to the use of reclaimed water. *Agricultural Water Management*, **71**, pp. 181–209, 2005.

[2]   Robinson, J., Cost benefit analysis of effluent re-use schemes: why water recycling projects fail to pass the test. Water recycling Australia: second national conference, Brisbane, 2003. CD ROM.

[3]   Blumenthal, U. J., Peasey, A., Ruiz-Palacios, G. & Mara, D., Guidelines for Wastewater Reuse in Agriculture and Aquaculture: Recommended Revisions Based on New Research Evidence. WELL Study, Task No. 68, Part 1. Water and Environmental Health at London and Loughborough (WELL), London, UK, 2000.
       http:/www.lboro.ac.uk/well/resources/well-studies/well-studies.htm.

[4]   Cunliffe, D. A., Bursill, D. & Hooy, T., Developing national guidelines on water recycling. Integrated Concepts in Water Recycling Conference, Wollongong, NSW, Australia, pp. 164–168, 2005.

[5]   National Research Council (NRC), Risk assessment in the Federal Government: managing the process, National Academy Press: Washington DC, 1983.

[6]   Haas, C. N., Rose, J. B. & Gerba, C. P., Quantitative Microbial Risk Assessment, John Wiley & Sons Inc.: New York, 1999.

[7]   Asano, T. & Sakaji, R. H., Virus risk analysis in wastewater reclamation and reuse. Chemical, water and wastewater treatment, eds. H. H. Hahn & R. Klute, Springer-Verlag: Berlin, Heidelberg. pp. 483–496, 1990.

[8]   Asano, T., Leong, L. Y. C., Rigby, M. G. & Sakaji, R. H., Evaluation of the California wastewater reclamation criteria using enteric virus monitoring data. *Water Science and Technology*, **26**(7–8), pp. 1513–1524, 1992.

[9]   Rose, J. B., Dickson, L. J., Farrah, S. R. & Carnahan, R. P., Removal of pathogenic and indicator microorganisms by a full-scale water reclamation facility. *Water Research*, **30**(11), pp. 2785–2797, 1996.

[10]   Shuval, H. I., Lampert, Y. & Fattal, B., Development of a risk assessment approach for evaluating wastewater recycling and reuse standards for agriculture. *Water Science and Technology*, **35**(11–12), pp. 15–20, 1997.

[11]   Tanaka, H., Asano, T., Schroeder, E. D. & Tchobanoglous, G., Estimating the safety of wastewater reclamation and reuse using enteric virus monitoring data. *Water Environment Research*, **70**(1), pp. 39–51, 1998.

[12]   Van Ginneken, M. & Oron, G., Risk assessment of consuming agricultural products irrigated with reclaimed wastewater: an exposure model. *Water Resources Research*, **36**(9), pp. 2691–2699, 2000.

[13]   Petterson, S. R., Ashbolt, N. & Sharma, A. A., Microbial risks from wastewater irrigation of salad crops: A screening-level risk assessment. *Water Environment Research*, **72**(6), pp. 667–672, 2001.

[14]   Fegen, N., Gardner, T. & Blackwell, P., Health risks associated with the reuse of effluent for irrigation—a literature review. State of Queensland Department of Natural Resources and Department of Primary Industries, 1998.

[15]   Shuval, H. I., Yekutiel, P. & Fattal, B., Epidemiological evidence for helminth and cholera transmission by vegetables with wastewater: Jerusalem—a case study. *Water Science and Technology*, **17**, pp. 433–442, 1984.

[16]   Fattal, B., Wax, Y., Davies, M. & Shuval, H. I., Health risks associated with wastewater irrigation: An epidemiological study. *Am. J. Public Health*, **76**, pp. 977–979, 1986.

[17]   Shuval, H. I., Investigation of typhoid fever and cholera transmission by raw wastewater irrigation in Santiago, Chile. *Water Science and Technology*, **27**(3–4), pp. 164–174, 1993.

[18]   Irving, L. G., Viruses in wastewater effluents (Chapter 7). Viruses and disinfection of water and wastewater, eds. M. Butler, A. R. Medlen & R. Morris, University of Surrey, Guildford, 1982.

[19]   Haas, C. N., Rose, J. B., Gerba, C. & Regli, S., Risk assessment of virus in drinking water. *Risk Analysis*, **13**, pp. 545–552, 1993.

[20]   Parkinson, A. & Roddick, F. A., Wastewater treatment effectiveness: a review. *Water*, **31**(5), pp. 63–68, 2004.

[21]   Fattal, B., Goldberg, T. & Dor, I., Model for measuring the effluent quality and the microbial die-off rate in Naan wastewater reservoir. *Journal of Handasat Maim*, **26**, pp. 26–30, 1996.

[22]   Schwartzbrod, L., Effect of human viruses on public health associated with the use of wastewater and sewage sludge in agriculture and aquaculture. World Health Organisation, Geneva. WHO/EOS/95.19, 1995.

[23]   Petterson, S. R., Teunis, P. F. M. & Ashbolt, N. J., B Modeling virus decay on salad crops using microbial count data. *Risk Analysis*, **21**(6), pp. 1097–1108, 2001.

[24]   US EPA, Guidelines for Reuse. EPA/625/R-92/004. Washington, DC. 247pp, 1992

[25]   López, S., Prieto, M., Dijkstra, J., Dhanoa, M. S. & France, J., Statistical evaluation of mathematical models for microbial growth. *International Journal of Food Microbiology*, **96**, pp. 289–300, 2004.

[26]   Rosebury, A. M. & Burmaster, D. E., Log-normal distribution for water intake by children and adults. *Risk Analysis*, **21**, pp. 99–104, 1992.

[27]   Vose, D. J., The application of quantitative risk assessment to microbial food safety. *Journal of Food Protection*, **61**(5), pp. 640–648, 1998.

[28]   Furumoto, W. A. & Mickey, R. A., Mathematical model for the infectivity-dilution curve of tobacco mosaic virus: experimental tests. *Virology*, **32**, pp. 224–233, 1967.

[29]   Ward, R. L., Bernstein, D. I., Young, E. C., Sherwood, J. R., Knowlton, D. R. & Schiff, G. M., Human rotavirus studies in volunteers: determination of infectious dose and serological response to infection. *Journal of Infectious Diseases*, **154**(5), pp. 871–880, 1986.

[30]   Vose D., (2000) Risk analysis: A quantitative guide, John Wiley & Sons Ltd: Chichester, 2000.

[31]   Haas, C. N., Acceptable health risk. Viewpoint. *Journal of the American Water Works Association*, **18**, pp. 8–10, 1996.

[32]   WHO (2004a). Quantifying public health risk in the WHO guidelines for drinking-water quality: a burden of disease approach.

[33]   WHO, Guidelines for drinking-water quality, 2004.

[34]   Carr, R. M., Blumenthal, U. J. & Mara, D. D., Health guidelines for the use of wastewater in agriculture: developing realistic guidelines, 2005. http://web.idrc.ca/es/ev-68330-201-1-DO TOPIC.html.

Chemical and ecotoxicological analyses to assess the environmental risk of the Garigliano River (central Italy)

N. Calace[1], B. M. Petronio[1], M. Pietroletti[1], E. Palmaccio[1], T. Campisi[2] & A. Iacondini[2]
[1]Department of Chemistry, University "La Sapienza", Italy
[2]Centro Ricerche e Servizi Ambientali Fenice S.p.A., Italy

Abstract

The aim of this paper was to assess the environmental risk of the Garigliano River on the Tyrrenean Sea. In particular we focused our attention on the chemical and ecotoxicological quality of the river. Nine stations (sediment) were analysed along the last 10 km before the sea for heavy metal content. Moreover, three ecotoxicological tests (*Vibrio fischeri* with Microtox®, *Pseudomonas fluorescens* DHase inhibition assay, *Pseudokirchneriella subcapitata* inhibition test) were carried out on sediment samples in order to evaluate the toxicity of the matrices. The principal components analysis (PCA) and clustering were performed in order to correlate all the data. The results showed that heavy metal content (Cu, Pb, Ni, Cd, Zn, Fe and Mn) is low in all stations; these data reflected the results obtained from ecotoxicological tests that showed no toxic matrices, except for one station. An integrated chemical and ecotoxicological approach applied on the Garigliano River found that actually its environmental impact is not hazardous for the Tyrrenean Sea.
Keywords: Vibrio fischeri test, Pseudomonas fluorescens test, algal test, heavy metals, Pseudokirchneriella subcapitata.

1 Introduction

In recent years, the assessment of the effect of sediment pollution on indigenous microflora has received more attention and an ecological interest [1]. Concentrations of contaminants in the environment are primarily determined by analytical chemical measurements, but often they do not provide direct information regarding biological effects of toxic compounds nor about the concentration available for microbial biodegradation [2]. The increasing in international regulations and the assessment of the potential risk caused by sediment pollution have focused on the need for rapid, reliable and accurate assays for soil and sediment environment. Using bioassays, the presence of toxic compounds and their biological and ecological risks can be determined. Moreover, among all the developed toxicity tests, bioassays with exogenous microorganisms or enzymes may be used to give information on the bioavailability and toxicity of the pollutants in soil and sediment [3, 4, 5].

Generally, regulations assume that acceptable concentrations for pollutants can be treated independently, even they are present in mixtures, but in many cases these assumptions may be uncorrected. Indeed, hazardous wastes sites often contain complex mixtures of pollutants which include both organic contaminants and heavy metals [6]. In particular, additive, synergistic or antagonistic interactions can take place when a target organism is exposed to mixtures of pollutants. Toxicity assessment of multiple combinations of different pollutants requires application of sensitive, rapid and reliable bioassays [7]. Among them, *Pseudomonas fluorescens* was successfully used in a new bioassay [8] to assess the ecotoxicity of heavy metals in soils [9]. Moreover, in order to obtain an ecological evaluation, two traditional bioassays were coupled to the new one: a test with the bioluminescent bacterium *Vibrio fischeri* (Microtox®) and an algal test with *Pseudokirchneriella subcapitata*. The aim of this work was to assess the environmental risk of the Garigliano River (Italy) on the Tyrrenean Sea. This study was carried out by means chemical analyses and ecotoxicological tests, in order to find also correlations between the two data.

2 Materials and methods

2.1 Samples collection

Sediments (0–10 cm) were collected in June 2004 with a van Veen grab sampler. The stations were sampled by the delta (station 1) of the river toward the hinterland to a distance of 1 km each other (overall 9 stations).

Sediments were immediately stored in polyethylene bags and frozen at -20°C. Before the analyses, the samples were lyophilised and homogenised.

2.2 Chemical analyses

2.2.1 Metal determination
Aliquots of sediment (0.20 ± 0.01 g) were introduced into PTFE vessels and 8 ml of concentrated HNO_3, 4 ml of 48% HF and 2 ml of concentrated H_2O_2 were added into vessels. The acid mixture was optimised in order to destroy completely the solid matrix. Then closed vessels with valve were introduced into a microwave oven working under the following conditions: 250 W, 5 min; 400 W, 5 min; 600 W, 10 min. Iron, copper, lead, manganese, zinc, nickel and

cadmium concentrations were determined by a Varian SpectrAA-10 atomic absorption spectrometer working with an air-acetylene flame.

The procedure was tested using two reference materials: IAEA-356 Polluted Marine Sediment and MURST-ISS-A₁ Antarctic Marine sediment.

2.2.2 Total organic carbon determination

Total organic carbon was determined by means of elemental analysis on sediment previously acidified with concentrated HCl to eliminate carbonates. Briefly, 100 mg of sediment was weighed out, acidified with 500 µl of HCl and then dried under an infrared lamp. The residue was again weighed and analysed using a Carlo Erba model EA11110 CHNS-O Element Analyser. The percentage carbon obtained from elemental analysis was recalculated for the original sediment and expressed as mg/g. The limit of detection (LOD) was 0.3%.

2.3 Toxicity tests

2.3.1 *Vibrio fischeri* test

The Microtox® Basic Solid Phase Test (BSPT) was performed according to standard operating procedure [10, 11] and the end point is the inhibition of light emission by the marine bacterium *V. fischeri*. Briefly, seven grams (± 0.01 g) of sediment were tested as suspensions prepared with 35 ml of diluent (35 g/l NaCl solution) and diluted to a series of 9 concentrations, in the incubator wells (Microtox® model 500 Analyser). Light readings were recorded at 5, 15, and 30 minutes, and, in this work, measures at 30 min were reported. Regression statistics of concentration (log C) on the gamma parameter (log Γ) were used to estimate the correlation which gives a nominal toxic effect. The software supplied by Azur Environmental calculated the EC50 value (g/l), and Toxicity Unit (TU, as 100/EC50). The greater the TU value, the greater the toxicity.

2.3.2 *Pseudomonas fluorescens* DHase inhibition assay

As screening test, DHase inhibition assay has been performed according to Guerra *et al.* [8] and Abbondanzi *et al.* [9]. The bacterium *P. fluorescens* ATCC 13525 was used after inoculum standardisation, at a concentration of 4-5 x 10^6 CFU ml^{-1}. The activity of dehydrogenase enzymes is linked to the respiratory and energy producing processes in the cell, and basically depends on the metabolic state of microorganisms. The dehydrogenase activity measures were carried out using 2,3,5-triphenyl tetrazolium chloride (TTC) as artificial electron acceptor. This salt is reduced by microbial activity to red coloured formazan, that can be determined with spectrophotometric measures (wavelength: 482 nm). After a 48-h incubation in the dark at 30°C, TPF was extracted with acetone for 2 h and its concentration was then determined spectrophotometrically. The test was conducted on total sediment matrix.

A garden soil was used as control soil, after chemical and chemical physical characterisations (80% sand, 20% silt and clay, 6.7% organic matter contents). The screening test was performed for every sediment sample, in order to estimate the Inhibition (I), calculated from TPF concentrations in samples and control:

$$\%I = \frac{(TPF_{control} - TPF_{sample})}{TPF_{control}}100$$

where TPFcontrol is the average of TPF concentration in control and TPFsample is the TPF average in sample (four replicates).

2.3.3 *Pseudokirchneriella subcapitata* inhibition test

Pseudokirchneriella subcapitata inhibition was performed as screening test and the green alga *P. subcapitata* (formerly known as *Selenastrum capricornutum*) was used following standard algal assay procedure [12, 13]. Cell growth inhibition was used as the endpoint in the toxicity experiments. Briefly, five grams (± 0.01 g) of sediment were suspended in 20 ml of algal culture (AAP) medium, without EDTA [13]. After 1h of shaking, the suspension was centrifuged at a 3200 rpm for 20 min and the surnatant was tested. The *P. subcapitata* culture was harvested at a cell density of 10^6 cells/ml, inoculated in surnatant and then incubated at 20±1°C under 5000-6000 Lux light. After 72-h incubation, the cell growths were estimated by manual counting method in samples and in control (ultrapure water), in order to calculated cell growth inhibition (I%), as for *P. fluorescens* DHase inhibition test.

3 Statistical analysis

The principal component (PCA) and clustering analyses were performed from Statgraphics plus 5.1 demo. PCA is a multivariate data reduction method that examines the variance patterns within a multidimensional dataset. The dimensionality of the dataset is reduced while retaining a major portion of the original information. This is accomplished by decomposing the correlation matrix of the variables of the data into a new set of axes, principal components, which define the directions of the major variances in the dataset. The principal components are linear combinations of the variables, comprised of three matrices that define the principal component: scores, loadings, and residuals. These matrices facilitate visualization of the relationships of the samples in the dataset and interpretation of the data. Clustering analysis supplies information about similarities between different variables. It was carried out by means of Ward's method with square Euclidean distance.

4 Results and discussion

Figure 1 shows the results of the two screening tests, using *Pseudomonas fluorescens* on sediment matrix and *Pseudokirchneriella subcapitata* on surnatant. For *P. fluorescens* DHase inhibition assay, the toxic effect was detected only in station 4 (21,8%), while for the other sampling points, the effect on test organism resulted as a no toxicity (inhibition in station 3 was < 10%, corresponding to a no toxic effect) or, mostly, a stimulation. The effect trend of *P. subcapitata* was mostly in according with *P. fluorescens*, except for station 1 and 2, and for station 3 which produced a stimulation effect in the algal test. In station 1 and 2, which are near the mouth of the river, the salinity was high (7 and 0.44 ‰ in station 1 and 2 respectively, against 0.10 ‰ in the other stations) and probably caused an adverse effect on test organism, which is a freshwater alga. The station 4 produced the higher inhibition on both test organisms (21,8% and 28.8% for bacteria *P. fluorescens* and alga *P. subcapitata*, respectively) and showed the higher toxic effect also with BSPT, using the marine bacteria *V. fischeri*, as shown in Figure 2 and in Table 1 (rank 1). In Table 1, a comparison between all the ecotoxicological tests was presented, using ranking method (1 stands for the highest effect, and 9 stands for the lowest effect). The order of sensitivity was bacterium *V. fischeri* > bacterium *P. fluorescens* > alga *P. subcapitata*. Moreover, a good agreement was found for station 4 that obtained the rank 1 for all the tests.

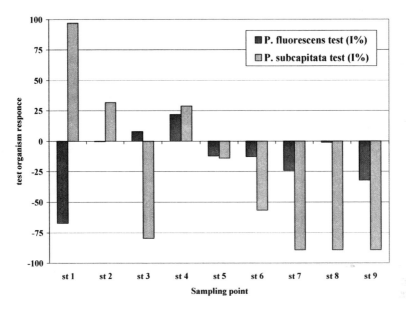

Figure 1:   Results of two screening tests.

The findings found by means of ecotoxicological tests could be related to the total organic carbon content and to the zinc, nickel and copper amount of the sediments (Table 2). Station 4 was indeed characterised by the highest organic carbon, zinc, copper and nickel amount probably due to anthropogenic input.

Principal Component Analysis (PCA) was applied to analyse the correlation matrix obtained from a (8 X 9) data matrix. The 8 variables were TOC, Ni, Cu, Cd, Zn, Fe, Mn and Pb. In the space of "eigenvectors", the dimensions were reduced to 2 principal axes, which account for about 82% of the total variance. The Varimax-rotated matrix obtained by the principal components showed that TOC, Cu, Zn, and Ni were bonded to the first principal component, while Fe, Mn and Pb to the second (Figure 3). Moreover stations 2, 3, 4 and 5 were described by the first principal component.

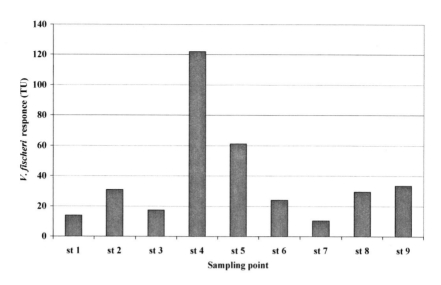

Figure 2:   Toxicity Unit results for the nine sampling points on Garigliano River.

Table 1:   Comparison of ranking of the three ecotoxicological tests, excluding the station 1 and 2 for *P. subcapitata* test. Rank 1: the highest effect; rank 9: the lowest effect.

Sampling points	*V. fischeri* test - ranking	*P. fluorescens* test - ranking	*P. subcapitata* test - ranking
st 1	8	9	/
st 2	4	3	/
st 3	7	2	4
st 4	1	1	1
st 5	2	5	2
st 6	6	6	3
st 7	9	7	5
st 8	5	4	6
st 9	3	8	7

This finding should be explained, by considering the associations of the chemical variables from different sources. The first principal component was attributable to an anthropogenic source while the second one to lithological source. On the other hand, this attribution was supported by taking into account that the Ausenta River, which is interested by several agricultural and urban activities on its riverbanks, flows into Garigliano River in front of the station 4. A clustering analysis of ecotoxicological and chemical data was carried out by means of Ward's method with squared Euclidean distance, highlighted three clusters having similarities (Figure 4).

Table 2:   Results of chemical characterisation (Total Organic Carbon content as mg/g, and total metal content as mg/kg of the sediments).

Sampling points	TOC(*)	Zn(**)	Mn(**)	Ni(**)	Pb(**)	Cd(**)	Fe(**)	Cu(**)
st 1	3,0	38,7	474,9	23,0	57,7	6,2	5687	5,0
st 2	16,0	90,4	519,6	38,1	59,8	2,4	5738	34,8
st 3	16,1	89,8	482,5	32,0	72,4	3,0	7565	40,2
st 4	16,8	107,2	430,1	39,6	60,9	2,7	8621	46,5
st 5	14,4	73,7	471,3	28,1	57,8	2,5	5310	21,6
st 6	12,1	71,9	583,6	31,3	62,4	2,7	14072	16,5
st 7	9,8	63,0	449,9	29,5	59,9	1,9	6723	19,9
st 8	2,1	61,2	679,8	18,6	90,6	1,9	15686	13,0
st 9	10,1	64,9	477,9	19,1	78,4	2,1	6092	19,9

(*) Relative standards deviation is less than 5% (five replicates).
(**) Relative standards deviation is less than 3% (six replicates).

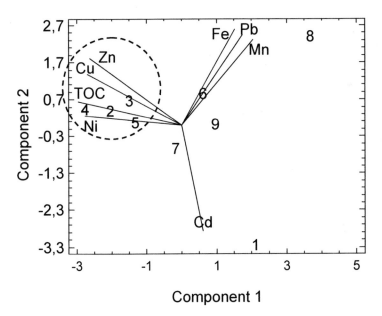

Figure 3:   Principal component analysis (PCA).

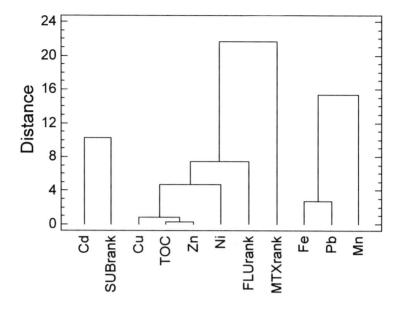

Figure 4: Clustering analysis (Ward's method and squared Euclidean distance). SUBrank, FLUrank and MTXrank stand *for P. subcapitata* test, *P. fluorescens* test and *V. fischeri* test, respectively.

One cluster of them represents the *V. fischeri* (MTXrank) and *P. fluorescens* (FLUrank) test data and TOC, Zn, Cu and Ni concentration highlighting the correlation between the toxic effect and the chemical data due to anthropogenic input.

V. fischeri sensitivity to heavy metals was well know and demonstrated in different studies [14, 15]. Considering *Pseudomonas fluorescens* DHase inhibition assay, the bacterium showed a good response in heavy metals soil and sediment bioassay, resulting more sensitive to heavy metals than to organic compounds toxicity effects, both singularly and in complex matrices [16]. Regarding *Pseudokirchneriella subcapitata* inhibition test, toxicity of heavy metals (i. e. Cd and Zn) to the green alga was demonstrated [17], confirming the clustering result for Cd.

5 Conclusion

An assessment of the environmental risk of the Garigliano River (Italy) was conducted on nine stations, sampled 9 Km back into the river from the delta. Only one stations (station 4) showed a significant toxicity effect to *Vibrio fischeri*, *Pseudomonas fluorescens* and *Pseudokirchneriella subcapitata* demonstrating a specific-spot contamination. Thus, integrated chemical and ecotoxicological approach applied on Garigliano River pointed out that actually its environmental impact is not hazardous for Tyrrenean Sea.

References

[1]   Carbonell, G., Pablos, M. V., Garcia, P., Ramos, C., Sanchez, P., Fernandez, C. & Tarazona, J. V. Rapid and cost-effective multiparameter toxicity tests for soil microorganisms. *The science of the total environment,* **247**, pp. 143-150, 2000.

[2]   Power, M., van der Meer, J. R., Tchelet, R., Egli, T. & Eggen, R.. Molecular-based method can contribute to assessments of toxicological risks and bioremediation strategies. *Journal of Microbiological Methods,* **32**, pp. 107-119, 1998.

[3]   Brohon, B., Delolme, C. & Gourdon, R. Complementarily of bioassays and microbial activity measurements for the evaluation of hydrocarbon-contaminated soil quality. *Soil Biology & Biochemistry,* **33**, pp. 883-891, 2001.

[4]   Torslov, J. Comparison of bacterial toxicity tests based on growth, dehydrogenase activity and esterase activity of Pseudomonas fluorescens. *Ecotoxicology and Environmental Safety.* **25**, pp. 33-40, 1993.

[5]   Meikle, A., Amin-Hanjani, S., Glover, L. A., Killham, K., & Prosser, J. I. Matrix potential and the survival and activity of a Pseudomonas fluorescens inoculum in soil. *Soil Biology & Biochemistry,* **27 (7)**, pp. 881-892, 1995.

[6]   A, Konopka, T. Zakharova, M. Bishoff, L. Olivier, C. Nakatsu & R.F. Turco. Microbial biomass and activity in lead-contaminated soil. *Applied and Environmental Microbiology,* **65 (5)**, pp. 2256-2259, 1999.

[7]   S. Preston, N. Coad, J. Townend, K. Killham, & G.I. Paton.. Biosensing the acute toxicity of metal interactions: are they additive, sinergistic, or antagonistic? *Environmental Toxicology and Chemistry,* **19 (3)**, pp. 775-780, 2000.

[8]   Guerra, R., Iacondini, A., Abbondanzi, F., Matteucci, C., & Bruzzi, L. A new microbial assay for the toxicity detection of contaminated soils. *Annali di Chimica. Annali di Chimica,* **92**, pp. 847-854, 2002.

[9]   F. Abbondanzi, A. Cachada, T. Campisi, R. Guerra, M. Raccagni, & A. Iacondini. Optimisation of a microbial bioassay for contaminated soil monitoring: bacterial inoculum standardisation and comparison with Microtox® assay, *Chemosphere,* **53 (8)**, pp. 889-897, 2003.

[10]   Azur Environmental. 1995. Microtox® Acute toxicity Basic Solid Phase Test. Microtox® Acute toxicity Basic Test procedures. Carlsbad, CA, USA.

[11]   Campisi, T., Abbondanzi, F., Casado-Martinez, C., DelValls, T.A., Guerra, R. & A. Iacondini. Effect of sediment turbidity and color on light output measurement for Microtox® basic solid-phase test. *Chemosphere,* **60(1)**, pp. 1715-1721, 2005.

[12]   USEPA, 1994. Short term methods for estimating the chronic toxicity of effluents and receiving waters to freshwater organisms. EPA/600/4-91/002 3rd edition – US Environmental Protection Agency, Cincinnati, Ohio.

[13]   Sbrilli G, Calamati E, Boccalini S, Bimbi B, & Pistolesi F. Effects of nutrients and salinity on the algal assay using *Pseudokirchneriella subcapitata* (Korshikov) Hindak. *Bull Environ Contam Toxicol.* **71(3)**, pp. 609-616, 2003.

[14]   Stronkhorst, J., Schipper, C., Brils, J., Dubbeldam, M., Postman, J., & Van De Hoeven, N. Using Marine Bioassays to Classify the Toxicity of Dutch Harbor Sediments. *Environmental Toxicology and Chemistry.* **22**, pp. 1535-1547, 2003.

[15]   Allen Burton Jr., G., Baudo, R., Beltrami, M., & C. Rowland. Assessing sediment contamination using six toxicity assays. *Journal of Limnology.* **60(2)**, pp. 263-267. 2001.

[16]   Abbondanzi, F., Cachada, A., Campisi, T., Castro Ruiz, A., Guerra, R., Raccagni, M., & A. Iacondini. Use of Pseudomonas fluorescens in a contaminated soil bioassay. *Proc. of the 8th International FZK / TNO Conference on Contaminated Soil.* CD version, 2003.

[17]   Koukal, B., Guéguen, C., Pardos, M., & Dominik, J. Influence of humic substances on the toxic effect of Cadmium and Zinc to the green alga Pseudokirchneriella subcapitata. *Chemosphere*, **53**, pp. 953- 961, 2003.

The use of TPH analytical data to estimate human health risk: practical approaches

B. Sarmiento, T. Goyanes, I. Coleto & N. De las Casas
URS Madrid, Spain

Abstract

This paper describes the three basic approaches that have been used to estimate potential human health risks posed by TPH contamination: the indicator approach, the surrogate approach and a mixed version.

Differences among methods are discussed in a case study: a former industrial area impacted with petroleum products, destined to be redeveloped for recreational use. Three exposure pathways have been considered: hydrocarbon vapor inhalation, ingestion and dermal contact. Firstly, only "indicator compounds" were evaluated. Next, the product was considered as gasoline in the Quantitative Risk Assessment. Afterwards, simple fractionation of hydrocarbon chains was introduced as the input parameter. Finally, the fractionation between the aromatic and aliphatic terms of each group of hydrocarbons was considered. Site-Specific Target Levels (SSTLs) for each pathway were calculated.

Results for different hypothesis have been evaluated from a technical and economic point of view. Cases in which input concentration for a compound was above soil saturation limit are also discussed.

Keywords: hydrocarbon, TPH, human health, indicator, whole product, TPH fraction, soil saturation, SSTL.

1 Introduction

Contamination of soils and groundwater by petroleum products can pose a risk to human health and environmental receptors. Petroleum products are complex mixtures containing primarily hydrocarbons. The toxicological evaluation of petroleum hydrocarbons is particularly difficult because these substances are present in the environment containing many hundreds of individual compounds, each with their own toxicological properties and environmental behavior. In addition, once a spill is released into the environment, changes in composition may occur as a result of physical, chemical and biological weathering processes. One of the parameters assessed for determining petroleum contamination is referred to as total petroleum hydrocarbon (TPH). TPH is defined as "the measurable amount of petroleum-based hydrocarbon in an environmental media" (CONCAWE 2003).

There are three basic approaches used to estimate potential human health risks posed by TPH contamination: the "Indicator" Approach, used mostly for the evaluation of the carcinogenic risks from TPH; the "Surrogate" Approach, which assumes that a single compound can characterize TPH; and a "Compromised Version", in which an intermediate approach between the Indicator and Surrogate methods is applied.

2   The indicator approach

This approach assumes that the toxicity of a petroleum mixture is characterized by the toxicity of one or more of the most toxic compounds. For sites contaminated by gasoline and jet fuel, the most often selected compounds are benzene, toluene, ethylbenzene and xylenes (BTEX). Polycyclic Aromatic Hydrocarbons (PAHs) are considered of concern when evaluating kerosene and fuel oils. ASTM follows this approach, and generally accepts it only for carcinogenic risks, considering mainly benzene and benz(a)pyrene as indicator compounds.

3   The surrogate approach

The Surrogate Approach assumes that a single surrogate compound can characterize the TPH. This approach can overestimate the risks, as benzene, which is a highly volatile and soluble compound and is assessed as a carcinogenic type A, is often considered as the surrogate compound for all aromatics. This approach has evolved to a fraction approach (see section 4).

A variant of the Surrogate Approach, the Whole Product Approach, is based on studies that consider the toxicity and mobility of the product as a whole. Most of these studies have been developed upon recent petroleum products, so risks posed by weathered substances can not been fully characterized.

4   The compromised version

At present, a compromise between the Indicator and the Surrogate Approaches is usually undertaken. Carcinogenic risk is estimated based on indicators (benzene, benzo(a)pyrene) and non-carcinogenic risk is calculated based on a number of TPH fractions. In this case, the surrogate would be an individual compound or a number of compounds within each TPH fraction that would be representative of the toxicity of the whole fraction. TPH can be divided into groups or fractions according to toxicity and transport properties. MADEP (1994) and TPHCWG (1999) have divided TPH mainly into aliphatic and aromatic compounds. The six carbon ranges identified by MADEP were based on differences in toxicity, while

TPHCWG established 13 fractions based on the "equivalent carbon" index, which is related to the expected environmental behavior of individual petroleum compounds. Conservative toxicity data were developed for each fraction, prioritizing mixture data. To avoid double counting, indicator substances must be subtracted from the corresponding mass fraction. Both, MADEP and TPHCWG, assume additivity of non-carcinogenic toxicity across the fractions. Fraction approach accounts for the age and weathering of the spilled product and allows the evaluation of one or more petroleum products.

5 Case study

A former hydrocarbon distribution facility will be decommissioned and the terrain will be redeveloped for recreational use. The main product stored was unleaded gasoline. During an environmental investigation some quantities of product were found on the surface soil, therefore a human health risk assessment was performed. The three approaches described above were developed.

5.1 Conceptual model

The facility is located on a former industrial area in the process of being dismantled. It is about 5,000 m^2. The Urban Plan contemplates the property as a future park.

Various hydrocarbon stains were found on the superficial soil at a depth of 20 cm. The largest stain was of 10 m length. The contaminated terrain is a fill material, consisting of gravel in a sandy-silty matrix. This material overlies a 10 m layer of low-permeability, natural clays. No groundwater was found at the site.

Users of the park (adults and children) were identified as potential sensitive receptors of the contamination detected. Three exposures pathways were considered: outdoor inhalation of vapors, accidental ingestion of soil and dermal contact with soil.

5.2 Procedures

The Quantitative Risk Assessment includes the following steps: Exposure assessment, Toxicity assessment and Risk characterization.

The exposure assessment estimates the type and magnitude of exposures to the chemicals of potential concern that are present at or migrating from a site. In this case study, the ASTM E-1739-95 Outdoor Model was used to estimate outdoor vapor concentration. The ingestion and dermal contact exposures were calculated by means of the equations presented in US EPA RAGs (p 6-40, 6-41). Exposure factors, site and model data are summarized in tables 1 and 2. The results of the exposure assessment are then combined with the chemical-specific toxicity information to characterize potential risks. Toxicity data applied in this assessment come from Integrated Risk Information System database (IRIS), the National Center for Environmental Assessment (NCEA) and TPHCWG. For carcinogens, the risk target level was established at 1.00E-05. Therefore any estimated risk over this value will indicate a potential threat due to the exposure to carcinogenic compounds. The non-carcinogenic effects are evaluated by comparing an exposure level over a specified time period with a reference dose derived for a similar exposure period. This ratio of exposure to toxicity is called a hazard quotient. The non-cancer hazard quotient target level is established as 1.00.

Table 1: Exposure factors.

Receptor input data			
Characteristics	Units	Child Resident	Source
Lifetime and body weight			
Lifetime	years	70	ASTM 1995
Body weight	Kg	15	ASTM 1995
Inhalation of outdoor air			
Exposure frequency for Outdoor Air events	events/yr	350	ASTM 1995
Exposure duration for outdoor air	years	6	ASTM 1995
Lung retention factor	-	1	ASTM 1995
Inhalation rate outdoors	m^3/hr	1.2	ECETOC 2001
Time outdoors	hr/day	24	Hypothesis
Ingestion of soil/ dermal contact with soil during leisure activities			
Exposure frequency for soils	events/yr	350	ASTM 1995
Exposure duration for soils	years	6	ASTM 1995
Ingestion rate for soil	mg/day	200	ECETOC 2001
Total skin surface area	cm^2	7640	ECETOC 2001
Fraction skin exposed to soil	-	0.52	ECETOC 2001
Soil/skin adherence factor	mg/cm^2	0.22	ECETOC 2001

Note: Only the child receptor was considered for this case study since it is normally the most sensitive receptor. For this purpose, maximum exposure factors have been taken into account.

Table 2: Site and box model parameters.

Unsaturated zone properties and source data for vapor model (gravel)			
Characteristics	Units	Value	Source
Total porosity	cm^3/cm^3	0.3	Site specific
Water content	cm^3/cm^3	0.1	Site specific
Distance from soil source to ground surface	m	0.2	Site specific
Fraction organic carbon in source	goc/g soil	0.002	Site specific
Soil bulk density	g/cm^3	1.7	Site specific
Box model parameters			
Height of box	m	2	ASTM 1995
Length of box (in direction of wind flow)	m	10	ASTM 1995
Wind speed	m/s	2.25	ASTM 1995

5.3 Developing approaches

5.3.1 Approach 1: indicator approach

BTEX and MTBE were considered as indicator compounds of the hydrocarbons present as, according to site historical data, the main product stored was gasoline. Samples were analyzed according to ISO 11423-1/CMA 3/E. Maximum concentration detected is included in table 3:

Table 3:   Input concentration for indicator compounds.

Compound	Input Concentration (mg/kg)
Benzene	26
Toluene	28
Ethylbenzene	22
Xylenes	67
MTBE	111
TOTAL	254

Risks levels are summarized in section 5.4. According to this approach, Soil-Specific Target Levels (SSTLs) were calculated for individual compounds. Laboratory costs for BTEX compounds are on the range of 96 €/sample.

Table 4:   Estimated composition of the mixture.

Compound	%	Estimated stain concentration (mg/kg)
Aliphatics	Aliphatics	Aliphatics
C5-C6	46	10,956
C6-C8	12	2858
C8-C10	7	1667
C10-C12	0.27	64
C12-C16	-	-
C16-C35	-	-
TOTAL	65%	15,546
Aromatics	Aromatics	Aromatics
C6-C7	2	452
C7-C8	19	4477
C8-C10	7	1736
C10-C12	7	1669
C12-C16	-	-
C16-C21	-	-
C21-C35	-	-
TOTAL	35%	8336.3

5.3.2 Approach 2: surrogate approach

The "Whole Product Approach" was developed in this example. The main product presented at the site was Gasoline. Samples were analyzed for TPH in accordance with standard ISO-CMA 3/R. The maximum concentration obtained was 23,818 mg/kg. The first column in Table 4 presents the average composition of a gasoline according to TPHCWG. In the second column, the estimated composition of the mixture (considering a total concentration of 23,818 mg/kg) is shown.

Risk levels are presented on section 5.4. SSTLs were calculated for the mixture, first considering only non-carcinogenic compounds and then considering the whole mixture. SSTLs for TPH were calculated by weighting individual fractions according to their composition in the total petroleum mixture and assuming their toxic effects are additive.

The normal laboratory price would be 56 €/ sample for obtaining the sum amount of TPH.

5.3.3 Approach 3: compromised version

Carcinogenic risk was estimated based on benzene as the indicator compound. Non-carcinogenic risk from the TPH was calculated based on fractions. Two cases were analyzed: Case A, where a simple division of TPH into chains was performed in the laboratory, without distinguishing between aliphatic and aromatic fractions (CMA 3/R method); and Case B, where this aliphatic-aromatic division was made (US EPA Method 8270). In case A, it was not possible to determine what percentage of TPH fractions belonged to aliphatic and which to aromatic compounds, therefore fractions have been duplicated in order to avoid underestimating the risk.

Analytical costs for Case A are 75 €/sample and Case B are 125 €/ sample, plus the 96 €/sample in both cases for benzene.

Table 5:   Cases contemplated on the third approach.

Case A		Case B	
Aliphatics	Concentration (mg/kg)	Aliphatics	Concentration (mg/kg)
C5-C6	115	C5-C6	90
C6-C8	1388	C6-C8	1360
C8-C10	600	C8-C10	204
C10-C12	362	C10-C12	145
C12-C16	7277	C12-C16	6782
C16-C35	14076	C16-C35	13,966
TOTAL	23,818 (100%)	TOTAL	22,547 (94.66%)
Aromatics	Concentration (mg/kg)	Aromatics	Concentration (mg/kg)
C6-C7	115	C6-C7	25
C7-C8	1388	C7-C8	28
C8-C10	600	C8-C10	396
C10-C12	362	C10-C12	217
C12-C16	7277	C12-C16	495
C16-C21	6887	C16-C21	105
C21-C35	7189	C21-C35	5
TOTAL	23,818 (100%)	TOTAL	1,271 (5.34%)

5.4 Results

Results for the three approaches considered are presented in table 6. Risk summary is considered for each pathway. The non-carcinogenic reference level is 1.00E+00 and 1.00E-05 for carcinogenic reference level (see section 5.2).

Table 6:   Estimation of the non-carcinogenic risk

Approaches	Ingestion	Dermal contact	Outdoor vapor inhalation
Indicator*	9.20E-02	3.70E-02	**4.80E+01**
Whole Product	**1.70E+00**	6.60E-01	**3.20E+00**
Case A: Aliphatic Fraction	**1.10E+00**	4.60E-01	1.70E-01
Case A: Aromatic Fraction	**8.70E+00**	**3.50E+00**	**2.00E+00**
Case B: real fractioning	**1.40E+00**	5.60E-01	4.70E-01

*In the indicator approach risks should not be summed as it is considered inappropriate to sum hazard indices unless the toxicological endpoints and mechanisms of action are the same for individual compounds. "Lack of sufficient toxicological information is an impediment to this procedure" (ASTM E-1739-95, p. 198). The sum was considered in this case study just to compare the results obtained with the other approaches considered.

Most of the risk results from the ingestion and vapor inhalation pathways.

Both Case B and Case A Aliphatics, are quite similar, as the real mixture is made of a 95% aliphatic compounds. On the other hand, risk values for Case A Aromatics are about four to six times higher than those obtained for the other two cases. This is due to the fact that aromatic compounds are, in general, more toxic and soluble than aliphatics. Moreover, a concentration of 23,818 mg/kg is being evaluated in the single case instead of the real aromatic concentration of 1.271 mg/kg, used in Case B (see table 5).

Results obtained for the Whole Product Approach are consequent with those obtained for the Compromised Version. For outdoor vapor inhalation, risks are higher in the Whole Product than for Case B due to a higher concentration of aromatics (see table 4). In the Indicator Approach, risks are 100% superior in comparison to Case B, because benzene is considered as an individual compound, whose inhalation reference dose is two orders of magnitude higher than that of its equivalent aromatic fraction C6-C7, considered in Case B. Moreover, according to TPHCWG the solubility and volatility of a compound decrease when a compound is present in the mixture when compared to its behavior when it is found pure. On the contrary, the risk values for the direct pathways are being underestimated in the Indicator Approach, as only a few compounds (BTEX and MTBE) were considered, and these compounds only sum 254 mg/kg instead of the 23,818 mg/kg of the total mixture (see Table 3).

Table 7:   Estimation of carcinogenic risks.

Approaches	Ingestion	Dermal contact	Outdoor vapor inhalation
Indicator*	2.0E-06	7.8E-07	**7.2E-04**
Whole Product	**2.70E-05**	**1.10E-05**	1.30E-04
Case A: Aliphatic Fraction	1.60E-06	6.20E-07	**2.80E-05**
Case A: Aromatic Fraction	1.60E-06	6.20E-07	**2.20E-05**
Case B: real fractioning	1.60E-06	6.20E-07	**2.80E-05**

No risk values exceeding the reference value were obtained for the direct pathways, except in the Whole Product Approach, in which estimated benzene concentration is about 452 mg/kg (corresponding to aromatics C6-C7, with a 2% of the total mixture) instead of the 26 mg/kg considered in the rest of approaches. The same level of risk was obtained for the direct pathways, as the TPH was not considered as a mixture. Risk levels for the vapor inhalation pathway where identified for all of the studied approaches. Risks values were higher when considering benzene as an individual compound instead of considering it as a part of a mixture.

The following table presents the clean-up levels estimated from the risks considered in each approach:

Table 8:   SSTLs for TPH / TPH with Benzene / Benzene.

Approaches	Ingestion+ Dermal contact (mg/kg)	Outdoor vapor inhalation (mg/kg)
Indicator	Benzene: 120 Ethylbenzene: 5,600 Toluene: 11,000 Xylenes: 11,000 MTBE: 2,000	Benzene: 0.37 Ethylbenzene: 82 Toluene: 18 Xylenes: 67 MTBE: 160
Whole Product	10,000 / 5,300 / 120	83 / 35 / 0.41
Case A: Aliphatic Fractions	15,000 / 14,000 / 120	RES / 380 / 0.42
Case A: Aromatic Fractions	2,000 / 1,900 / 120	300 / 210 / 0.41
Case B: real fractioning	12,000 / 11,000 / 12	RES / 460 / 0.48

The most restrictive SSTL was obtained for benzene vapor inhalation in the Indicator Approach (0.37 mg/kg). On the other hand, when benzene is considered as a part of a mixture, the SSTLs increase depending on the composition of the mixture.

The application of the Whole Product Approach could result in higher costs of remediation and very difficult to obtain clean up goals (83 mg/kg for TPH).

Case A of the Compromised Approach cannot be considered as an appropriate solution as risks are overestimated compared with Case B (an SSTL of 12,000 mg/kg could be applied instead of 210 mg/kg if benzene were not in the soil). Results become similar when considering benzene, although they are much more restrictive for Case A.

Note that for the third approach, in Case A Aliphatic and Case B the SSTLs exceed the residual concentration for any of the chemicals evaluated as part of the particular mixture considered (RES). This means that there will be no risk at any given concentration, except when considering benzene.

5.5 Considerations to soil saturation

Soil saturation concentration is the theoretical soil concentration at which the solubility limits of the soil pore water, the vapor phase limits of the soil pore air and the adsorptive limits of the soil particles have been reached.

Considering only vapor inhalation outdoor in case B of the fraction approach, it would be possible to leave 23,818 mg/kg of TPH in soil, as there will be no risk since, theoretically, volatile emissions will not increase above this level. But it is difficult to accept that such a concentration could be left in the soil. MADEP recommends a "ceiling value" of 500–1,000 mg/kg in sites contaminated by gasoline considering odors and esthetic criteria. TPHCWG establishes values from 5,000 to 10,000 mg/kg for sites affected by crude oils and when benzene is not present.

5.6 Conclusions

The implementation of the Compromised Approach can be considered as the most appropriate for the evaluation of risks posed by petroleum hydrocarbons. Decomposition of the mixture between aliphatic and aromatic chains (Case B) should be undertaken as the lack of knowledge in Case A can result in an expensive overestimation of risks. Due to higher laboratory cost for Case B it may not be possible to perform this type of analysis on every sample in restricted budget investigations, but it should be recommended at least for the most representative samples of the contamination detected.

The Indicator Approach, as expected, was appropriate when evaluating carcinogenic risks, although a slightly overestimated SSTL for benzene was obtained. Nevertheless, the risks for the non-carcinogenic compounds were underestimated.

The Whole Product Approach overestimated both carcinogenic and non-carcinogenic risks in this case study, as the composition of the product detected did not correspond to the gasoline considered.

References

[1] ASTM Standard E1739-95 *Guide for Risk-Based Corrective Action Applied al Petroleum Release sites,* American Society for Testing Materials, Philadelphia, 1995.
[2] ASTM Standard E2081-00 *Standard Guide for Risk Based Corrective Action,* American Society for Testing Materials, Philadelphia, 2000.

[3] CONCAWE Report no 3/03 *Guideline for Risk-Based Assessment of Contaminated Sites (revised)*, European Oil Industry, Brussels, 2003.

[4] MaDEP *Interim Final Petroleum Report: Development of Health Based Alternative to the Total Petroleum Hydrocarbon (TPH) Parameter*, Massachusetts Department of Environmental Protection, Boston, 1994.

[5] MaDEP Characterizing Risks Posed by Petroleum Contaminated Sites: Implementation of the MADEP VPH/EPH Approach. Draft for Public Comment, Massachusetts Department of Environmental Protection, Boston, 1997.

[6] TPHCWG, *Total Petroleum Hydrocarbon Criteria Working Group Series (Volumes 1,2,3,4,5),* Amherst Scientific Publishers, Amherst, Massachusetts, 1997-1999.

[7] US EPA EPA540/1-89/002 *Risk Assessment Guidance for Superfund Volume I, Human Health Evaluation Manual (Part A) Interim Final*, Office of Emergency and Remedial Response, U.S Environmental Protection Agency, Washington 1989.

Advanced computer-multi-media technology and direct mental health delivery

D. Segal[1] & D. A. Gordon[2]
*[1]Department of Behavioural Sciences,
The College of Management Academic Studies Division, Israel
[2]Department of Psychology, Ohio University, U.S.A.*

Abstract

Computer multi media rapid developing technology provides new possibilities for mental health delivery in the form of direct psycho-educational intervention and prevention with clients, as well as training professionals. It is now possible to integrate computer multi media technology and clinical interventions, and develop intervention and training programs that are efficient and involve relatively minimal or no face-to-face contact with therapists. Such interventions, unlike traditional psychotherapeutic methods, could be at low cost and quickly disseminated to clinics and social agencies. Accumulating supportive research is showing moderate to large effect sizes in using an interactive computer multi media program for addressing clinical problems. The article addresses advantages of implementing psycho-educational intervention via advanced technology in clinical practice by following the case study of the Parenting Wisely (PW) intervention program.
Keywords: multimedia, intervention, mental health, parenting, psycho-educational, parenting, technology.

1   Introduction

Mental health delivery structures have been significantly changing over the past few years. These changes could be attributed to; 1) theoretical paradigm shifts, 2) rising cost of mental health treatment that generates pressure to design and conduct cost-effective interventions [1], and 3) rapid technological development as more mental health professionals are getting familiar and comfortable with the opportunities embedded in the utilization of advanced technology.

WIT Transactions on Biomedicine and Health, Vol 9, © 2005 WIT Press
www.witpress.com, ISSN 1743-3525 (on-line)

In a meta-analysis of 100 studies, McNeil and Nelson [2] found substantial effects of interactive videodisk instruction on cognitive and performance measures, with a .53 mean effect size across age groups (college students, military personnel, sales persons), instructional content, and environment. These studies were conducted in military, industrial, and higher educational settings, and they have shown that interactive videodisk instruction reduces instruction cost and time [4,5,6]. In addition, this form of instruction has been shown to lead to greater practice time than did other methods; users find the experience very enjoyable. Interactive videodisk instruction has been found to be more effective than traditional lectures, reading, and passive viewing of videotapes; and it produces greater effect sizes than does computer-based instruction (.69 vs. .26) [7,8].

It is now possible to integrate computer-multimedia technology and clinical interventions. Such integration could mean more efficient and relatively short interventions with a low number of face-to-face contact hours with therapists. Furthermore, integrative interventions could resolve major difficulties in reaching targeted at-risk population or reaching therapeutic goals in comparison to classical therapy practice as depicted in table 1 where we summarize the differences between therapy, as practiced in community settings, and the technological approach used in interactive CD-ROM training program. Design of valid contents and procedures for intervention and professional-training programs should be thoroughly planned. Based on our experience we identified several areas for consideration for program planning:

1. Targeted change.
2. Target population.
3. Technical concerns.
4. Personnel responsible for intervention implementation.
5. Scientific considerations
6. Methods of dissemination & further program development.

1.1 Case study overview – the Parenting Wisely

Throughout this article we refer to our practical experience using the Parenting Wisely interactive CD-ROM parent-training program. The program combines the powerful effects of teaching parenting skills via videotaped modelling [9] with the responsiveness of a computer program [10]. Each user's responses determine the subsequent content and feedback that he or she receives, much like an interaction with a therapist. The PW program presents the parent with nine different problem situations that are common in many families. When a problem is selected, a short video plays in which actors illustrate the problem. After the initial problem situation is presented, a screen appears that prompts the parent to select the method he or she normally uses (from a list of three solutions) to respond to the child's problematic behaviour. The parent then watches as his or her selected solution is played out in the video. After the video segment is completed, the computer provides the parent with feedback in the form of a question and answer session. This feedback prompts the parent to think about the response he or she chose, as well as reasons why the response was effective or ineffective. Through the question and answer sections, the parent is taught parenting skills. If an effective and adaptive method of dealing with the problem was not selected, the program prevents the parent from progressing to a new problem until the correct solution is chosen, viewed, and critiqued. After the correct solution has been chosen, a short review quiz (with feedback) is presented. This quiz allows parents to practice the newly learned skills. Upon completion of the quiz, the parent then advances to a new problem situation.

Table 1:   Comparison of therapy and interactive CD-ROM.

Therapies[1]		Interactive CD-ROM	
1.	Verbal descriptions of targeted skills	1.	Detailed verbal and visual examples of targeted skills
2.	Judgment by therapist	2.	No judgment by computer
3.	Client defensiveness main obstacle to progress	3.	Minimal client defensiveness
4.	Client discloses performance errors	4.	Client recognizes performance errors by actors
5.	Feedback on performance errors is infrequent and indirect	5.	Client actively seeks feedback on performance errors performed by actors in the program
6.	Client rarely asks for repetition of unclear advice	6.	Client can repeat any portion of the program at any time
7.	Often pace is selected by therapist	7.	Pace always selected by client
8.	Infrequent reinforcement of good performance practices	8.	Frequent reinforcement of good performance practices
9.	Focus on therapist-client relationship	9.	Exclusive focus on teaching targeted skills
10.	Considerable therapy time and cost devoted to resistance	10.	Little of program time devoted to resistance
11.	Difficult to improve therapist skills	11.	Relatively easy to improve program structure and content

[1]Therapy as commonly practiced in community settings. Empirically validated treatments, which have just begun to penetrate community practice, may share some of the features listed under Interactive CD-ROM (such as demonstration of effective parenting practices).

2 The 6-point consideration protocol

Following we address the 6 point planning protocol, based on our experience from planning, researching, implementing, and disseminating the PW program.

2.1 Targeted change

Interventions with cognitive-behavioural, psycho-educational, emphasis are suitable for the clinical-computer integration. In such an orientation the targeted change in clients is defined as change in knowledge, thought process, and behaviour. These areas of functioning are measurable and concrete. They could be quite easily addressed through computer technical operations.

Interactive multimedia technology allows users to determine pacing, sequence and selection of learning content. These interactive features accommodate different users' responses and permit them to choose different pathways throughout their learning process (e.g., exit any part of the program whenever they desire or choose to review other content in the program). Since this type of learning is deductively structured with enriched and contrived experience, it presumably allows learners to take responsibility for their learning [11], which in turn facilitates the learning of new material and exploration of new ideas [12].

A content validation model is depicted in figure 1, modified from Goldstein's [13] and Ford, Quinones, Sego and Sorra's [14] training evaluation models. This model could serve as a guideline for developing intervention programs. In the PW example, it consists of two dimensions: parenting skills identified from the empirical literature and parenting skills represented in the intervention program. Valid content of the program is affirmed if the intervention only contains critical and relevant skills identified from the research (i.e., intervention content relevance shown in quadrants A and D). An intervention program would be considered content deficient or contamination if the intervention omitted crucial skills (shown in quadrant B) or included irrelevant skills (shown in quadrant C).

2.2 Target population

It has been argued that clients prefer to interact with a machine rather than a human therapist when instructional knowledge and its practice are a primary requirement for behavioural change [15]. This preference may be attributed to the non-judgmental nature of computers which encourages clients to learn tasks thoroughly or repeat difficult segments of content at their own pace. Nevertheless, programs should address level of education and language proficiency of prospective clients. PW was designed for use by all parents and all personnel who work with children, their parents, and their families. Because it was developed to appeal to low income families, it was written on a fifth-grade reading level. When PW's narrator option is chosen, all text is read aloud. This enables parents who cannot read, or have minimal reading ability, to benefit from the program as well.

PW is easy to use, even for those who have little or no experience with computers. In most cases, we have found that, if a staff person starts the PW program for the parent and shows the parent how to use the mouse, the parent is able to complete the program on his or her own. PW prompts the parent to select his or her level of computer ability. It then proceeds with instructions based on computer literacy.

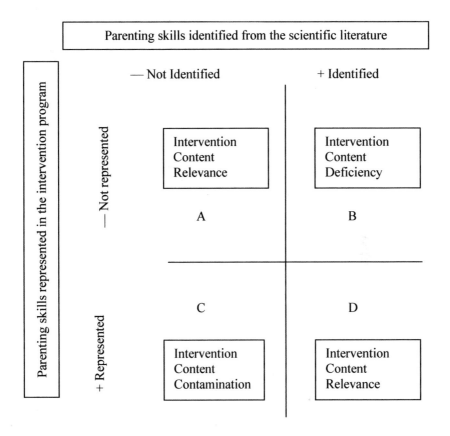

Figure 1:   Conceptual content validation model.

2.3 Technical concerns

Rapid advances in multi-media technology have been providing us with user-friendly non-expensive software and hardware for program development. When considering development of new intervention programs one must address the cost of program development in terms of content and media. The cost will vary significantly if, for example, one includes video scenes to illustrate targeted problems or desired behaviour. Another important consideration is the cost for the end-user. In contrast to just 15 years ago, many people own computers. Intervention programs should be disseminated through social agencies where a computer can be dedicated for client use.

2.4 Personnel responsible for intervention implementation

One of the main objectives in implementing psychological interventions via multi-media technology is the self-help format. Therefore, professional personnel should be minimally involved in program implementation. Their responsibility should be restricted to the basics of helping the client feel at ease with the first step with the program. Some multi-media interventions could, and maybe should, be relevant for training professionals. In both cases special technical training should be planned to minimal length and complexity.

Since we designed PW to be used by parents with little or no staff involvement (other than brief staff contact to boot up the program), training or professional experience in the use of the PW program is not required. Clinical training and experience can be useful, however. A professional with clinical experience can assess the needs of the family and tailor his or her recommendation of PW to a particular family. Clients are more likely to use a program when a trusted professional recommends it.

In addition to use by therapists, PW is used as the curriculum for parent education classes, as an adjunct to traditional family therapy, as curriculum for high school family living skills courses, etc. Some agencies have used PW with parents in substance abuse treatment centers and some with incarcerated parents. Courts have used PW as an alternative to other punishments. The various professionals implementing this program are counsellors, case managers, home visitors (nurses, child protective service personnel, probation officers) case workers, child care workers, extension agents, police, and teachers. Therefore, it is recommended that a program is versatile so it could be used by a variety of professionals and environments.

2.5 Scientific considerations

Issues such as content validation and intervention evaluation need to be meticulously addressed (e.g.; therapeutic effect and the overall human-computer interaction). Evaluation is critical with any type of intervention. A comprehensive evaluation is particularly challenging to researchers and practitioners in the discipline of human-computer interaction. Given its interdisciplinary nature, a comprehensive evaluation of human-computer interaction requires relevant (i.e., valid) and reliable criteria assessing multiple aspects such as mental abilities (e.g., effects on learning speed, recall accuracy, or reasoning), physiological capabilities (e.g., effects on visual acuity, visual field, auditory sensation), interface designs (e.g., ease of use), psychological reactions (i.e., anxiety, or resistance to technology), behavioural changes, and so on [16].

In studies we conducted, table 2, we demonstrate how the PW intervention was evaluated by three types of criteria: 1) users' reaction to the program (i.e., reaction criteria), 2) knowledge acquisition from the program (i.e., learning criteria), and 3) behaviour transfer to outside of the intervention (i.e., behaviour criteria).

Table 2:   Comparison of studies of Parenting Wisely.

Study	Participants (n)	Site	Design	Follow Up Period	Child Problem Behaviour PW Effect Size (Cohen's d)
Lagges & Gordon [17]	Teen parents of infants and toddlers (62)	School	RA to treatment and control	2 months	.67[4]
Gordon & Kacir [18]	Parents of delinquents	Community and University	Treatment and matched control	1, 3, 6 months	.59[2], .76[3]
Kacir & Gordon [19]	Parents of problem adolescents (38)	University	RA to treatment and control	2, 4 months	1.2[2]
Woodruff, Gordon, & Lobo [20]	Parents of 9-13 year olds	Home	RA to 2 treatment groups	2, 6 months	.37[2]
Rolland Stanar, Gordon, & Carlston [21]	Parents of 11-13 year olds	Home and school	Treatment and matched control	3, 6, 9 months	.63 to .88[2]
Segal et al. [22]	Parents of 11-18 yr olds (42)	Community mental health and juvenile Detention	RA[1] to 2 treatment groups	1 month	.78[2], 1.27[3]

[1] = RA: Random Assignment
[2] = Eyberg Child Behaviour Inventory
[3] = Parents Daily Report
[4] = Parental response to hypothetical problem behaviour

Our research studies have shown that PW is effective at reducing child problem behaviours, improving family functioning, reducing maternal depression, improving parent knowledge of positive parenting skills, and increasing parent use of such skills. In all the studies conducted on PW, parents who used the program reported overall satisfaction and found the teaching format easy to follow. They also found the scenarios realistic, the problems depicted to be relevant to their families, and the parenting skills taught reasonable solutions to those problems. The parents felt confident they could apply the skills in their families. These findings may help explain why parents were willing to spend two to three hours in one sitting using the program, and why improvements in child behaviour were evident a week after parents used the program.

In addition to the data we presented, we know of approximately 25 independent evaluations of PW in community settings in the US and in the UK underway currently. Continuation of supportive empirical research is critical for establishing credibility of integrated technology-intervention programs.

2.6 Methods of dissemination and further program development

Disseminating a psycho-educational intervention that is based on advanced technology (Level III) requires special considerations. This approach to intervention is still regarded as unusual for most practitioners in the field of psychotherapy. Many barriers block the path of even the most vigilant technology supporter (e.g. the lack of available equipment and funding to purchase, update, and maintain equipment; the lack of technological expertise; and the lack of training on how to implement the use of technology within specific fields) [23]. The use of technology among mental health providers is particularly challenging, as the mental health profession holds many views about the nature of change that must be altered for successful implementation of technological resources. Therefore, innovative programs will, most likely, be approached with some suspicion by agencies and individual clients. Therefore, dissemination requires extra effort.

Professional conferences should be actively utilized to demonstrate the technology for the purpose of exposure. Multimedia presentation in addition to the usual presentation of the program's content and research findings is highly recommended.

The internet is a viable place today for demonstration and dissemination due to its rapid data-transfer advancements. Programs should be designed to work on internet platform and as such could be considered an internet-based intervention [24] (see: www.familyworksinc.com). It is quite feasible to use governmental agencies that publish and disseminate information on mental health practices, including website listing. In our case governmental agencies such as SAMHSA, CSAP, OJJDP, and the Centers for the Application of Prevention Technologies (CAPT) were quite relevant.

An essential step to foster dissemination is continued contact with agencies that might be interested or have purchased the intervention program. By staying in contact with a variety of agencies using the program, developers can incorporate their feedback and research results into improvements to the program. This can be done regularly and inexpensively, via upgrades to the program. Changing the CD-ROM is a much less daunting task than that faced by developers of traditional programs who wish to introduce changes, following initial training, in the practices of service providers. Agencies should be asked of what additions to this technology they would like to see, and notify them when these improvements or new programs are available. From our experience, this feedback loop has resulted in further development and expansion of the program as well as more inquiries about it.

References

[1]   Hoyt, M. F. & Austad, C. S., Psychotherapy in a staff model health maintenance organization: Providing and assuring quality care in the future. *Psychotherapy: Theory, Research, Practice, Training, 29*, pp. 119 129, 1992.

[2]   McNeil, B. J., & Nelson, K. R., Meta-analysis of interactive video instruction: A 10-year review of achievement effects. *Journal of Computer-Based Instruction*, 18 (1), pp. 1 6, 1991.

[3]   Bosco, J., An analysis of evaluations of interactive video. *Educational Technology*, 26, pp. 7 17, 1986.

[4]   Cohen, V. B., Interactive features in the design of videodisc materials. *Educational Technology*, 24, pp. 16 22, 1984.

[5]   Fletcher, J. D., Effectiveness and cost interactive videodisc instruction in defense training and education (Report No. P-2372). *Institute for Defense Analysis,* 1990.

[6]   Kacir, C., & Gordon, D.A., Parenting adolescents wisely: The effectiveness of an interactive videodisk parent-training program in Appalachia. *Child and Family Behavior Therapy*, 21 (4), pp. 1 22, 1999.

[7]   Fletcher, J. D., Effectiveness and cost of interactive videodisc instruction in defense training and education (Report No. P-2372). *Institute for Defense Analysis,* 1990.

[8]   Niemiec, R., & Walberg, H.J., Comparative effects of computer-assisted instruction: A synthesis of reviews. *Journal of Educational Computing Research, 3*, pp. 19 37, 1987.

[9]   Webster-Stratton, C., Kolpacoff, M., & Hollinsworth, T., Self-administered videotape therapy for families with conduct-problem children: Comparison with two cost-effective treatments and a control group. *Journal of Consulting and Clinical Psychology, 56*, pp. 558-566, 1988.

[10] Bosco, J., An analysis of evaluations of interactive video. *Educational Technology*, 26, pp. 7 17, 1986.

[11] Cohen, V. B., Interactive features in the design of videodisc materials. *Educational Technology*, 24, pp. 16 22, 1984.

[12] Hapeshi, K, & Jones, D. M, Interactive multimedia for instruction: A cognitive analysis of the role of audition and vision. *International Journal of Human-Computer Interaction, 4*, pp. 79 99, 1992.

[13] Goldstein, I. L., *Training in Organizations* (3rd Ed.). Pacific Grove, CA: Brooks/Cole Publishing Company, 1993.

[14] Ford, J. K., Quinones, M. A., Sego, D. J., & Sorra, J. S., Factors affecting the opportunity to perform trained tasks on the job. *Personnel Psychology, 45,* pp. 511 527, 1992.

[15] Burda, P. C., Starky, T. W., & Dominguez, F., Computers administered treatment of psychiatric inpatient. *Computers in Human Behaviors, 7,* pp. 1 5, 1991.

[16] Faulkner, C., *The Essence of Human-Computer Interaction.* New York, NY: Prentice Hall, 1998.

[17] Lagges, A., & Gordon, D. A., Use of an interactive laserdisc parent-training program with teenage parents. *Child and Family Behaviour Therapy,* 21, pp. 19 37, 1999.

[18] Gordon, D. A., & Kacir, C. D., Effectiveness of an interactive parent training program for changing adolescent behavior for court-referred parents. Unpublished manuscript, Ohio University, Athens, 1998.

[19] Kacir, C., & Gordon, D.A., Parenting adolescents wisely: The effectiveness of an interactive videodisk parent-training program in Appalachia. *Child and Family Behavior Therapy,* 21 (4), pp. 1 22, 1999.

[20] Woodruff, C., Gordon, D.A., & Lobo, T. R., Reaching high-risk families through home-based parent training: A comparison of interactive CD-ROM and self-help parenting programmes. Unpublished manuscript, Ohio University, 2000.

[21] Rolland-Stanar, C., Gordon, D.A., & Carlston, D., Family violence prevention via school-based CD-ROM parent training. Unpublished manuscript, Ohio University, 2001.

[22] Segal, D., Gordon, D. A., Chen, P. Y., Kacir, C. D. & Gylys, J., Development and evaluation of a parenting intervention program: Integration of scientific and practical approaches. *International Journal of Human-Computer Interaction,* 15, pp. 453 468, 2003.

[23] Gordon, D.A., & Rolland-Stanar, C., Lessons learned from the dissemination of Parenting Wisely, A Parent Training CD-ROM. *Cognitive and Behavioral Practice,* 10, pp. 312-323, 2003.

[24] Gordon, D.A., Parent training via CD-ROM: Using technology to disseminate effective prevention practices. *The Journal of Primary Prevention,* 21, (2), pp. 227 251, 2000.

Pollutant and noise impact on child morbidity

C. Linares[1], J. Díaz[2], R. García-Herrera[2], A. Tobías[3] & A. Otero[1]
[1]*Departamento de Medicina Preventi, Facultad de Medicina,
Universidad Autónoma de Madrid*
[2]*Departamento de Física del Aire, Facultad de Ciencias Físicas,
Universidad Complutense de Madrid*
[3]*Departamento de Estadística, Universidad Carlos III de Madrid*

Abstract

The aim of this paper is to analyse the effects of the urban air pollutants and noise levels on daily emergency hospital admissions of children less than ten years of age in Madrid. Poisson Regression Models were used to quantify the associations. Meteorological variables, influenza epidemics, pollen concentrations and trends and periodicities were used as controlling variables. The main results obtained were the detected relationship ($p<0.05$) between emergency hospital admissions due to organic causes and noise levels and PM10. Significant statistical associations were detected also for pollen concentrations, for cold temperature and for the difference in pressure. The results obtained suggest that particularly PM10 and noise levels are risk factors for the daily emergency hospital for organic causes.
Keywords: air pollution, children's health, emergency hospital admissions, noise levels, time series analysis.

1 Introduction

A growing body of evidence has demonstrated that children's susceptibility to environmental hazards is remarkably different to adults [1]. Children are more vulnerable than adults to environment factors because children are growing and their rapidly developing organ systems are particularly vulnerable, moreover children have a longer life expectancy than adults, giving long latency agents time to work alone or in combination [2]. Between the burdens of environmental risks that children are exposed to, outdoor air pollution is responsible about 6.4%

of deaths from all causes among children aged 0-4 years in the European region [3]. After extended epidemiological studies on outdoor air pollution as a risk factor for morbidity and mortality on general and older population [4], latest studies [5] indicate that the consequences of air pollution are not spread equally among the population, particularly over children's health. Children may have greater exposure than adults to airborne pollutants, this fact is mostly the consequence of their higher exposure level due to their small size and weight. Children breathe more rapidly and inhale more air per breath compared to adults and they spend more time outdoors being physically active, moreover their breathing zone is lower than adults so they are more exposed to vehicle exhausts and heavier pollutants that concentrate at lower levels in the air [6]. Their immune systems and developing lungs are still immature, so irritation or inflammation caused by air pollution is more likely to obstruct their narrower airways [7].

On the other hand, little attention has been paid to the role of environmental noise as risk factor in urban environments. Noise levels can also be considered an environmental pollutant and in the last decade an increasing number of studies are focusing on the role of environmental noise on health [8, 9], between them, there are really few studies analyzing the impact of noise on children. Children may be more annoyed or otherwise adversely affected by noise than adults, in part because they have less well-developed coping responses and are often less able to control their environments. Noise can adversely affect children, the most well-know and most serious consequences of noise are hearing damage and tinnitus, but noise also provoke stress response in children that includes increased heart rate and increased hormone response. Noise can disrupt sleep and thus hinder needed restoration of the body and brain and high noise levels can negative affect children's learning and language development, can disturb children's motivation and concentration and can result in reduced memory and in reduced ability to carry out more or less complex task [10]. One of the main problems when trying to evaluate the role of environmental noise on health is the scarcity of proper measurements of noise levels adequately representing the real exposure to noise [11]. This has lead to a lack of studies including environmental noise levels as input for the behaviour of health variables. Previous studies [12] do not control the synergic effect which can be originated by air pollutants of chemical origin, thus leading to uncertainties when assessing the noise attributable effects [13].

Nowadays, very few studies have considered the effect of noise and air pollutants together over children morbidity to point out a statistically association between them, after controlling for other potential explanatory variables also related with emergency hospital admissions. In this paper, a time series approach is performed to analyse the effects of the principal urban pollutants (PM_{10}, O_3, SO_2, NO_2, NO_x) and noise levels over daily emergency hospital admissions of children less than ten years of age in Madrid (Spain) for organic causes since 1995 to 2000. Another variables as pollen concentration, meteorological variables and flu epidemics have been into consideration as control variables.

2   Methodology

As dependent variable, the series of daily emergency hospital admissions for children younger than ten years old has been computed during the period of January 1, 1995 to December 31, 2000 (2,192 days). This data serie, was supplied by the "Gregorio Marañon" Hospital of Madrid. Causes of admission were defined according to the *International Classification of Diseases, 9th Revision* [14], were grouped as total organic disease causes (ICD-9: 1-799). On the other side, independent variables analyzed were: Air pollutants (PM_{10}, O_3, SO_2, NO_2, NO_x) and daily noise levels. As covariables were analysed meteorological variables and daily levels of pollen (*Poaceae sp.*).

The air pollutants variables have been computed as daily average values and have been provided by the City Council. Daily mean concentrations of nitrogen oxides (NO_x), sulphur dioxides (SO_2), particles with a median aerodynamic diameter of < 10 μm (PM_{10}) and ozone (O_3) were considered, as furnished by Madrid's Municipal Automatic Air Pollution Monitoring Grid.

Acoustic pollution variables were provided by a real-time acoustic pollution network. Diurnal equivalent Level (Leqd) (including the 08-22h period), Night equivalent Level (Leqn) (including the 22-08h period) have been considered. Total daily values for the 24h period (Leqt), have also been considered. Data were provided by the Madrid City Council Noise Pollution Measurement Network.

Meteorological variables included in the models (maximum daily temperature, minimum daily temperature, median daily temperature, pressure and relative humidity at 7 a.m.) were provided by the Spanish National Institute of Meteorology, from the Madrid-Retiro observatory of reference, because of its convenient location in the vicinity of the "Gregorio Marañon" Hospital.

A new variable called "difference in pressure" (dP) was created and included in the models. It was defined as: $dP = P_t - P_{t-1}$, where P_t represents the pressure on the day in question and P_{t-1}, the pressure on the preceding day, so this new variable represents the following:

if $dP<0$ $P_t<P_{t-1}$ means cyclonic trend

if $dP>0$ $P_t>P_{t-1}$ means anticyclonic trend

Pollen data were drawn from the Madrid Regional Health Authority Palinology Network. Information was collected on the daily average levels of *Poaceae* pollen, which is one having highest allergenic potential in Madrid [15].

In previous papers [16], a V-relationship between temperature and emergency in-patients was established, with a minimum daily emergency admissions or comfort value of temperature. Maximum temperature has been used because the maximum daily temperature shows a significant relationship with child mortality, which is not the case for the minimum daily temperature [17]. In the case of ozone, a similar behavior pattern was observed [16]. These previous results have been found in morbidity for general population.

With regard to SO_2, analysis of scatter-plots obtained in previous papers [18], recommended the use of a log transformation for it before entering the models.

The rest of the variables have been used without any previous transformation due to their linear behavior [17]. Fast Fourier Transform method [19] was used to identify trends and periodicities through spectral density function analysis. This led to the introduction of dummy variables to control periodicities, as annual; biannual and three-month seasonalities and also trends. Additionally, influenza epidemics were described through, covariables computed as 1 if it was an epidemic day and as 0 otherwise. To control weekly variation dummy variables for weekdays were introduced in the models.

To eliminate analogous periodicities and autocorrelations a pre-whitening procedure [20] was performed. The cross-correlation function (CCF) between the residuals of the pre-whitened series was computed.

Poisson Regression Models were used in order to describe the association between daily emergency admission and the independent variables, through a step-by-step procedure. In the first step, the individual effect of all the environmental variables was assessed, taking into account the control covariables. Since the environmental variables exhibit a significant degree of colineality, a model describing their joint effect was obtained. Goodness-of-fit was evaluated through simple (ACF) and partial autocorrelation functions (PACF) of the residuals, using as well the Akaike´s information criteria [21]. The environmental variables influence on daily emergency hospital admissions was assessed through the attributable risk (AR), assuming that the whole population was exposed to its effects. In this way, attributable risk can be easily computed as follows: $AR = (RR-1)/RR$ [22], where RR is the relative risk obtained by Poisson models. The analysis was carried out using S-Plus 2000 statistics pack.

3 Results

The descriptive statistics for emergency hospital admissions in children under ten years old and for meteorological and pollutants variables for the study period are shown in Table 1. It should be noted that organic causes show significant decreasing trend. Respect air pollutants, they showed annual seasonality and seven days periodicity and only pollen and noise levels show an increasing trend.

Scatter-plot diagrams of the different independent variables and hospital emergency admissions for organic causes, showed a linear relationship without threshold for PM_{10}, NO_x, NO_2 and a logarithmic relationship for SO_2 (as previously commented). Ozone (O_3) troposphere levels fit a quadratic curve when related to hospital emergency admissions; minimum admissions occurred when ozone was at a concentration of 50 $\mu g/m^3$, that value served as the basis for defining high and low ozone and it corresponds with 95 percentile of the daily mean concentrations values of ozone in the studied period:

$$O_3h = O_3 - 50 \ \mu g/m^3, \text{ if } (O_3) > 50 \ \mu g/m^3$$
$$O_3l = \ 50 \ \mu g/m^3 - O_3, \text{ if } (O_3) < 50 \ \mu g/m^3$$

For noise levels and pollen concentrations and organic causes a threshold is observed in both. These thresholds are 65 dB (A) for Leqd (Figure 1) and about 300 grains/m^3 for pollen concentrations.

Table 1: Statistics for emergency hospital admissions in children under ten years old and environmental variables in Madrid (1995-2002).

	Max	Min	Mean	S.D.	Trend	Periodicity
Organic	21	0	7.0	3.0	Yes ↓	Annual, 3 months, 3-4 days
Tmax (°C)	39.5	1.1	20.0	8.2	Non	Annual, 5 days
Tmin (°C)	25.4	-3.4	10.4	6.2	Non	Annual, 3 days
Hr (%)	100	31	73.7	14.8	Non	2-3 days
P (mb)	956.9	916.5	940.4	6.2	Non	7-15 days
PM_{10} ($\mu g/m^3$)	109	6	33.4	13.7	Yes ↑	Annual, 7, 4-5, 3 days
SO_2 ($\mu g/m^3$)	113	5	22.0	14.0	Non	Annual, 7, 4-5, 3 days
O_3 ($\mu g/m^3$)	76	2	28.2	15.2	Non	Annual, 7,4-5, 3 days
NO_2 ($\mu g/m^3$)	144	23	64.8	17.1	Non	Annual, 7, 4-5, 3 days
NO_x ($\mu g/m^3$)	617	35	150.1	77.6	Non	Annual, 7 , 4-5, 3 days
Pol(grain/m^3)	552	0	13.5	39.4	Yes ↑	Annual, 6 & 3 months, 3 days
Leqd (dBA)	73.7	56.2	68.4	1.7	Yes ↑	Annual, 7, 2-3 days
Leqn (dBA)	71.8	55.9	63.4	1.4	Yes ↑	Annual, 7, 2-3 days
Leqt (dBA)	71.3	57.2	66.4	1.4	Yes ↑	Annual, 7 , 2-3 days

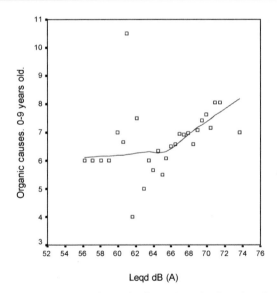

Figure 1:   Scatter-plot diagram of Leqd (diurnal equivalent level of noise) and emergency hospital admissions for organic causes in the group of 0 to 9 years old.

Respect temperature, a V-shaped distribution was observed with a minimum daily emergency admissions or confort value of 33°, indicating the existence of admissions peaks related to low and high temperatures. To control the temperature effect, two additional variables were used, defined as:

$$Tcold = 33 \text{ °C} - Tmax, \text{ if } Tmax < 33 \text{ °C}$$
$$Thot = Tmax - 33 \text{ °C}, \text{ if } Tmax > 33 \text{ °C}$$

Table 2 shows the cross-correlation function outputs between environmental variables and emergency hospital admissions for organic causes, after the prewhitening process. Figure 2 shows the CCF for Leqt versus organic causes. Table 3 shows the results for the Autoregressive Poisson Regression Models that describe the association between daily emergency admissions by organic causes, in which can be observed that Leqt and PM_{10} are the variables with main attributable risk. Temperature showed statistically significant associations with emergency hospital admissions only when Tcold was considered, no effect was found due to Thot. The effect of cold was in long-term effect.

Table 2: Lags with significant pre-whitened CCF values between organic causes emergency hospital admissions and environmental factors.

Variables	Organic Causes
Tmax	10 (negative coefficient)
PM_{10}	0
NO_x	Without relation
Leqt	3
Pollen	4

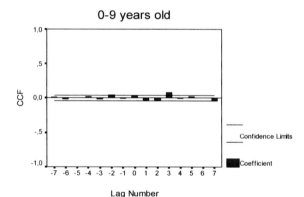

Figure 2: Cross correlation function between Leqt versus emergency hospital admissions for organic causes in the group of 0 to 9 years old.

Table 3: Statistically significant variables in Poisson Regression Models.

Factor (Lag)	RR (95% CI)	AR(%)
$PM_{10}(0)$[I]	1.02 (1.01 1.03)	2.1
Tcold (10)[II]	1.00 (1.00 1.01)	0.5
Leqt (3)[III]	1.02 (1.01 1.04)	2.4
Pollen (4)[IV]	1.01 (1.00 1.01)	0.9
dP (2)[V]	1.01 (1.00 1.01)	0.5

[I] RR for an increase of 10 $\mu g/m^3$ in the PM_{10} concentration.
[II] RR for each degree of Tmax (maximum temperature is less than 33°C).
[III] RR for an increase of 1 dB(A) in Leqt.
[IV] RR for an increase of 10 grain/m^3 in the Pollen concentration.
[V] RR for a decrease of 1mb in dP.

4 Discussion and conclusions

The relationship detected through the scatter plot diagrams between the air pollutants and children emergency hospital admissions is similar to that obtained in others studies that analyze the effects of the air pollutants in general population [18], and similar to that detected over children mortality [17]. About the pattern detected for ozone concentrations and maximum temperature, indicating the existence of admissions peaks related to low and high ozone concentrations and the existence of two branches of temperature called Thot and Tcold, are comparable to the values detected in morbidity for general population in Madrid [16] but not reported until now in children morbidity. Moreover concerning to the relation found in the scatter plot with noise levels and children hospital admissions that establish a strong increase about a level of 65 dB (A), two previous papers centred in Madrid City, establish this identical level for morbidity in general population too [13, 23]. The relation found for pollen levels it also has been detected previously in Madrid over daily number of asthma emergency room admissions and high levels of *Poaceae* pollen that suggests their implication in the epidemic distribution of asthma, during the period coinciding with their abrupt release into the environment [24].

The results of cross-correlation functions (CCFs) found that daily Tmax is the best indicator for thermal impact [17]. Cold temperature give rises to bronchoconstriction, which can enhance previously existing pulmonary diseases, leading to casualties in the short-medium term.

The association found between air pollutants and emergency hospital admissions in this group of age for PM_{10} levels in the short-term are also coherent with the results obtained by others authors [25], which reported the short-term effect (0 and 3 days lag) of this pollutant and its relationship with circulatory and respiratory diseases.

About noise levels, a relationship between Leqt and organic causes was established at short-term (lag 3). The results obtained suggest that the associations indicating the short-term effects of exposure to high noise levels are non spurious and point out that the current levels of environmental noise have a considerable epidemiological impact on children emergency hospital admissions [8, 9]. The association at lag 3 for *Poaceae* pollen concentrations has been reported also, as previously commented in asthma hospital emergencies in the metropolitan area of Madrid [23]. This is line with the biological mechanisms of allergens, since the clinical consequences of a given pollen load increased as the pollination season progressed.

About difference of pressure that appears as statistically significative in the models, its behaviour is similar in another previous study about general population and mortality in Madrid [26]. This pattern means that an anticyclonic trend is associated with an increasing of children emergency hospital admissions due to organic causes.

For last, the results obtained for the Autoregressive Poisson Regression Models that describe the association between children daily emergency admissions and the environmental variables are according to the associations obtained in the CCFs. The relative risk and the attributable risk are similar to those reported for other studies in children [27, 28].

The results obtained suggest that the urban air pollution, particularly PM_{10} and noise levels, are risk factors for the daily emergency hospital admissions of children less than ten years of age in Madrid for organic causes. Hence, the importance of this study does not lay simply in the establishment of a relationship between air pollution and hospital admissions. Rather, it lies in the quantification of this relationship; by establishing models capable of diagnosing and forecasting for hospital management purposes. On the other hand, it is well-known that traffic is the major source of air pollutants and noise levels in urban areas, but despite the important contribution of traffic sources to reduced urban air quality, relatively few studies have evaluated the specific effects of traffic-related air pollution over children health. Moreover, respect noise levels; Madrid is a city with an unacceptable high background noise level. In this sense, a reduction of the noise levels could be accompanied by a possible decrease in the number of children emergency admissions in Madrid due to organic causes. So it must be emphasized that traffic appears to be one of the main environmental risk factors for children health in Madrid.

.....Although these environmental risks are not the leading cause of death or morbidity in children in the developed world, it seems interesting to know how affect children's health, because there is increasingly strong evidence that air pollution and high noise levels are associated with nontrivial increases in the risk of death and chronic diseases in children, moreover, what is important to realize is that this is an modifiable risk.

Acknowledgement

The authors gratefully acknowledge the support of this study to the ISCIII (Red de Centros C03/09).

References

[1]   Landrigan PJ, Suk W, Amler RW. Chemical wastes, children's health, and the Superfund basic research program. Environ Health Perspect, 107: 423-427, 1999.

[2]   Fact sheet EURO/05/04. Study on environmental burden of disease in children: key findings. WHO Europe.

[3]   Valent F, Little D, Bertollini R, et al. Burden of disease attributable to selected environmental factors and injury among children and adolescent in Europe. Lancet, 363: 2032-2039, 2004.

[4]   Katsouyanni K, Touloumi G, Samoli E, et al. Confounding and effect modification in the short-term effects of ambient particles on total mortality: results from 29 European cities within the APHEA2 project. Epidemiology, 12: 521-31, 2001.

[5]   Schwartz J. Air Pollution and Children's Health. Pediatrics, 113: 1037-1043, 2004.

[6] Children's Environmental Health Project. Respiratory health effects. Canadian Association of Physicians for the Environment. 2000.

[7] Air Pollution and Children's Health. A fact sheet by Cal/EPA's Office of Environmental Health Hazard Assessment and The American Lung Association of California. November, 2003.

[8] Ising H, Lange-Asschenfeldt H, Lieber GF et al. Effects of long-term exposure to street traffic exhaust on the development of skin and respiratory tract diseases in children. Schriftenr Ver Wasser Boden Lufthyg, 112: 81-99, 2003.

[9] Ising H, Kruppa B. Health effects caused by noise: evidence in the literature from the past 25 years. Noise Health, 6(22): 5-13, 2004.

[10] Health effects of noise and perception of the risk of noise. National Institute of Public Health. Dinamarca, 2001. Edited by Marie Louise Bistrup.

[11] Passchier-Vermeer W, Paschier W. Environ Health Perspect, 106: A222-A223, 1998.

[12] Babisch W, Ising H, Gallacher JEJ et al. Traffic noise and cardiovascular risk. Outdoor noise levels and risk factors. Arch Environ Health, 43: 407-414, 1998.

[13] Díaz J, García R, Tobías A et al. Noise levels in Madrid: association with emergency hospital admissions. Environmental Health Risk. WIT Press, 2001.

[14] Commission on Professional and Hospital Activities. The international classification of diseases (9th Rev.: Clinical Modification). Ann Arbor, MI: Author, 1978.

[15] Galán I, Tobías A, Banegas JR et al. Short-term effects of air pollution on daily asthma emergency room admissions. European Respiratory Journal, 22: 802-808, 2003.

[16] Díaz J, Alberdi JC, Pajares MS et al. A Model for forecasting emergency hospital admissions effect of environmental variables. J Environ Health, 64: 9-15, 2001.

[17] Díaz J, Linares C, García-Herrera R et al. Impact of temperature and air pollution on the mortality of children in Madrid. J Occup Environ Med, 46: 768-774, 2004.

[18] Díaz J, García R, Ribera P et al. Modelling of air pollution and its relationship with mortality and morbidity in Madrid, Spain. Int Arch Occup Environ Health, 72: 366-376, 1999.

[19] Box GEP, Jenkins GM & Reinsel C. Time Series Analysis, Forecasting and Control. Englewood Cliffs: Prentice Hall, 1994.

[20] Makridakis S, Wheelwright SC & McGee VE. Forecasting methods and applications. Wiley and Sons. San Francisco, 1983.

[21] Akaike H. A new look at statistical model identification. IEEE T Automat Contr, 9: 716-722, 1974.

[22] Coste J & Spira A, Le proportion de cas atribruable en Santé Publique: definition(s), estimation(s) et interprétation. Rev Epidemiol Santé Publique, 51: 399-411, 1991.

[23] Tobías A, Díaz J, Saez M et al. Use of Poisson regression and Box-Jenkins models to evaluate the short-term effects of environmental noise levels on daily emergency admissions in Madrid, Spain. Eur J Epidemio, 17: 765-771, 2001.

[24] Tobías A, Galán I, Banegas JR et al. Short-term effects of airborne pollen concentrations on asthma epidemic. Thorax, 58: 708-710, 2003.

[25] Wong TW, Lau TS, Yu TS et al. Air pollution and hospital admissions for respiratory and cardiovascular diseases in Hong Kong. Occup and Environ Med, 56: 679-683, 1999.

[26] González S, Díaz J, Pajares MS et al. Relationship between atmospheric pressure and mortality in the Madrid Autonomous Region: a time-series study. Int J Biometeoro, 45:34-40, 2001.

[27] Kim J, Smorodinsky S, Lipsett M et al. Traffic-related air pollution nears busy roads. Am J Resp Crit Care, 170:520-526, 2004.

[28] Gehring U,Cyrys J, Sedlmeir G et al. Traffic-related air pollution and respiratory health during the first 2 years of life. Eur Respir J, 19(4):690-698, 2002.

Some nanotechnology risks

J. A. Donovan
University of Massachusetts at Amherst, USA

Abstract

By analogy with known toxins (pollutants, quartz, and asbestos) some nanomatter may be toxic. Nanomatter is formed by manipulating atoms and molecules into new, useful materials that are on the same size scale as virus cells. The properties of nanomatter differ from macromatter with the same chemistry, and depend on its size (two of the reasons for all the excitement). Some nanomatter already exists from natural processes, but engineered nanomatter may (probably will) change our lives more than the industrial revolution. However, because these are **new** materials their <u>properties</u> and their interaction with the <u>environment</u>, and their effect on <u>health</u> are unknown. What is known by analogy and the few toxicology reports on nanomatter will be reviewed. Because of the significant potential benefits and equally significant potential risks the public needs to be informed and involved in the policy discussions concerning nanotechnology.
Keywords: nanotechnology, benefits and risks, size dependence, societial effects.

1 Introduction

Nanotech (NT) *promises* to change the way we live. How? By making things on the scale of atoms and molecules and exploiting their properties. Governments, companies, and venture capitalists throughout the world, big and small, are pouring money into nanoscience and NT. In 2004 funding of nano research and development was $8.6 billion [1] most of it coming from the governments of at least 30 countries. The U.S. in 2005 will spend about $2.5 bill compared to $1.6 bill in 2004. The contribution of the U.S. government in 2005 will be almost $ 1 billion [2]. The world wide annual industrial production of nanoproducts in 10-15 years is estimated to be greater than $1 trillion, and will require about 2 million NT workers [3]. Is it worth it? Will the positive effects outweigh the negative?

NT promises, according to its supporters, to radically transform the treatment of cancer, increase the efficiency of electronic devices such as solar cells, clean up the environment, enhance food supply etc. To date these are promises, but there are nanoproducts, some old some new, in the stores: tires and photocopier toner, wrinkle and stain resistant fabrics, reinforced tennis rackets, tennis balls that do not loose their bounce, sunscreen and ultra-violet screening, anti-bacterial and medical applications that incorporate nanoparticles (NP), cosmetic products, joint cream that professional athletes are using, etc. These incrementally improved products are just the beginning. Eventually disruptive technologies (technologies that displace older technologies) will emerge, therefore it is important for the scientist, engineer and layperson to begin to understand NT. It is too early to predict how disruptive NT will be, but not too early to be concerned about how it will affect our health, environment, and safety, economy, security, etc. Will there be a backlash, like occurred with genetically modified food, biotechnology, and nuclear energy? The best and only way to avoid such a backlash is to have open discussion, open literature, open procedures that the public can study and understand and choose to support or not to.

2 Nanotechnology and society

The chosen assumption of the body politic in the past has been that science and engineering have been good for society; recently this assumption has been challenged, for example genetically modified food, cloning, stem cell research, wind energy, etc. As pointed out recently in SCIENCE [4] that many of these areas of research and the technology based on it clash with certain human beliefs and values. NT raises issues that challenge some of these human values and health issues. First is the *toxicity* of NP, with little data available the issue is unresolved. The second concerns of the relationship of between man and nature, because of the potential to manipulate life at the nanoscale it probably will challenge traditional values. These concerns and other similar ones raise questions for the funding agencies and society.

Michael Crichton in his new book, **State of Fear** [5] writes, "The intermixing of science and politics is a bad combination, with a bad history" [6]. However, there is no way for NT and politics not to mix because it's funding is mostly from taxes. In the future industrial support will grow and make a more significant contribution than now. This direct and strong link with taxes gives the public the *right and responsibility* to influence the future of NT.

State of Fear was <u>not</u> about NT (but about climate change). His previous book, **Prey** [7] focused on "nanobots", self-replicating nano-scale machines, which get out of control. It alerted and alarmed some readers, and prompted discussion of the benefits and the risks and the responsibility of developing these technologies. **Prey** is science fiction that concerns the clash of technology with human nature. This is one way for the public to get information about NT, but if it is the primary way it could polarize the public against NT.

Recent surveys in the U.S. and U.K. found that between 10 and 20 per cent of the population had heard of NT. These 10 to 20 percent have high hopes that it will cure disease, but fear that it will lead to a loss of privacy. They are not much concerned that nanobots will take over the world. But, they worry the most that industry will not be honest about the risks to human health [8]. To avoid this mistrust from developing more people need to become involved in the public discussion of NT. As NT becomes better known through the commercial products based on NT the risk to NT is misunderstanding. It is important that the public be openly informed about the positive contribution that it will make to our and our children's lives. But, it is equally important that the public be informed about the risks of NT. NT will not be successful by only doing good engineering research [9]. Therefore, the US government has started funding significant research on the risks of nanoresearch to the health, environment and security. And, it intends to communicate this information with the public.

3   Simple Introduction to Nanoscience

To begin to understand and appreciate the benefits and risks of NT it is necessary to know that we are talking about particles or aggregates of matter that are between 1 and 100 nanometers, or 10^{-9} to 10^{-7} meters. That is the length of 10 aligned hydrogen or four gold atoms up to the diameter of a virus. So these are small particles, in fact so small that the number of atoms on the surface is comparable to the number in the total particle. For example, consider a gold particle: with a diameter of 1.3 nm would contain about 64 atoms and all the atoms would be on the surface. This solid particle would melt at about 200 °C. The normal melting point of bulk gold is 1064.4 °C.

The atoms, of any size solid, that are on the surface have more energy than atoms that are in the interior of the particle. This is why liquid drops tend to form spheres to minimize the surface energy by minimizing the ratio of surface area to bulk volume. Because NP have a large ratio of surface atoms to bulk atoms, they are high energy particles. Macroscopic gold is one of the most inert elements known; but when the particles are less than 5 nm in diameter gold is a catalyst, which depends on a high energy surface to interact with the reacting species [10]. The melting point of this 5 nm particle would be about 830 °C.

Another property of the gold particle that changes as a function of size is color: 100 nm gold particles appear golden, but 50 nm particles appear green, and if they were only 25 nm they would be red.

The above description highlights two important characteristics of nanomaterials: 1) they are high energy, highly reactive particles, and 2) their properties are a function of their size. Only their melting point and color were described, but most of their properties such as electrical, magnetic and mechanical are functions of their size. This is the difference between macro and nano materials: the properties of macro materials do not change with size, those of nano do. Therefore, nanomaterials are **new** materials with different properties than their macro equivalent with the same chemistry. Many nanomaterials, according to today's nomenclature, have been around for years. The gold particles described above were used to make stained glass, and vehicle tires are black because they contain manufactured NP of carbon black. They also occur naturally from fires, in the casein micelles in milk, wear debris from tires, and from vehicle exhaust. We have been living with NP for a very long time, but what is different is that new engineered nanoparticles are being made in many laboratories and many different countries. It is estimated that about 130 nano-based products have been introduced to the market. So the potential for exposure to nanoparticles, in the laboratory or plant and in public places will increase significantly in the near future.

4   Risks

Because our knowledge is insufficient a formal risk assessment is not possible. To fill in the knowledge gaps a new discipline: nanotoxicology is developing [11] and a new scientific journal, Nanotoxicology, will begin publication in the UK this summer. What do we know?

The current assumption is that nanotechnologies based on free NP, that can become airborne, are the potential, imminent threat. NP that are dispersed in a liquid, for example, colloids are included since the liquid may evaporate and the NP become airborne. NP that are fixed to a surface or in a solid matrix have a lower priority. However, as NT develops the same questions need to be asked as for free NP.

Natural or biological nanosystems, such as viruses are abundant in nature, and the cellular processes are nanoscale processes. Nanobiotechnology genetically, atomically or molecularly modifies these systems or processes, or in other words manipulates life at the nanoscale; at the moment these systems are not receiving the attention they deserve, but they will as nanotoxicology matures.

Nanosystems, built up by self assembly (development of three dimensional periodic arrays such as crystals, folding of proteins, the pairing of DNA, etc.) can mimic natural systems, and can be self-replicating. The current assumption, with good basis, is that these built up n-systems will require 5-10 years more development and can be controlled, so for the time being higher priority is being put on free NP. But, eventually more safety research will have to be done to conceive, develop, understand, access their risk, and control these self-replicating systems.

The research on air pollution is relevant to free NP; this work initiated when the primary cause of 4000 deaths in London in 1952 was attributed to smog. Smog is a high concentration of particles in the nanometer size range from combustion processes, fossil fuel power plants, incinerators, diesel engines, etc. This research showed that ultrafine particles caused the increased mortality, and non-toxic substances when on the order of nanometers may cause a toxic response [12]. Finer particles have a larger percentage of surface sites (higher energy) that can attach other toxic atoms or molecules, and serve as transport agents. They are generally more reactive and can produce free radicals that damage tissue.

Studies concerned with the effect of the inhalation of quartz dust demonstrated that their toxicity is related to the surface area of the particles and their surface activity. The toxicity of asbestos depends on the length and diameter, and surface activity of the particle. With both quartz and asbestos the harmful affects depend on the dose. All of us have some quartz and asbestos in our lungs, but they become toxic only after the accumulation of a critical dose [13].

Research continues to try to identify the relative contribution of surface area and surface activity. There is no generally accepted metric to measure dose because the mechanisms of how the fine particles cause respiratory and cardiovascular problems are not well understood. However, researches in nanotoxicology agree that the toxicity of nanomaterials, for which there is no accepted standard for quality and purity, cannot be based on the toxicity of bulk materials of the same chemistry.

Eva Oberdorster reported recently at the annual meeting of the American Chemical Society that carbon NP, buckyballs or fullerenes, could damage the cell membranes of the brains of large mouth bass [14]. The water fleas were also killed by the addition of the buckyballs to the water. Buckyballs are one of the NP receiving a lot of the attention of nanoscientists. They are made up of only carbon atoms that form a hollow structure that resembles a soccer ball. They are believed to have applications for drug delivery, environmental remediation, and in cosmetics. Also, it was reported by V. Colvin [15] that 1.5ppm of buckyballs in water killed one-half of E-coli bacteria that were present. The mechanisms and implications of these results have not been worked out.

These buckyballs and other carbon NP have been around for a while: they were found in an ice core 10,000 years old indicating their natural existence [16]. These same researches showed that carbon nanotubes, similar to buckyballs, are produced by methane combustion sources: kitchen gas stove tops, furnaces, power plants, etc. What is different is that with the manufacture of NP their concentration in the environment probably will become much higher. This means that the dose the population could receive might be much higher.

Gunter Oberdorster, professor of Toxicology at the University of Rochester, has been studying how the body interacts with ultrafine particles for years focusing on smog. Recently he has studied how NP accumulate, therefore they must be able to easily move which is not true for larger particles, in the cavities, lungs and brains of rats, and worries if this could lead to brain damage or harmful inflammation [17]. He is developing a model to predict the toxicity of NP. This is a significant scientific challenge because the chemical (and other) properties are a function of their size. This will not be the evolution of a model, but the creation of a new model for new materials, that will require new information and scientific understanding.

A recently published paper by Lam et al. [18] concluded that carbon nanotubes can be more toxic than quartz, and that toxicity of NP cannot be extrapolated from existing data for particles of similar chemistry. And, a paper by Warheit et al. [19] supports this conclusion. In addition its data suggest that the pulmonary toxicity, caused by carbon NP, is by a new mechanism, not observed before with other toxic dusts.

Preliminary work by one of the UK's leading toxicologists, Howard [20] suggests that gold nanoparticles can move from mother to the fetus by passing through the placenta. The mother rat was injected with gold particles, and then the fetus was examined for the presence of gold particles. Dark particles were observed but they have not been identified as gold particles.

Zinc oxide and titanium oxide are both used in some kinds of sunscreens and cosmetics. And, a coat of titanium oxide about 15 nm thick is placed on window glass and the glass becomes "self-cleaning." The oxide absorbs the sunlight, produces a photocatalytic reaction that breaks down the dirt and it washes off with the next rain or by being rinsed with water. The adsorption of the sunlight is one of the reasons that they are added to cosmetics or sunscreens. If the NP oxide is adsorbed into the skin cells, how will the particles affect the health of the cells if they are exposed to light? The answer is unknown, and the related question: Do NP get adsorbed by the skin? has not been answered. There is concern that NP could be adsorbed by injured skin and some data that they can be preferentially adsorbed at hair follicles [21], but there is no data showing adverse effects of exposure to NP.

One of the big hopes for NT is improved drug delivery and disease diagnoses. One of the NP considered for this is a cadmium selenide quantum dot that might segregate to diseased tissue, and allow identification of this tissue. However, a recent paper suggests [22] that the dots are soluble and the released cadmium would be poisonous. More work is required on its toxicity and great caution before initiating tests with humans.

Finally, how about our food supply? Some people claim that molecular food manufacturing will provide unlimited food, without farms, and without farmers. We are not there yet. The earliest applications will come with food packaging and sensors, which determine the quality of the contained food [23].

For example, it has been a long time goal to have plastic beer bottles. Plastic bottles fail because oxygen diffuses through the container spoiling the beer. Reinforcement with nano-clay particles makes the bottle stronger, but more importantly traps the oxygen (slows its transport) and increases the shelf life so that it is feasible to package beer in plastic bottles.

Other nano-additives are already available and being sold. The advantages of these additives are that they are adsorbed more easily by the body and they have a longer shelf life. Are they safe? No body knows. Do you know if your food contains nano-additives? No; because there are no requirements to list nano-ingredients on the label.

5 Summary

NT will revolutionize our life, even if only some of the claims come true. But, NT is based on new, manufactured materials that have properties radically different from normal sized materials. Therefore, a hazards analysis cannot be done because the necessary database does not exist. However, there is enough data to know that great caution is necessary with regard to NP in the environment. The immediate goal of NT should be to start with the Recommendations of the Royal Society, their report [13] is the most thorough available. Or in brief 1) develop a technological basis for formal and complete safety analysis, and 2) develop better understanding of the nanostate as a basis for the engineering design of nanoproducts. This must include an open information policy so the public knows the good and bad of NT, and develops trust with this new exciting technology.

References

[1]   Loder, N., *Small Wonders*, The Economist, Jan. 1, 2005.
[2]   Giles, J., Growing nanotech trade hit by questions over quality, *Nature*, **432**, 791, 2004.
[3]   Roco, M.C. International Strategy for Nanotechnology J. of Nanoparticle Research, **3**, 353-360, 2001.
[4]   Leshner, A. I., Where Science Meets Society, *Science*, 302, 815, February 11, 2005.
[5]   Creichton, M., *State of Fear*, HarperCollins, New York, 2004.
[6]   *Hotting Up*, The Economist, 73, February 5, 2005.
[7]   Creichton, M., *Prey*, HarperCollins, New York, 2002.
[8]   Cobb, M. D. & Macoubrie, J., Public Perceptions About Nanotechnology: Risks, Benefits and Trust. *J. of Nanoparaticle Research*, **6**, 395-405, 2004.
[9]   Roco, M. C., Broader Societal Issues of Nanotechnology. *J. of Nanoparticle Research*, **5**, 181-189, 2003.
[10] Cortie, M. B. & van der Lingen, E., *Material Forum*, *26*, 1-14, 2002.
[11] Donaldson, K., Stone, V., Tran, C.L. Kreyling, W. & Borm, P. J. A., Nanotoxicology, *Occupational Environmental Medicine*, **61**,727-728, 2004.
[12] Donaldson, K., Stone, V., Clouter, A., Renwick, L. & MacNee, W. *Ultrafine Particles*, *Occup.* Environ. Med. **58**, 211-216, 2001.
[13] *Nanoscience and Nanotechnologies*, The Royal Society and the Royal w, Academy of Engineering, 36, July 2004March 30, 2004.
[14] Service, R. F., *Buckyballs Bad for Fish*, Science
[15] Service, R. F., *Nanotechnology Grows Up*, Science, **304**, 1732-1734, June 18, 2004.
[16] Murr, L. E., Soto, K.F., Esquivel, E.V., Bang, J.J., Guerrero, P.A., Lopez, D.A., & Ramirez, D.A., *Carbon Nanotubes and Other Fullerene-Related Nanocrystals in the Environment*, JOM, **56**, 28-31, 2004.
[17] Taylor, P., *Tiny Tech Could Be Big Health Problem*, DrugResearcher.com, August 4, 2004
[18] Lam, C-W, James, J. T., McCluskey, R. & Hunter, R. L., *Pulmonary Toxicity of Single-Wall Carbon Nanotubes in Mice...*Toxicological Sciences, **77**, 126-134, 2004.

[19]   Warheit, D. B., Laurence, B. R., Reed, L. L., Roach, D.H., Reynolds, G.A. M., & Webb, T. R., *Comparative Pulmonary Toxicity Assessment of Single-wall Carbon Nanotubes in Rats,* Toxicological Sciences, **77**, 117-125, 2004.

[20]   Howard, V., *British Scientist: Nanoparticles Might Move From Mom to Fetus*, Smalltimes, Jan. 14, 2004.

[21]   Shim, J., Seok Kang, H., Park, W. –S., Han, S.-h., Kim, J., &Chang, I. – S., *Transdermal Delivery of Mixnoxidil With Block Copolymer Nanoparticles,* **97**, 477-484, 2004.

[22]   Mullins, J., *Safety Concerns Over Injectable Quantum Dots,* New Scientist, **181**, 10, February 28, 2004.

[23]   The ETC Group, *Down on the Farm,* November 2004.

Hazardous material transport accidents: analysis of the D.G.A.I.S. database

S. Bonvicini & G. Spadoni
Department of Chemical, Mining Engineering and Environmental Technologies, Bologna University, Italy

Abstract

In this paper results are presented and discussed about the analysis of the data of hazardous materials road transport accidents reported by the Canadian database D.G.A.I.S. (*Dangerous Goods Accident Information System*). The records of the database have been subdivided first of all on the basis of the transport phase to which they belong; then they have been classified by the accident typology and, for each type, by its primary cause. Subsequently accidents with hazmat release have been grouped considering the physical state of the spilled substance, in order to determine, basing on the leaked mass, the release categories and their occurrence probabilities. Finally the post-release event trees have been drawn and quantified for flammables. This work has allowed on one hand to determine the major causes of accidents and thus the actions to adopt for reducing the accident frequencies; on the other hand it has been possible to extract data for transport risk analysis, also suggesting useful improvements for bettering the quality of the information recorded by accident databases.
Keywords: accident database, event tree, flammables, hazardous materials, road transport, spill, tank truck.

1 Introduction

The analysis of an accident database can be performed with two aims. One of these is surely that of "learning from experience" ([1, 2]), that is first of all to understand what are the causes of an accident, in order to pre-emptively undertake those safety measures which will lower the probability it will occur again, and, further, to comprehend what actions have been adopted (or should have been adopted) to limit the consequences of the accident once it has happened, in order to face in a suitable way a similar situation which will occur in the future. To confirm this teaching purpose of the databases, in some of them there is a special field for the "learned lessons".

The second reason justifying the examination of a database is that of extracting information useful for quantified risk analysis [3]. Referring to the transport of dangerous goods, useful data are, for instance, the probability that an accident is followed by a release of the shipped chemical, the probability the release being continuous or instantaneous, the probability density distribution of the released mass, the probability of each possible final outcome.

Very often, if transport specific information is not available, these data are obtained from the databases reporting accidents occurred in fixed facilities, like production plants or warehouses. In fact in the process industry it has become routine to collect data about accidental events; indeed the companies with more plants have internal databases for storing and processing these data [1].

However, it is necessary to notice that the equipment of a plant are of a greater variety than those used for transport and also different from them; further the accidents which can occur in a facility are very different from those of a transport vehicle. For this reason for transport risk studies it would be better to use data obtained from accidents occurred during transport.

The analysis of the database D.G.A.I.S. (*Dangerous Goods Accident Information System*) [4], where information about transportation accidents occurred in Canada is reported, has been performed in order both to determine the main causes of accidents and to extract data for risk analysis. In Italy (and indeed in Europe) there are no transport specific databases. Though, since the Canadian transportation system is very different from the Italian one, because of both the infrastructures and the features of the vehicles, caution should be used when applying Canadian data for Italian case studies.

2 The D.G.A.I.S. database

The D.G.A.I.S. database is part of a Canadian national program for public safety in the transport of dangerous goods [5]; this program has been developed by TDG (the *Transport Dangerous Goods Directorate*) of *Transport Canada*.

When an accident occurs, the person responsible of the transport or a delegate of him has to compile a form called DOR (*Dangerous Occurrence Report*), which is then sent to TGD. In this form information is collected about the site and the data of the accident, the transport modality, the type of vehicle, the involved chemicals, the accident causes and consequences.

The accidents records, stored in files, are available on a yearly base; in this research data of 13 years, from 1988 to 2000, have been examined. For each year there are two files: the "accidents file" and the "substances file". In each "accidents file" there are so many records as the accidentals occurrences happened in the year to which the file refers to; in the "substances file" there are so many record as the substances involved in the accidents occurred during the year. Since more chemicals can be involved in a single accident, each record of an "accident file" is in relation with one or more records of the "substance file".

The research has focused on on-land and in-bulk transportation; in this paper results of the road accidents are reported. 3282 accidents record have been examined, referring to 3431 substance record. The accident records have been subdivided first of all on the basis of the transport phase to which they belong; then they have been classified, for the main transport phase, taking into account the accident typology and its primary cause. Further accidents with hazmat release have been grouped considering the physical state of the substance, in order to determine, basing on the spilled quantities, the release categories and their occurrence probabilities. Finally, further distinguishing the substances on the basis of their hazardous properties, the post-release event trees have been drawn and quantified for flammables.

The categories used for each classification do not always match with those of D.G.A.I.S.; in fact in some cases the classes of the database have been grouped together in order to obtain more meaningful and statistically valid results.

Unfortunately the records are often incomplete, that is many fields have not been filled in; as a consequence, for some classifications only a small number of records has been available, thus affecting the statistical validity of the extracted data.

3 The analysis of the road accidents

First of all it has been necessary to determine the transportation phase to which the accident records belong. Three main phases have been taken into account: *en-route transit*, *loading/unloading*, *rest* in a parking area. The distribution of the accidents among these categories is reported in fig. 1.

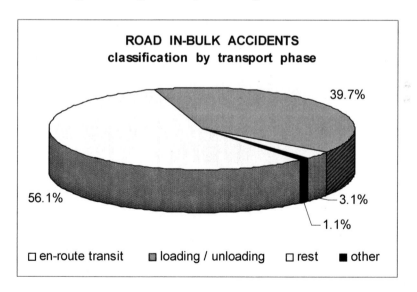

Figure 1: Classification of accidents by phase of transport.

It is possible to notice that more than half of the accidents (i.e. 56.1%) occurs during *en-route transit*; a smaller group occurs during the *loading/unloading* operations (with a valued of 39.7%); finally the percentage of the accidents happened during *rest* in a parking area or in another transport phase is negligible at all.

Generally tank trucks are loaded and unloaded inside the plant limits under the responsibility of the plant personal; thus the risk of these operations, which are part of the numerous activities performed inside the factory, is usually quantified in the plant risk assessment. Further at plants there is generally a specifically trained emergency team and also specific tools for facing an abnormal situation. For this reason the *loading/unloading* operations, though they pertain to a tank truck, do not really concern the transport process and thus they have not been considered further in this work.

Focusing on the *en-route transit*, the accident typologies have been investigated, considering four accident types: *collision* (with a vehicle or a generic obstacle), *turn-over*, *run-off-road* and *spontaneous leak* form the tank (for instance due to corrosion or from a not perfectly closed valve). The results of this classification are reported in fig. 2.

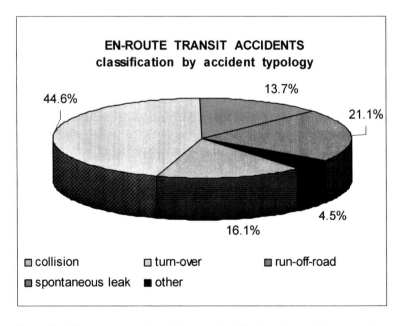

Figure 2:   En-route transit accidents: classification by accident typology.

It is possible to notice that, in addition to the traffic accidents, like the *collision*, the *turn-over*, the *run-off-road,* which occur also to vehicles not shipping dangerous goods, the category of the *spontaneous leaks* (i.e. of the non accident-induced spills) has a great relevance. Subsequently for each accident typology referring to the *en-route transit*, the primary accident cause has been investigated, assuming four primary causes: *human error, vehicle failure, tank failure, external event*. For *human error* a wrong action or an omission of the driver is intended (for instance wrong manoeuvres; the non-respect of traffic lights, right of ways, speed limits; grinding halts; driving behaviours not suitable to the road pavement and/or the atmospheric conditions; bad psycho-physical situations of the driver) or an error of the person who has loaded the vehicle (like the overfilling of the tank; the imperfect closure of a valve; the omission of the introduction of specific reaction inhibitors). *Vehicle failure* stands, for instance for a break-down of the truck, the rupture of an axle, the burst of a tire, the malfunctioning of the braking system. Finally examples of *tank failures* are leaks due to corrosion, bad welds, cyclic stress, construction defects, overpressure. *External events* are, for instance, an obstacle or a fire on the road, adverse meteorological conditions, vandalism. The results of this classification are summarized in fig. 3.

From this figure it results that for all accident typologies *human error* is the main accident cause, followed by *external events*; for spontaneous leaks also the *tank failure* is important. For *collision, turn-over* and *run-off-road* events, which occur independently of the transported good, it would be very useful to know the probability an accident being followed by a release; unfortunately the information reported by records does not allow to extract this value. Indeed this datum has a great relevance, since the release frequency, which enters all risk studies, is generally obtained by multiplying the accident frequency and the release probability conditioned to the occurrence of the accident.

Another information which would be important to know is weather a release is continuous or instantaneous; this information too is missing in nearly all records. Though in some records the quantity of spilled substance is reported; this datum has been analysed separately for the liquids and the liquefied pressure gases.

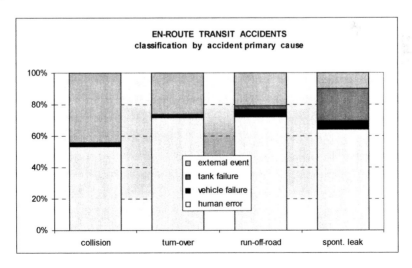

Figure 3: En-route transit accidents: classification by accident primary cause.

Generally liquids are shipped at ambient conditions of pressure and temperature, while liquefied gases are transported at their vapour pressure at ambient temperature. The different pressure values of liquids and liquefied gases strongly influences the release rate (and thus also the totally released mass) and for this reason a separate classification has been performed for these two types of fluids. Results, referring to 220 liquid records and to 1897 liquefied pressure gas records, are graphed in fig. 4.

It is possible to notice that for liquefied gases all spills are lower than 1 t (ton), while for liquids the spilled quantities are greater, thus allowing the definition of three release categories: 0–1 t, 1–10 t and 10–100 t.

This fact can be justified by considering the major resistance of the tanks for pressurised chemicals (like those used for liquefied gases) with respect to those designed for atmospheric transports (like those used for liquids). In fact, taking into account that there are no great differences in the tank capacities, the major strength of a pressurized tank determines that accidental holes on this tank will have minor dimensions than those on a pressurized tank: for this reason, though the major pressure, the total released quantity for liquefied gases is smaller than for liquids. In addition the occurrence probability of the release categories becomes lower for greater holes, and this fact too confirms that small leaks are more probable than big ones, as usually assumed in risk analysis studies.

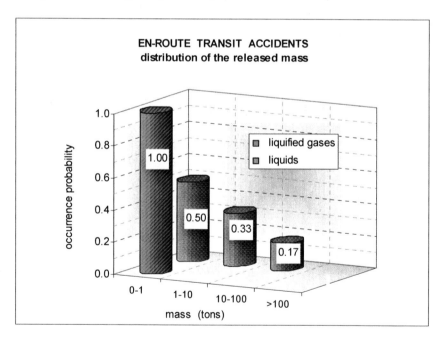

Figure 4: En-route transit accidents: probability density distribution of the released mass.

For flammable substances it has been possible to draw and quantify also the post-release event trees, distinguishing between liquids and liquefied gases, since the final outcomes of spills involving flammables depend on the storage conditions. In both cases a small number of record has been used for this classification (1844 for liquids; 128 for liquefied gases), since in the major part of the records where a release is reported, no information is given on the final scenario.

In addition for some of these records it has been necessary to make some assumptions in order to assign the outcome reported by the record to a specific final scenario of the event tree; for instance, some records contain the generic information "fire,", without specifying what kind of fire has occurred; though, by reading the information reported in the record, in some cases it has been possible to presuppose a specific type of fire.

The event tree for flammable liquids is reported in fig. 5. It is possible to note that the immediate ignition probability is equal to 0.03, which is also the value of the delayed ignition probability, thus giving a total ignition probability equal to 0.06. Further in the case of delayed ignition of a plume evaporated from a pool, it is more probable that there is an explosion (i.e. a VCE, vapour cloud explosion, with probability 0.84) than a simple flash-fire (probability 0.16).

It's worth noticing that, when performing a transport risk analysis for flammable liquids, it is generally assumed that the final outcome of a delayed ignition is a pool-fire. This assumption implies considering that, also in case of a catastrophic tank truck rupture, the rate of evaporation is so low as to form a very small plume, which does not extend beyond the contour of the pool. Instead from fig. 5 it emerges that the delayed ignition of a plume can produce different and more hazardous scenarios than the pool-fire, and that the delayed ignition probability (equal in percentage value to 0.5%+2.4%=2.9%) is similar to the immediate ignition probability. In addition the fact that the VCE is more probable than the flash-fire is not justifiable; in fact, though the VCEs are favoured, with respect to flash-fires, by the presence of obstacles which obstruct the area occupied by the plume, the poor information reported in the database does not allow to further investigate the influence of this aspect.

In particular the quantified event tree of fig. 5 refers to flammables with a flash-point temperature in the range -18°C–23°C; though the probabilities of the event trees of flammables with higher flash-point (and consequently less hazardous) are similar, so that the event tree of fig. 5 can be adopted for all flammable liquids. This fact is difficult to justify, since one could expect that the total ignition probability becomes smaller while increasing the flash-point temperature.

In the case of liquefied gases it would be necessary to consider two event trees, one for continuous leaks and one for instantaneous releases, since the final outcomes are different in these two cases [3]; unfortunately the fact that no information is given in the records about the spill being continuous or instantaneous has not allowed this analysis and only a total event tree has been quantified, which is reported in fig. 6.

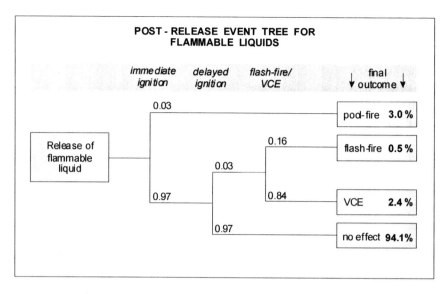

Figure 5:   Post-release event tree for flammable liquids.

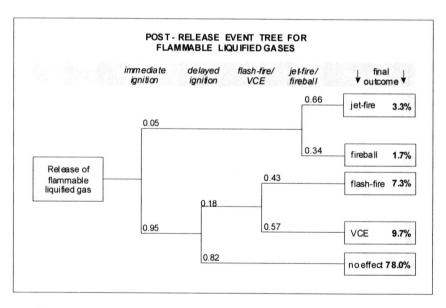

Figure 6:   Post-release event tree for flammable liquefied pressure gases.

The percentage total ignition probability is equal to 22.0%, that is greater than the total ignition probability of the liquefied gases, thus confirming the major flammability of liquefied gases with respect to liquids [1].

The probability of occurrence of the VCE and the flash-fire (equal, respectively, to 0.43 and 0.57) are not dissimilar as in the case of liquids. This fact too is difficult to justify, since the explosion is advantaged, with respect to a simple fire, by the internal turbulence of the cloud, which is surely greater in the case of a plume formed by liquefied gases having at the source a jet, than in the case of a plume developed from an evaporating pool. In addition the fact that the VCE and the flash-fire have similar occurrence probabilities is in contrast with the hypothesis usually assumed in risk analysis, that is to consider negligible the probability of occurrence of the VCE, taking equal to 1, once a delayed ignition occurs, the probability of the flash-fire [6].

4   Conclusions

The main result which has emerged form the analysis of the accident primary causes is the great incidence, for all accident typologies, of human error, which varies between 53.2% and 72.2%.

In the case of spontaneous leaks the error generally occurs while loading the tank truck, and thus is not directly attributable to the shipping company. Though it has to be noticed that the compliance with specific procedures about the handover and acceptance of vehicles, when they are consigned from the sending company to the carrier, in order to verify, for instance, the quantity of chemical which has been loaded (that is the compliance with the filling degree established by regulation), its pressure and temperature conditions, the effective closure of the filling valves and the absence of leaks, could greatly reduce the number of spills which are detected during transport. On the other hand the sudden detection of spills avoids that leaking vehicles began to move, with the hazard that, also because of the strains due to the movement, the leak becomes greater.

A smaller but not negligible percentage of spontaneous leaks is due to the tank failure, that is to the rupture or usury or malfunctioning of the shell of the tank and of the various components of the its equipment, like for instance, the corrosion of the shell, the faulty closure of valves, the wear-out of the gaskets. Since the tank of a truck is not very different form the tanks inside chemical plants, its failure frequency depends on its constructive features, on its time in life and on the period after which the tank is subject to maintenance in order to verify the resistance to pressure and the good functioning of all the servicing equipment. For lowering the occurrence frequency of the spontaneous leaks due to the tank failure, it could be necessary to intensify the tank inspections, in order to detect in advance those components which have to be repaired or substituted.

Indeed the contribution of human error is high for all accident typologies, that is not only for spontaneous leaks, but also for transport accidents; the majority of the traffic accidents is due to the non-compliance with the procedures for driving tank trucks shipping hazardous chemicals. A more rigorous respect of the existing regulations and an increase of the information and training activities for hazmat drivers could drastically lower the occurrence of road accidents.

Looking at the probability data extracted from D.G.A.I.S. for transport risk analysis studies, it is necessary to notice that the information reported by the database is often incomplete and generic, thus not allowing to obtain all data which would be necessary for calculations. To increase the number of the records used for the various classifications, it has been necessary to assign the records with generic information to specific categories trough the adoptions of some hypothesis. In addition sometimes it has not been possible to fully understand and justify the differences in the value of some data.

Though the numeric values which have been extracted are uncertain for the above mentioned reason, it seems better to use these data for transportation risk analysis instead of information derived from plants, since data from factories refer to accidents occurred in a totally different context.

At a conclusion of this research, the necessity has become evident to undertake specific initiatives, at a European level, to develop complete and detailed databases for the collection of information about hazmat transport accidents, also in order to obtain reliable data for transportation risk analysis.

References

[1] Lees, F.P., Loss Prevention in the Process Industries. Butterworth-Heinemann: Oxford, 1996.
[2] Kletz, T., Learning from accidents, Butterworths: London, 1988.
[3] CCPS, Guidelines for Chemical Transportation Risk Analysis. AIChE: New York, 1995.
[4] D.G.A.I.S., Dangerous Goods Accident Information System. Canada, 2000.
[5] http://www.tc.gc.ca/tdg/menu.htm
[6] TNO, Department of Industrial Safety, Guidelines for quantitative risk assessment (Purple Book, CPR18E). Sdu Uitgevers: The Hague, 1999.

Radiological risks in the construction and operation of alpine tunnels

M. De Salve[1], M. Esposito[2], P. Gozzelino[1] & M. E. Parisi[3]
[1]Department of Energetic, Turin Polytechnic, Italy
[2]U-series s.r.l, Italy
[3]LTF SAS

Abstract

The construction of long tunnels for railway transport poses the problem of the evaluation of the environmental impact and the reduction and prevention of risks for the workers and for the population. Important risks are connected with the presence of natural ionizing radiation produced by radionuclides such as Uranium, Thorium, Radon and their daughters. The main pathway of the workers exposure includes both external and internal irradiation risks. LTF (Lyon Turin Ferroviaire SAS) has performed a predictive evaluation of the radiological risk from the analysis of litotypes found during the boreholes. This work is connected with the project for the railway connection between Turin-Lyon and is carried out with the collaboration of Turin Polytechnic, LTF SAS and the U-series laboratory in Bologna. The purpose of this study is the acquisition of the information and data necessary for the evaluation of the radiological risk in the region affected by the works for the railway connection, with particular attention to the areas with workers and/or local people. The results obtained allow us to classify the litotypes for the disposal, to estimate the radioactivity sources, considering the permeation properties, and to carry out an analysis of the correlation between radioactivity concentrations in the litotypes and the water sources influenced by the digging.
Keywords: radiological risk, external irradiation, Uranium, Thorium, Radium and Potassium-40.

1 Introduction

The Italian territory is bordered in the north by a chain of Alps which needs to be crossed in order to reach other European countries. Therefore, the studies regarding the territory (characteristics, structures, naturally occurring elements, and so on) play an important role in planning and designing new communication strategies. The primary objective of the present study is the acquisition of information and data necessary for the forecast of the radiological risk in the region affected by the work for the railway connection. This information on terrestrial radiation and radioactivity is of extreme importance with regards to health.

Considerable attention has been given to possible exposure of humans to ionizing radiation from external and internal environmental sources. Therefore, the determination of radioisotope concentrations in the rocks found during the excavation can supply important data. The main pathway of the workers exposure includes both external and internal irradiation. External irradiation is due to gamma ray emissions from the natural radionuclides present in rocks (Uranium and Thorium families and Potassium-40). Internal irradiation is caused by radon inhalation (^{222}Rn and ^{220}Rn) and by inhalation of radioactive powders produced during the excavation. Radon is a noble gas which is easily emanated from soil and rocks and can be carried, from ground water, up to a great distance. If the excavation intercepts the ground waters, the radon gas is quickly released into the air posing a significant risk for the workers. It is very important to understand the distribution of the natural radioisotopes in order to classify the quality of the air in the tunnel. Finally, it is important to emphasize that the excavation could alter the flow of the groundwater which could modify its chemical composition because it has flown over different rocks with a different speed. In order to evaluate radiological risks it is very important to focus on Radium because, in ground water, it is a subject of both practical and scientific importance. The practical importance stems from the human health risks associated with both the ingestion of Ra [1] and the inhalation of Rn and its daughter products ([1] and [2]). These risks have prompted European and national regulations concerning the maximum total alpha and beta activity concentration in drinking water [3]. The scientific importance derives largely from the potential applications of Ra isotopes in tracing the mechanisms and rates of water-rock interaction and element transport in aquifers ([4] and [5]). The information from such scientific studies can lead to an improved understanding of the factors controlling water quality and can be useful in establishing better strategies for the use and protection of under-ground water resources.

This study was undertaken to estimate the radiation hazard indices in sedimentary and not rocks from the Val Susa Region and to predict the effective dose received by workers from only external irradiation during underground operations. The evaluation of the global effective dose which workers are exposed to needs to consider inhalation of radon and long-lived radioactive dust and it is the scope of this work.

2   Radiological risks

Measurement of natural radioactivity in ground is very important in order to determine the amount of change in the natural background activity which may occur over time, as a result of any radioactive release. Monitoring of any release of radioactivity to the environment is important for environmental protection. Radon (^{222}Rn) is a radioactive noble gas, so an inert gas, (half-life 3.82 d) produced naturally by the decay of radium in soils and rocks. It has been hypothesised that ^{222}Rn transfers from bedrock to groundwater via an alpha recoil process followed by diffusion. ^{222}Rn is normally transferred, according to the normal use of water, from water to air by out-gassing, especially if the water is agitated or heated.

All significant exposure pathways need to be considered and these include the following:

- Direct exposure to external radiation from the rock material;
- Internal dose from inhalation of airborne radionuclides, including radon progeny;
- Internal dose from ingestion of drinking water.

The pathway analysis has four parts: (1) source analysis, (2) environmental transport analysis, (3) dose/exposure analysis, and (4) scenario analysis.

Source analysis addresses the problem of deriving the source terms that determine the rate at which radioactivity is released into the environment. This rate is determined by the geometry of the zone, the concentrations of the radionuclides present, the ingrowths and decay rates of the radionuclides, and the removal rate by erosion and leaching.

Environmental transport analysis addresses the problems of identifying environmental pathways by which radionuclides can migrate from the source to a human exposure location and determining the migration rate along these pathways. The gamma-ray radiation hazards which are due to the specified radionuclides U, Ra, Th and K were assessed by many different indices, often embedded in national regulations to prevent the use of high radioactive building materials. Some studies about the indices have been done by some authors [6], [7] and [8]. The final index has been suggested to the European Commission [7] for use in future directives. The index is described as follows:

$$I=\frac{C_{Ra}}{300}+\frac{C_{Th}}{200}+\frac{C_{K}}{3000} \tag{1}$$

where C_{Ra}, C_{Th}, C_{K} are, respectively, in Radium, Thorium and Potassium activity concentrations in Bq/kg, and the coefficients are the concentrations of the same isotopes, in Bq/kg, which provide a dose like 1 mSv/y. When the activity index is less than 1 in all materials used for a standard room (dimensions of 5x4x2.7 m, with homogeneous wall 20 centimetres thick, without opening) it is unlikely that the people in this room will receive an exposure in excess of 1 mSv/y. Moreover, when the activity index is less than 0.5, the material can be used without any restriction to the quantity of the final use of the building. Nevertheless this activity index is not intended for dose evaluation, but only for the safe use of a building material. When applied to the walls of underground cavities, the activity index is an effective way to evaluate the radiological risk for workers. The evaluation of the index I for the mucking during the excavation of tunnels gives a criterium for disposal or final use. The total outdoor air absorbed dose rate, D (nGy/h) due to the mean activity concentrations of ^{238}U, ^{232}Th and ^{40}K (Bq/kg) in soils and rocks, is calculated using the formula of Beck et al. [10] and UNSCEAR [11]:

$$D = 0.427 \, A_U + 0.622 \, A_{Th} + 0.0432 \, A_K \qquad (2)$$

Beck et al. derived this equation for calculating the absorbed dose rate in air at a height of 1.0m above the ground from measured radionuclide concentrations in environmental materials.

The value of the quotient of effective dose equivalent rate to absorbed dose rate in air is 1 for photons [12]. This value applied equally to males and females and to indoor and outdoor environments.

In a working environment like a tunnel the occupancy factor is 1 for 2000 hours/year, the annual effective dose equivalent from terrestrial gamma-radiation is found to be:

$$D_a = 2000(h/y)*D \, (nGy/h)*1 \, (Sv/Gy) \qquad (3)$$

3   Materials and methods

The underground of Val Susa region has been investigated till 915 m of depth by drilling. Thirty boreholes have been done to represent the entire Val Susa along the proposed tunnel alignment. All the carrots found (about 7000 m in depth) have been classified in 12 main litotype groups cited in table 1.

Table 1:   Litotype groups found in Val Susa.

Litotype groups	length [m]	%
Calcareous schist	2049.4	29.17
Gneiss	1126.45	16.03
Mica schist	801.90	11.41
Detrital deposit	585.5	8.33
Schist	384.00	5.46
Marble	440.80	6.27
Serpentine	131.10	1.87
Prasinite	78.55	1.12
Quartzite	77.25	1.10
Dolomite	88.20	1.25
Mylonite	12.80	0.18
Limestone	11.70	0.17

The object of the study is the choice of a representative number of samples to characterize, at best, the natural radioactivity present in the rocks found in the area. Fifty samples belonging to litotypes mentioned in table 1 (three for every main group and one for every secondary) have been chosen and measured by gamma-ray spectroscopic analysis. The samples are collected in their natural form and ground to fine powder, dried and sealed in cylindrical polyethylene containers of 5.5 cm diameter and 11 mm height. The spectrometer consists of 3 HPGe p-type (relative efficiency 10%, 20% and 30%) coupled with 16384 multicanale. The ^{238}U activity was measured from the ^{234}Th gamma ray at 63.4 KeV, the ^{226}Ra activities were estimated from ^{214}Pb (295.2, 351.9 keV) and ^{214}Bi (609.3, 1120.3 keV). The gamma-ray energies of ^{212}Pb (238.6 keV), ^{228}Ac (338.4, 911 keV) and ^{208}Tl (583.2 keV) were used to measure the concentration of 232Th, while the ^{40}K activity was determined from the 1460.7 keV emission. Measurements were conducted following Italian standards UNI 10797 [13].

4   Results and discussion

Table 2 shows the activities in Bq/kg obtained from the gamma-ray spectroscopic analysis and estimated doses D and D_a.

Results indicate that the area under investigation has a normal level of natural background. Also, ^{40}K shows high concentration but still within the natural background level values. These values are considered to be at a typical level for the ground samples from this area. Figure 1 shows the values found for the activity radiological index.

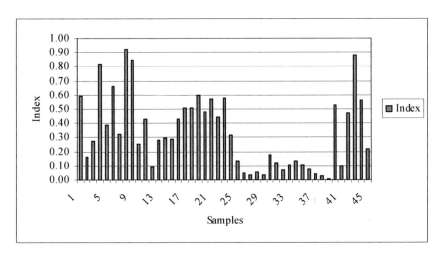

Figure 1:   Activity radiological index.

In figure 1, the numbers represent the samples shown in table 2 where the reference litotype and activity are reported.

All the samples have a radioactivity index less than 1. The starting safety conditions of excavation activities should be good for the workers. The annual effective dose equivalent calculated reaches 0,2 mSv/y, < 1 mSv/y Italian normative limit [12] for the workers who are not at risk, but it is important if we consider that the external irradiation is negligible compared with the internal irradiation caused by radon and radioactive powders inhalation.

Therefore, the workers should be exposed to a dose more than 1 mSv/y with non-sufficient mechanical ventilation and lowering powder concentration. Further studies on Radon emanation from rocks and groundwater in the area concerned with the tunnel, can help to calculate the radiological risks during the excavation activities.

Table 2: Results obtained from gamma-ray spectroscopic analysis and using the eqns. (2) and (3).

N°	Litotype	U-238 [Bq/kg]	Ra-226 [Bq/kg]	Th-232 [Bq/kg]	K-40 [Bq/kg]	D [nGy/h]	D_a [mSv/y]
1		40 ± 30	19 ± 4	34 ± 5	1080 ± 130	84.88	0.170
2		15 ± 6	16.2 ± 1.5	7.0 ± 1.7	210 ± 20	19.83	0.040
3		20 ± 7	21 ± 4	12.9 ± 0.8	430 ± 40	35.14	0.070
4		34 ± 12	55 ± 7	85 ± 6	630 ± 50	94.60	0.189
5	Gneiss	25 ± 8	23 ± 3	26 ± 3	550 ± 50	50.61	0.101
6		60 ± 30	35 ± 4	50 ± 3	890 ± 110	95.17	0.190
7		33 ± 17	17 ± 2	28 ± 2	390 ± 50	48.36	0.097
8		70 ± 40	58 ± 4	76 ± 6	1040 ± 120	122.09	0.244
9		50 ± 8	50 ± 8	50 ± 2	1280 ± 150	107.75	0.215
10		15 ± 6	18 ± 2	20 ± 3	280 ± 30	40.12	0.080
11		26 ± 4	26 ± 4	29 ± 6	600 ± 70	37.59	0.075
12	detrital deposit	6.8 ± 1.7	6.8 ± 1.7	4.4 ± 0.7	133 ± 19	30.94	0.062
13		31 ± 13	20 ± 5	21 ± 2	320 ± 40	55.06	0.110
14		20 ± 4	20 ± 4	22 ± 2	360 ± 40	11.39	0.023
15		13 ± 6	13 ± 6	12 ± 3	560 ± 70	37.21	0.074
16		30 ± 5	30 ± 5	31 ± 3	520 ± 70	54.56	0.109
17		26 ± 5	26 ± 5	30 ± 5	820 ± 100	65.19	0.130
18		23 ± 8	29 ± 4	34 ± 2	720 ± 60	62.07	0.124
19		31 ± 6	31 ± 6	34 ± 6	980 ± 120	76.72	0.153
20	Mica schist	30 ± 9	27.7 ± 0.9	34 ± 2	660 ± 50	62.47	0.125
21		34 ± 10	35 ± 4	40 ± 2	760 ± 60	72.23	0.144
22		17 ± 7	22 ± 4	27 ± 2	710 ± 60	54.73	0.109
23		29 ± 4	29 ± 4	36 ± 2	910 ± 110	74.09	0.148
24		32 ± 9	33 ± 3	28.8 ± 0.9	188 ± 18	39.70	0.079
25		9 ± 5	16.4 ± 1.6	5 ± 2	168 ± 16	14.21	0.028
26		9 ± 4	11 ± 2	< 1,4	< 9	5.10	0.010
27	Marble	< 4	5.4 ± 0.9	< 1,4	38 ± 6	2.51	0.005
28		12 ± 5	14 ± 3	1.1 ± 0.2	< 9	6.20	0.012
29		5 ± 2	6.7 ± 1.2	1.1 ± 0.4	24 ± 4	3.86	0.008
30		< 50	48 ± 8	2.4 ± 0.7	13 ± 4	2.05	0.004
31		< 7	3.6 ± 1.3	1.6 ± 0.4	300 ± 20	13.96	0.028
32	Prasinite	< 7	5 ± 2	3 ± 2	117 ± 13	6.92	0.014
33		< 17	< 7	2.4 ± 0.7	210 ± 30	10.56	0.021
34		< 40	10 ± 4	9 ± 2	160 ± 20	12.51	0.025
35	Calcareous shist	25 ± 13	8.0 ± 1.7	4 ± 3	170 ± 20	20.51	0.041
36		6 ± 3	8.4 ± 1.9	8.72 ± 0.14	26 ± 4	9.11	0.018
37		< 30	< 5	< 4	10 ± 5	2.92	0.006
38	Serpentinite	n.r.	< 3	< 3	n.r.	1.87	0.004
39		n.r.	< 2	< 0,6	n.r.	0.37	0.001
40		50 ± 30	31 ± 7	34.0 ± 1.5	760 ± 90	75.33	0.151
41	Chloritic schist	< 30	7.1 ± 1.3	10.8 ± 1.2	61 ± 11	9.35	0.019
42		40 ± 19	23.0 ± 2.0	26.8 ± 1.3	790 ± 90	67.88	0.136
43	Quartzite	90 ± 50	87 ± 13	87 ± 12	460 ± 60	112.42	0.225
44		21 ± 6	23.4 ± 1.3	33 ± 6	970 ± 80	71.40	0.143
45	Quartz	19 ± 7	21 ± 5	28.0 ± 1.5	33 ± 8	26.95	0.054

This result shows no problem about the radiological risk in the disposal or the final use of the mucking for the known litotype.

Acknowledgements

This work was supported from LTF sas in the framework of collaboration of department of Geo-resources and land, Turin Polytechnic (Prof. M. Patrucco).

References

[1]   National Academic of Science (NAS), *Health Risks of Radon and Other Internally Deposited Alpha Emitters*. National Academy Press, Washington, DC, 1988.

[2]   NAS/NRC, Health Effects of Exposure to Radon. National Academy Press, Washington, DC, 1998.

[3]   DLgs n° 31 del 2/2/2001.

[4]   Dickson, B.L., *Radium in ground water. In: The Environmental Behavior of Radium*, vol. 1 (Chapter. 4-2) International Atomic Energy Agency (IAEA), Vienna, pp. 335±372, 1990.

[5]   Ivanovich, M. & Harmon, R.S., *Uranium-Series Disequilibrium: Applications to Earth, Marine, and Environmental Sciences*, 2nd ed. Clarendon Press, pp. 631±668, 1982.

[6]   Abbady, A.G.E., Estimation of radiation hazard indices from sedimentary rocks in Upper Egypt, *Applied Radiation and Isotopes*, **60**, 111-114, 2004.

[7]   Sroora, A., El-Bahia, S.M., Ahmedb, F. & Abdel-Haleemc, A.S., Natural radioactivity and radon exhalation rate of soil in southern Egypt, *Applied Radiation and Isotopes*, **55**, 873-879, 2001.

[8]   Bossew, P., The radon emanation power of building materials, soils and rocks, *Applied Radiation and Isotopes*, **59**, 389-392, 2003.

[9]   Directorate-General Environment, Nuclear Safety and Civil Protection, European Commission, Radiological Protection Principles concerning the Natural Radioactivity of Building Materials, Radiation protection 112, 1999.

[10]   Beck, H.L., Decompo, J. & Golgogak, J., In-situ Ge(Li) and Na(Tl) gamma ray spectrometry. Health and Safety Laboratory AEC (HASL), Report 258, New York, 1972.

[11]   United Nations Scientific Committee on the Effects of Atomic Radiation Ionizing Radiation (UNSCEAR): Sources, Effects and Risks of Ionizing Radiation. United Nations, New York, Annex A, B, 1988.

[12]   DLgs n° 230 del 17/03/1995 modified by DLgs n°241 del 26/05/2000.

[13]   UNI 10797, Natural radionuclides in the building materials– Determination with gamma spectrometry - high resolution, 1999.

Section 2
Air pollution

Local and global impact considerations on the turbo gas combined cycle

P. Baggio[1], A. Cemin[1], D. Cocarta[1,2], A. Gasparella[3]
& M. Ragazzi[1]
[1]*University of Trento, Italy*
[2]*Technical University of Bucharest, Romania*
[3]*University of Padua, Italy*

Abstract

Studies on the impact on public health from macro and micro pollutants released from significant punctual sources have shown a remarkable development during the last years. These depend on the possibility of associating information on each pollutant to multiple pathways of exposition of the population present in the area of interest. In the field of energy generation the implementation of turbo-gas plants has not always have found a favourable welcome from the local population, nevertheless they have shown improvements compared to conventional systems. The present work wants to analyse in details some aspects related to the most recent debates on this topic, in particular pointing out the role of the introduction of a selective catalytic reduction for the removal of NOx from the off-gas of the turbo gas plants. Aspects related to ammonia release, the secondary particulate formation and the heavy metal release (in particular Vanadium) are dealt with, both in terms of global balance and in terms of local balance. At a local scale, the present work is faced with the role of the various methods of pollutant release (off-gas velocity, temperature, stack height).
Keywords: environmental impact, gas turbine, incineration, selective catalytic reduction.

1 Introduction

Production in the electric energy sector is based more and more on the realization of the new turbo gas combined cycle or the conversion of existing plants to this technology. Thanks to the contained costs of management, elevated flexibility and continuity of exercise, the turbo gas combined cycle guarantees high-performance production and lower polluting emissions in comparison to coal plants and combustible oil plants.

Concerning this last aspect some scientific works have recently underlined that, also using a less polluting fuel, these kinds of plants can constitute a source of impact for the environment though this does call for some cognitive closer examinations.

The purpose of the present work is to analyze some aspects of these plants from the point of view of the impact on the environment and on the health of the population in order to assess technological interventions of mitigation.

2 The turbo gas combined cycle plants

For the thermal power plants adopting the turbo gas combined cycle (CCGT) natural gas is used as fuel.

Currently this technology constitutes a valid solution for the conversion of old plants burning coal or combustible oil.

In the case of the turbo gas combined cycle plants the natural gas is mixed with compressed air in the combustion chamber and the off-gas produced from the combustion at high pressure and temperature are expanded in a gas turbine (turbo gas) that, rotating, operates an alternator for the generation of electric energy.

The products of the combustion at elevated temperature exiting the gas turbine are subsequently sent to a steam generator. The off-gases cooled by the process of thermal exchange go to the stack while the water that crosses the reheating system of the steam generator is vaporized. The steam is used for operating a steam turbine which is connected to an alternator. The steam at low pressure exits the turbine and is condensed in a special reheating system (condenser). The cycle is closed with a pump which sends the condensed water to the steam generator.

Currently this kind of plant is receiving remarkable interest, both in Europe and in non-European countries, for the high production efficiency that can be more than 55% and the low management costs. Moreover, partial heat released from the condenser can be used for applications of district heating (cogeneration). In conclusion, this approach results in one of the less pollutant systems among those that use fossil fuels for the generation of electric energy.

3 NO$_x$ emissions from a CCGT power plant

On a global basis, the relevance of the emissions of a power plant with respect to other emission sources of a specific region can be considered. Some data are reported for the CCGT power plant of Sermide (Mantova), in the North of Italy.

The plant is composed of two CCGT lines, respectively for 760 MW and 380 MW of electric power. The plant is allowed to work up to 8760 hours per year. Considering a technical availability of around 7500 hours the energy production is 8550 GWh$_e$ per year while the natural gas consumption ranges from 5.1–5.2 million Sm^3. The incidence of the plant in terms of NO$_x$ emission at the authorised limit concentration (50 mg/Nm^3) is around 2317 t per year. This amount is compared in Figure 1 with the NO$_x$ emissions from other sources in the Lombardia Region, while in Figure 2 in the Mantova Province. The available data were reported for the year 2001 in the INEMAIR database [7]. The 2003 electricity final consumptions were 62570 GWh$_e$ and 3620 GWh$_e$ for the considered Region and Province respectively [5].

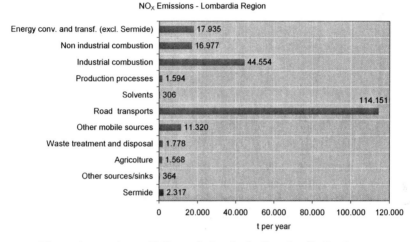

Figure 1: Annual NO$_x$ emission in the Lombardia Region.

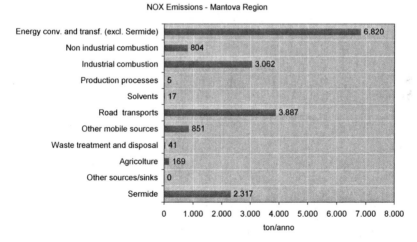

Figure 2: Annual NO$_x$ emission in the Mantova Province.

As can be seen, the considered plant emissions are very much lower than the regional ones from the road transport sector or from the industrial combustion. The NO$_x$ emissions from the energy conversion sector (excluded Sermide plant), which included in 2001 power plants for an electric power of 6805 MW besides to district heating plants, refineries, etc., were 17935 t.

The energy conversion sector assumes a significant relevance on a provincial scale.

As a general consideration, the NO_x emission from a medium to large size CCGT contributes up to a few percent of units to the total emissions on a regional basis while the relevance on a provincial basis is comparable to the emissions of a single sector of industry or road transport.

4 The CCGT plants atmospheric emissions and health effects

The main pollutants from the turbo gas plants belong to the macro pollutants category. Those that are more interesting from the point of view of the health risk and for the emission quantities into the atmosphere are the carbon monoxide and the nitrogen oxides. Ammonia emission appears if the plant is equipped with a system of selective catalytic reduction (SCR) for the nitrogen oxide removal. The existence of the micro pollutants in the atmospheric emissions can be both of organic nature (for instance, polycyclic aromatic hydrocarbons) and of inorganic nature (heavy metals). The quoted micro pollutants, besides having a high level of toxicity, generally have a long lifetime (in the order of years) and once introduced into the environment their dangerousness does not diminish with time. So, it is therefore important to verify that the emissions allow one to respect the most stringent targets of environmental quality.

Recently, because of the more and more frequent exceeding of the reference levels foreseen by the standards of air quality for the particulate matter in urban areas, attention to the problem of the secondary particulate has grown. This is not constituted of fine particles emitted directly from the plant but of particulate matter formed in the atmosphere following photo chemical reactions beginning from precursors, typically nitrogen oxides, sulphur oxides and ammonia. One of the remarks of the opponents of the SCR systems is the presence of ammonia releases and the consequent formation of secondary particulate. As we will see, the problem must be faced with the development of a cost-benefits balance. A second remark concerns the presence of Vanadium emissions that would be released by the catalyst of the SCR systems. This aspect should also be treated with a more correct approach, that keeps in mind the released quantities and the multiple pathways impact, with the aim of assessing which is the concentration limit to be authorized (if it is necessary to state it).

Presented below is a comparative example among an incineration plant for municipal solid waste (MSWI) and a CCGT plant both of great dimensions. The data used for the comparative balances are certified by the environment protection agency. The two plants are supposed to release the pollutants through stacks of the same height and temperatures. As a first approximation, in this paper the hypothesis that the dilution of the pollutants in the atmosphere has the same characteristics is made. The incineration plant for MSW has a net generation of 320 GWh_{el}/y while the CCGT can supply 8550 GWh_{el}/y. It can be noted the different role of the two plants in terms of generators of energy.

In Table 1 the amounts of emitted macro pollutants are presented comparatively. As can be noticed, the quantity of NO_x emitted by the thermo power plant is one order of magnitude higher than the amount emitted by the waste incineration plant. So, the importance of locating the plants in climatologically favorable areas and of assessing the environmental pressure in order to avoid exceeding the daily limit of NO_x in ambient air is clear (in fact NO_x is already a potential problem for incineration plants located in polluted areas and with a low dilution level).

Table 1 also reports a comparison between the two plants in terms of emitted heavy metals. Concerning the used data for the CCGT plant sector, it must be specified that in other plants higher values for Vanadium (also one order of magnitude) and lower values for Nickel (also one order of magnitude) were measured. As can be observed, for some cases the differences between the two plants are of some orders of magnitude.

In consideration of the heavy metals cancer potency emitted by the MSW incinerator the risk is driven by Cd. The other heavy metals contribute to the risk, but their dangerousness is of one or more orders of magnitude lower.

Table 1:   Comparison between pollutants.

		MSWI	CCGT	
macro pollutants	NO_x	206.8	1966.5	t/y
	CO	48	128.3	t/y
	TOC	1.4	3.7	t/y
heavy metals	V	0.8	183.8	kg/y
	Cd	0.3	4.3	kg/y
	Tl	0.3	4.3	kg/y
	Cr	0.8	17.1	kg/y
	Ni	2.8	2659.1	kg/y

In fact, the pollutants of interest can be expressed as equivalent Cd through the ratio between their cancers potencies. For example, with reference to the risk by inhalation, Nickel is 16 times less dangerous than Cadmium and even if the emitted amount is around 9 times higher, the order of magnitude of the risk does not change.

In the present comparison the CCGT plant is assumed to have a similar release modality, from which the following considerations are reached. The most recent studies of health risk applied to MSW incineration underline that for operational values, the maximum individual risk from Cd results about 10^{-8}. From that it is deduced that for the CCGT plants the carcinogenic risk is driven by Nickel and it can be attended of about 10^{-6}. In fact, it one order of magnitude is lost because of the higher amounts (4.3 against 0.3 kg/y of Cd); a factor 16 is gained for the dangerousness of Nickel in comparison to Cadmium, but a factor around 900 is lost because of the different amounts. In consideration of the adopted approximation it is clear that there is a need for closer examination in order to verify the respect of the limit of 10^{-6} given by the World Health Organization.

Concerning BaP (Benzo(a)pyren), such a pollutant will soon be considered a tracer of the presence of other carcinogenic PAH. In fact, according to a recent Directive (2004/107/CE), an ambient air value of 1 ng/Nm^3 will be fixed. In the case of this paper, the concentration in the flue gas resulting from the CCGT is equal to 1µg/Nm^3. In order to comply with the quoted Directive, the atmospheric dilution of the stack flue gas must guarantee a dilution higher than 1000 times. A modeling verification is necessary.

The CCGT quality as an energy generator is underlined if the pollutants emission factors are expressed in comparison with the generated kWh (Table 2). However, Vanadium and Nickel result in counter tendency.

The turbo gas plant contribution to the secondary particulate (PM$_{2.5}$) formation is an aspect that requires additional studies. In recent months the first data of qualitative characterization of the PM$_{10}$ have been issued. Such data will be useful to clarify which is the thermo power plant role to this concern. Concerning the primary particulate, there is a lack of unitary vision. Studies showing significant PM releases [1, 2] have been followed from studies [6] demonstrating an equivalence among input and output concentrations.

Table 2:   Comparison between the emission factors.

		mg/kWh MSWI	mg/kWh CCGT
macro pollutants	NO$_X$	646.25	230
	CO	150	15
	TOC	4.375	0.435
heavy metals	V	2.625	21.5
	Cd	0.875	0.5
	Tl	0.875	0.5
	Cr	2.625	2
	Ni	8.75	311

5   The SCR issue

The selective catalytic reduction is the best available technology for the reduction of NO$_x$. It involves the ammonia injection in the combustion products before a catalytic bed.

The process catalysts can be constituted by titanium oxide (carrier material), vanadium oxides and tungsten (active elements). The SCR systems have a wide diffusion in environmentally aware regions like California, but they are still not very diffused in Europe. One of the reasons for opposition of this system is the presence of an ammonia slip that can be responsible of the formation of secondary particulate.

The optimal operating temperature depends on the type of catalyst. The range of operation is 180–260 °C for Platinum and 300–455°C for Vanadium. This range of temperature must be respected for two main reasons: 1) if the temperature goes down under the first range considered, it also lowers the efficiency of the reaction and in this way it also increases the ammonia release from the stack; 2) if the temperature increases too much the catalyst looses its proprieties.

The convenience of the SCR is demonstrable from the following considerations: starting from a quantity of 50 mg/Nm^3 of NO$_x$, the addition of NH$_3$ can decrease the concentration to 5 mg/Nm^3 of NO$_x$ with a release of 5 mg/Nm^3 of NH$_3$. The conversion coefficients in secondary particulate vary, but the available information on it allows one to state that, even taking into account the contribution of NH$_3$ to the secondary particulate, the advantages of SCR are clear. Considering the ratio of dangerousness of the considered pollutants equal to 6.8 (value obtained as the ratio between the exposure levels for Ammonia and NO$_x$ according to EPA: 3200 µg/m^3 and respectively 470 µg/m^3 - Inhalation Reference Exposure Level), it is evident that the substitution of NH$_3$ with NO$_x$ gives a lower environmental toxicity.

In order to assess the convenience, the costs of the flue gas cleaning system of the nitrogen oxides must be compared with the external costs of the pollutants (or to the environmental, social and economic costs). This type of approach is used with the target of individualizing the environmental sustainability of the use of a SCR system. The environmental costs (EC) can be considered from the European Commission ExternE method [3] (expressed in Euro/t of NO$_x$ emitted into the atmosphere), comparing them with the costs (CT) for the nitrogen oxides removal system: the resulting EC/CT ratio is around 1.1. Therefore the installation of a SCR system appears justified.

Another reason for concern is the possible release of Vanadium as an element of the catalyst: as it has been seen that in reality Vanadium is already present in trace amounts in natural gas.

6   Conclusions

The CCGT plants fed by natural gas undoubtedly result in a "clean" way of energy production. This does not cancel the importance of analysing some aspects with reference to their global and local impact. In particular, it is necessary to verify the carcinogenic risk from heavy metals emissions, (already present in natural gas), the contribution to the environmental background with reference to the new Directive 2004/107/CE (for Cd, Ni, BaP) and the role in the secondary particulate balance. Finally the opposition to the installation of SCR for the removal of the nitrogen oxides is not acceptable, as the obtainable benefits overcome the disadvantages.

References

[1]   N. Armaroli, C. Po: Emissioni da centrali termoelettriche a gas naturale. La letteratura corrente e l'esperienza statunitense. La chimica e l'Industria – Chimica e….Ambiente, May 2003.

[2]   N. Armaroli, C. Po: Centrali termoelettriche a gas naturale Produzione di articolato primario e secondario. La chimica e l'Industria – Chimica e....Ambiente, November 2003.

[3]   European Commission, in "Research and Development ExternE Externalities of Energy - Vol X: National Implementation"1999.

[4]   Eurosea http://www.eurosea.net/turbogas/ciclo.htm.

[5]   GRTN, National balance of electric energy 2003 http://www.grtn.it.

[6]   Macchi E.: Impatto ambientale dei cicli combinati alimentati a gas naturale, con particolare riferimento alle emissioni di polveri sottili (environmental impact of CCGT, with particular reference to PM emissions). Technical University of Milan. November 2004 – Italy.

[7]   Regione Lombardia: Piano di Risanamento della Qualità dell'Aria - INEMAR (INventario EMissioni ARia), data 2001 updated to 2003 – Italy.

Assessing vulnerability of low-income communities to indoor air pollution in South Africa: towards the development of a vulnerability index

M. Binedell
Division of Water, Environment and Forestry Technology,
CSIR, South Africa

Abstract

Health Risk Assessment (HRA) is a valuable tool for determining the potential human health risk associated with environmental exposures to hazards. HRAs are, however, limited in that they do not allow an assessment of other factors which may render people more vulnerable. Low-income (and often marginalised) communities are subjected to multiple environmental exposures and often lack the coping mechanisms that enable them to resist, cope with and manage their exposure to hazards. This paper presents the components of a proposed vulnerability index that could be used to assess levels of vulnerability of low-income communities that are exposed to indoor air pollution. A number of social, biophysical and service-related factors which are particularly relevant to the South African context have been considered and are discussed further.
Keywords: vulnerability, household risk factors, indoor air pollution.

1 Introduction

Traditional health risk assessments aim to determine the probability and magnitude of risks to human health from exposure to a particular hazard. These assessments consider some of the characteristics of an exposed population, such as age and length of exposure, and include these into the assessment of risks. However, there are a number of other physical, social, economic and built environment factors which may influence the magnitude of adverse health effects (particularly for low-income households) that are not accounted for in traditional risk assessments.

The purpose of this study was to develop an index for assessing vulnerability of low-income households to indoor air pollution. The index was designed to incorporate vulnerability risk factors which not only heighten one's exposure to indoor air pollutants but also contribute to the household's ability to cope with indoor air pollution and the effects thereof. This paper discusses the components of the vulnerability index and explains their relevance to the South African context.

2 Background

The study area of Cato Crest is an informal settlement located a few kilometres from the central business district of the city of Durban, located on the eastern seaboard of South Africa. It is one of the most densely populated informal settlements in Durban and consists of an informal network of dirt roads and pathways amongst a number of self-constructed dwellings. Service provision is lacking and houses are poorly constructed. Most households share pit latrines and water pipes [1]. Overcrowding, a high crime rate, unemployment and a high prevalence of HIV/AIDS are some of the key problems facing this community. In addition, the lack of electricity in the area necessitates the use of kerosene (paraffin) which has been linked to a number of health effects in exposed individuals [2]. A health risk assessment conducted in the community demonstrated high risks to human health from kerosene combustion, used mainly for cooking purposes [3].

3 Vulnerability and risk

Wisner [4] (in his study of Tokyo's urban poor) called for the inclusion of social variables when assessing vulnerability of urban groups. He states: "socio-economic status, occupation and nationality have a marked effect on access to information and services as well as on resources available to people for self-protection and recovery. Certain status, occupation and nationality groups suffer increased vulnerability because their capacity to cope and to recover has been diminished" [4, p27]. He further states that there is evidence to show that people with certain social characteristics are more likely than others to be affected by lack of resources and the lack of access to these resources.

Within the field of disaster management, much has been done to develop, test and validate tools, methodologies and other instruments for factoring issues related to social equity (including gender analysis) into risk management at the local level [5, 6]. According to the International Strategy for Disaster Reduction (ISDR) some phases in risk assessment are weak and therefore people's strengths and abilities, their susceptibilities, socio-economic status and gender should be considered [6]. They suggest that people's risk perceptions and the socio-economic and environmental context within which they live should be incorporated, and are essential in the identification of risk scenarios [6].

In the ISDR disaster management assessment, two elements are essential in the formulation of risk: the probability of occurrence for a given threat – the HAZARD; and the degree of susceptibility of the element (community) exposed to that source – VULNERABILITY. Coupled with this is the growing interest in the positive capacities of people to cope, withstand and recover from the impact of a hazard.

The development of comprehensive risk assessments thus far focuses on conventional hazardous phenomena such as windstorms, earthquakes and floods; but the approach can also be applied to assess the risk and vulnerability to human-induced environmental hazards of indoor air pollution.

It is therefore imperative that risk assessments should incorporate dimensions of physical, social, economic and ecological vulnerability. Although the complexity of the environmental change process makes assessing and measuring human vulnerability highly speculative [7], an attempt to 'factor in' vulnerability into the risk assessment equation provides an assessment which may be more socially acceptable. The inclusion of vulnerability and capacity assessment in risk assessments is a move forward to better understanding the full risk to human health and well-being.

4 A vulnerability index for indoor air pollution

4.1 Methodology

The methodology used to derive variables of vulnerability in this study was systematic and consisted of a series of three filters. They were: A literature survey of the concepts of urban poverty and vulnerability; primary vulnerability data collected from households in Cato Crest; and the development of vulnerability indicators. The variables (or indicators) are specifically relevant to the South African context as well as to an informal settlement community who is exposed to an environmental factor such as indoor air pollution [8].

4.2 Components of the vulnerability index

The indicators and measures which were derived through the above approach were grouped within six broad themes. These themes, indicators and measures are shown in Table 1.

The section which follows provides a description of each of the themes and indicators which form part of the vulnerability index. It should be noted that this index has been specifically developed for the South African context and more specifically for the assessment of vulnerability of low-income, informal communities to indoor air pollution. Scoring and weighting of each variable in the index and the possible aggregation of variables into a single vulnerability score, is the subject of ongoing research. It is therefore not discussed further in this paper.

Table 1:   Indicators and measures as components of a vulnerability index [8].

	THEME	INDICATOR	MEASURES (Environmental, social & economic)
1	Demographics	Gender	Ratio of males to females per household Gender of household head Percentage of males older than 18yrs
		Age	Age of household head Average age of household
2	Livelihoods	Unemployment rate	Percentage unemployed of employable age (>18yrs)
		Income distribution and dependency	Monthly household income Per capita income Percentage of household contributing to household income
		Dependency on care	Ratio of adults to dependents (Ratio of children >15yrs:<15yrs) Number children under 15yrs who do not go to school
		Levels of education	Percentage of household achieving grade 10 (of potential age)
3	Physical exposures	Overcrowding	Number of people per square metre Number people per household
		Air pollution	Percentage of household sleeping in cooking area Percentage windows which open
		Waste	Frequency of removal Cost of service
4	Externalities	Building materials	Presence of damp Type of materials
5	Services	Access to water supply	Number litres accessed per day Proximity to source Reliability Cost of service
		Quality of water	Potability
		Sanitation services	Type of toilet Private or shared facilities Odour problems Cost of service
6	General health	Food and nutrition	Percentage of nutritional problems recorded at clinic
		Other diseases	Number of household members with pre-existing respiratory problems Prevalence of HIV/AIDS in the community/area Prevalence of diarrhoeal diseases in the community Prevalence of Tuberculosis in the community/area

5   Vulnerability themes and indicators

5.1   Demographics

Demographic indicators of **gender** and **age** can reflect vulnerability in low-income households as these variables influence a household's access to resources and health care. Social exclusion and vulnerability in South Africa follow gender and racial lines, with certain groups of the population (such as rural people, women and the youth) more vulnerable to social exclusion than others [9].

Rakodi *et al* [10, p156] found that "women household heads were thought to be vulnerable because they have had poorer access to education and have as a result lower literacy rates. They own limited productive assets, especially land and have limited access to credit than men. They tend to be ignorant of their rights and thus exploited and discriminated against in economic activities".

Rakodi *et al* [10] goes on to state that young people in low income groups have been described as "helpless, frustrated and dangerous" due to the fact that they lack practical training necessary to secure employment. The age profile of households provides a measure of the potential for the household to access employment and therefore sufficient income to sustain their livelihoods. Households with many young children are more dependent on others for care and may limit the caregiver from involvement in economic activities which would generate income.

The presence of adult males in the household may contribute to a sense of safety. Conversely, the absence of males, especially in areas where there is civil unrest or violence, may contribute to a household's insecurity. This may affect their sense of well-being and contribute to their anxiety and mental stress. In addition, it could worsen indoor air pollution because people keep their windows closed, thereby limiting ventilation.

Gender and age are visible issues in Cato Crest, with 42% of the surveyed households run by female heads. Female-headed households also contained other siblings and a number of dependent children, whilst some male headed households had fewer dependents and higher household income. In Cato Crest the mean age of households is 28 years of age with 15% of households run by pensioners (people over 60 years of age). Another important gender-related issue is the high prevalence of HIV/AIDS amongst females aged 15 to 35 years, indicating that females in this age group are more vulnerable to infection [11].

5.2   Livelihoods

Unemployment, income distribution, dependency on care and education are the four indicators used in this study to determine livelihood status of households. According to the literature [10, 12, 13, 14], the **rate of unemployment** is an important determinant of urban poverty and vulnerability. Unemployment and lack of income can also prevent a household from accessing the required food and nutrition for maintaining a healthy body and can contribute to the more rapid progression from HIV infection to AIDS [15].

Income distribution and economic dependency are regarded as the highest measures of poverty. The extent of income poverty in Cato Crest is high, with only half the number of households maintaining a per-capita income above the poverty line [1]. Unemployment and the resulting lack of income can forcibly increase levels of exposure to pollutants through the use of cheaper and 'dirtier' fuels. Increased exposure can result from the use of non-electrified energy sources such as kerosene, as well as through extended exposure times in the home as opposed to the work environment where indoor air pollution may not be as great a hazard.

The issue around **dependency on care** in this study arose through the identification of a number of young children in the household who were not at school. While questions on child care were not asked in this study, it is expected that these children were dependent on another family member or caregiver to care for them. This creates a large burden on the caregiver who could be otherwise free to pursue economic activities.

According to the World Health Organization [16], lack of **education** limits the ability of the poor to identify and take appropriate action to improve their health and secure their basic needs. Education at the household level gives an indication of the potential for individuals to enter the formal employment sector based on a recognised level of education.

5.3 Physical exposures

Overcrowding, air pollution and waste disposal are included as indicators of vulnerability related to physical exposure. **Overcrowding** is responsible for unsanitary conditions and can allow for the prolific spread of disease. Both poor ventilation and inadequate sized housing aids the transmission of diseases such as tuberculosis, influenza and meningitis. Crowding has been noted as a direct health factor in a number of health studies [17]. Risks of household accidents may increase and the burden to safeguard children from fires and stoves becomes greater. Overcrowding has also been recognised as having an influence on quality of life [2].

Crowding was one of the first issues to be identified in the household survey in Cato Crest. Eighteen percent of households consisted of more than 5 members per house, with the average household size being 3.69 members [1]. This is high considering that most houses in Cato Crest and many other informal settlements consist of only one room

Air pollution is a common environmental hazard affecting people living in unserviced settlements. Apart from not having the option of electrification as an energy source, informal households lack the income to pay for electrical appliances and therefore rely on cheaper methods for cooking and heating which use 'dirtier' fuels such as kerosene or coal. Poorly designed stoves and smoky fuels further exacerbate the problem. One of the dangerous pollutants which arise from kerosene combustion, nitrogen dioxide, has been shown to be associated with increased susceptibility to respiratory infection [18].

Unsanitary conditions caused by uncollected **waste** encourage the proliferation of disease. Burning and dumping problems in informal settlements seem to be related to the lack of adequate waste removal services [2]. People living in unserviced settlements are also exposed to disease-carrying vectors such as rats, mice and flies which proliferate in uncollected waste and refuse. These conditions may contribute to a greater burden of disease and a reduced ability of the body to recover from these diseases, particularly in immuno-compromised individuals.

5.4 Externalities

Low-income communities are exposed to a variety of hazards which arise from both the type of building structure they live in as well as the location and condition of the house. **Building materials** contribute to water leakages and the development of mould leading to poor respiratory health and allergic responses. [2, 17]. Lack of windows (or small windows) leads to poor ventilation which prevents harmful pollutants from being dispersed.

According to the United Nations [19], poor living conditions are associated with poverty, homelessness, poor health, social exclusion, family instability and insecurity, violence, environmental degradation, and increased vulnerability to disasters.

Apart from household building materials, informal settlements are often found on marginalised land next to hazardous waste sites, industrial areas or quarries. Lack of facilities associated with these informal settlements compound the risk to environmental hazards and prevent the community from gaining access to knowledge (through the provision of libraries and information centres).

5.5 Services

Lack of services in low-income communities can contribute to environmental degradation and exposure of individuals to a variety of health hazards. **Access to water, quality of water** and **sanitation services** has been considered.

In Cato Crest, no households collect water from rivers or streams as they have access to piped water, mainly to a shared tap or water carrier. Contamination of water supplies is a particular problem in areas where sanitation facilities, waste disposal services and wastewater removal systems are absent. Water contaminated by sewage may expose users to a wide range of diseases such as cholera or typhoid, with infants and children being particularly vulnerable. Apart from the risk of infectious water-borne diseases, standing water around standpipes can allow proliferation of mosquitoes, a vector of the malaria parasite.

Access to adequate, reliable and safe **sanitation** has been used as a good universal indicator of human development [19] and is one of the eight elements of primary health care. It is therefore a significant indicator of potential risk of disease. In Cato Crest, 91% of households have access to pit latrines (half of whom share with neighbours) amounting to an average of 8 users per latrine.

5.6 General health

Food and nutritional deficiencies, incidence of respiratory disease, prevalence of HIV/AIDS and other communicable diseases are important health issues facing low-income communities. Moser [20] includes an individual's access to adequate nutrients and healthcare as one of the most important determinants of well-being.

Low-income communities often lack the resources to purchase or grow the necessary spectrum of foods which will provide the household with a well-balanced diet. Nutritional deficiencies and the inadequate intake of certain micronutrients can lead to malnutrition and the lowering of resistance to certain diseases [21]. Studies have shown that people with a vitamin C deficiency may be more susceptible to impaired air quality, as vitamin C inhibits the oxidation reactions of nitrogen dioxide (NO_2) in the body [22]. Long-term malnutrition has also been shown to increase susceptibility of the developmental effects of toluene – a pollutant emitted during kerosene combustion [22].

People with pre-existing **chronic respiratory problems** are more susceptible to exposure to NO_2 and other respiratory toxicants. Studies have shown that NO_2 can increase susceptibility to respiratory infection making children and infants in particular, more susceptible to viral and bacterial attack through inhalation, causing an increased incidence of diseases [18]. For example, tuberculosis impairs the ability of the lung to eliminate particulates and the air borne toxicants which bind to particulate surfaces. This condition therefore increases a tuberculosis sufferer's susceptibility to lower levels of air pollution [21].

Individuals with **pre-existing diseases** are more susceptible to additional hazards. Furthermore, vulnerable communities often do not have access to vaccines and anti-bacterial/viral drugs which makes them more vulnerable to infection, and increases the length of recovery from an existing illness. In this study, the prevalence of diarrhoeal diseases and tuberculosis has been chosen to represent the potential pressure that may exist in households exposed to the additional hazard of indoor air pollution.

Diarrhoea is a symptom of infection from a variety of water-borne diseases caused by a number of micro organisms affecting the intestinal tract. The incidence of diarrhoea has been associated with unserviced households which are reliant on untreated water sources.

Tuberculosis (TB) is the most frequently notified disease in South Africa and is rising with the proliferation of HIV/AIDS [23]. A strong correlation exists between the presence of HIV/AIDS and the presence of TB in individuals. Distribution of TB in South Africa indicates strong geographical and racial disparities being influenced strongly by socio-economic status [24].

The burden of HIV/AIDS is heavy on low-income households. It is recognized as a driver of vulnerability (in that it affects a person's immune defence mechanisms) as well as a consequence of vulnerability (in that HIV infection and the onset of AIDS are perpetuated by a variety of physical, social and economic determinants of low-income livelihoods) [15]. The onset of AIDS in an HIV-positive individual can be accelerated by exposure to high levels of nitrogen dioxide arising from combustion of fuels such as kerosene [18]. Socio-economic impacts of HIV/AIDS include lowered life expectancy, dependency on care for the sick, dependency on care for infants and children, and an increased social stigma associated with HIV status. In Cato Crest, HIV prevalence has increased from 41.4% in 1999 to 45.3% in 2000 with the highest prevalence in the 20 to 29 year age group [11].

6 Summary

The purpose of this study was to generate a vulnerability index that can be used to assess levels of vulnerability of low-income communities exposed to indoor air pollution. The variables in the index have been selected based on available literature of the direct or indirect influence of that variable on heightening vulnerability or provision of coping mechanisms. Local issues were included, ensuring relevance to the South African informal settlement context.

Several important points need to be made regarding the index. Firstly, the index may be used to measure vulnerability of a community or household at a particular point in time as people's vulnerability may change over time. Secondly, selection of many of the variables relies on subjective judgement and many assumptions have been made. This paper discusses the components of the vulnerability index and explains their relevance to the South African context. Further work is required on the weighting and possible scoring of each vulnerability factor in order to derive a single score of vulnerability. This would facilitate the integration of traditional health risk assessment results with a vulnerability assessment – ensuring that 'true risk' is assessed.

Acknowledgements

The author wishes to thank Elizabeth Muller and Mamopeli Matooane for their contributions to this paper and to the community of Cato Crest.

References

[1]   Vermaak, K., Gumede, S., Dallimore, A. and Stewart, R. Cato Manor environmental study, Report no. P8-2, CSIR, Durban, 2001.
[2]   Thomas, E.P., Seager, J.R., Viljoen, E., Potgieter, F., Rossouw, A., Tokota, B., McGranahan, G. and Kjellen, M. Household environment and health in Port Elizabeth, South Africa, Urban Environment Series Report no. 6, Stockholm Environment Institute, South African Medical Research Council and Sida, 1999.
[3]   Muller, E. Quantification of the human health risks associated with kerosene use in the informal settlement of Cato Manor, Durban, Unpublished master's thesis, University of Natal, Durban, 2001.
[4]   Wisner, B., Marginality and vulnerability. *Applied Geography*, **18(1)**, pp. 25-33, 1998.
[5]   Kotze, A., A new concept of risk. *Risk, sustainable development and disasters: Southern perspectives*, ed. A. Holloway, Periperi publications, University of Cape Town, Cape Town, 1999.
[6]   ISDR, Living with risk: A global review of disaster reduction initiatives, preliminary version, International Strategy for Disaster Reduction, 2002.

[7]   UNEP, *Global Environment Outlook 3: Past, present and future perspectives*, Earthscan Publications Ltd., London, 2002.

[8]   Binedell, M.L., The whole is greater than the sum of its parts: Cumulative risk of indoor air pollution and urban vulnerability in Cato Manor, South Africa. Masters Thesis. University of Natal, Durban, 2003.

[9]   Department of Social Development. State of South Africa population report, 2003. Online. http://population.pwv.gov.za/state.htm.

[10]   Rakodi C., Gatabaki-Kamau, R. & Devas, N., Poverty and political conflict in Mombasa. *Environment and Urbanisation*, **12(1)**, pp. 153-170, 2000.

[11]   Smith, A., HIV/AIDS statistics, Department of Virology, University of Natal, Durban, 2001.

[12]   Amis, P., Making sense of urban poverty. *Environment and Urbanisation*, **7(1)**, pp. 145-157, 1995.

[13]   Wratten, E., Conceptualising urban poverty. *Environment and Urbanisation*, **7(1)**, pp. 11-36, 1995.

[14]   Moser, C., Asset vulnerability framework: Reassessing urban poverty reduction strategies. *World Development*, **26(1)**, pp. 1-19, 1998.

[15]   Zawaira, F., HIV/AIDS: The unmitigated disaster, *Risk, sustainable development and disasters: Southern perspectives*, ed. A. Holloway, Periperi publications, University of Cape Town, 1999.

[16]   WHO, Health and sustainable development: Meeting of senior officials and ministers of health, summary report, Johannesburg, 2002.

[17]   Al-Khatib I., Ju'ba A., Kamal N., Hamed N., Hmeidan N. & Massad S., Impact of housing conditions on the health of the people at al-Ama'ri refugee camp in the West Bank of Palestine. *International Journal Environmental Health Research*, **13(4)**, pp. 315-326, 2003.

[18]   Law, E., Quantification of the human health risks of NO_2 pollution in Johannesburg and Cape Town, CSIR Report ENV-P-I-99010, Pretoria, 1999.

[19]   UN, Indicators of sustainable development: Guidelines and methodologies, United Nations, 1995. Online. http://www.un.org.za/esa/sustdev/indisd/isdms2001/isd-ms2001isd.htm

[20]   Moser, C., Urban social policy and poverty reduction. *Environment and Urbanisation*, **7(1)**, pp. 159-171, 1995.

[21]   Rios R., Poje V.G. & Detels R., Susceptibility to environmental pollutants among minorities. *Toxicology and Industrial Health*, **9(5)**, pp.797-820, 1993.

[22]   Oosthuizen, R. and John, J., Trends in air quality and health, CSIR Report ENV- P- I- 2002-003, Pretoria, 2002.

[23]   HST, South African health review, Health Systems Trust, 1996. Online. http://www.hst.org.za/sahr

[24]   DACE, Mpumalanga State of the Environment Report, Department of Agriculture, Conservation and Environment, Mpumalanga, 2003.

Air pollution of PM10 with radionuclide Cs-137 in Kuwait City, Kuwait

H. Tang[1], D. Al-Ajmi[1] & X. Shen[2]
[1]Kuwait Institute for Scientific Research, CTBTO
[2]International Monitoring System Division, CTBTO

Abstract

Kuwait City is surrounded by deserts. PM10 is a problem for this city. Statistical studies show that the percentage of violations of the Kuwait government's PM10 standard is high. Cs-137 is a man-made radionuclide produced through nuclear fission. It has very high fission yield, and has a 30.1 years' half-life. From a non-radiological hazards point of view, no potential health effects are known for Cesium. However, large oral doses of the material may cause gastrointestinal disturbances. A large amount of Cs-137 was released into the atmosphere from nuclear tests in early 1950's and 1960's, and from nuclear accidents in the past. The International Commission on Radiological Protection has set up exposure standards for many radionuclide elements.

In cooperation with the Centre of Monitoring Research, USA and the International Monitoring System Division, the Preparatory Commission for the Comprehensive Nuclear-test-ban Treaty Organization, Kuwait Institute for Scientific Research has operated a radionuclide monitoring station in Kuwait City for many years. It has been discovered that Kuwait City has the highest Cs-137 activity concentrations and largest range of concentrations among the CTBTO monitoring stations from 1995 to 1999. This study found from April 2004 to February 2005, the average concentration of Cs-137 in Kuwait City was about the same level of the average concentration from 1995 to 1999 although the monthly average of Cs-137 concentrations had changed. This paper will detail the measurement results, and discuss the health effects.
Keywords: radionuclide, Cs-137, health effect, particle, PM10.

1   Introduction

There is radiation all around us and we cannot eliminate radiation from our environment. Radioactive materials that decay spontaneously produce ionizing radiation, which has sufficient energy to strip away electrons from atoms or to break some chemical bonds. Any living tissue in the human body can be damaged by ionizing radiation. The most common forms of ionizing radiation are alpha and beta particles, or gamma and x-rays. These radiations are from consumer products, security devices, foods, food containers, medical procedures, naturally occurring processes, nuclear test, nuclear power plant emissions etc.

In the atmosphere, one of the radiation sources is particulate phase. The particulate phase can be divided into two major groups according to sizes: corse particles PM10 and fine particles PM2.5.

Radiation effects human health not only directly from a source beaming out and striking the exterior of a body, but also from particles becoming lodged inside the body and exposing internal organs as the radionuclides decay. There are three main routs of exposure to radiation: inhalation, ingestion and direct exposure.

There are many natural radionuclides such as K-40, Be-7, Pb-212, Ac-228, Bi-212, Tl-208 etc. For example, K-40 can be found from Banana. Radon is always in the air that man breathes. Indoor concentrations of Radon are typically 2 – 10 times those in outdoor air.

Cs-137 is a man-made radionuclide product through nuclear fission. It has very high fission yield, and has a 30.1 years' half-life. From non-radiological hazards point of view, no potential health effects are known for Cesium. However, large oral doses of the material may cause gastrointestinal disturbances. A large amount of Cs-137 was released into the atmosphere from nuclear tests in early 1950's and 1960's [1–4] and from nuclear accidents in the past. International Commission on Radiological Protection has set up exposure standards for many radionuclide elements.

Cooperated with Centre of Monitoring Research, USA and International Monitoring System Division, Preparatory Commission for the Comprehensive Nuclear-test-ban Treaty Organization (CTBTO), Kuwait Institute for Scientific Research (KISR) has operated a radionuclide monitoring station in Kuwait City for many years. It is well known that Kuwait City is surrounded by deserts, and PM10 is a problem for this city. Statistic studies show that the percentage of violation of Kuwait government PM10 standard is high. Unfortunately it has been further discovered that Kuwait had the highest Cs-137 activity concentrations and largest range of concentrations among the CTBTO radionuclide monitoring stations in the world from 1995 to 1999 [5]. Our study found that from April 2004 to March 2005, the average concentration of Cs-137 in Kuwait was still about the same level as from 1995 to 1999 although the monthly average concentrations were changed. This paper will detail the measurement results, and discuss the health effects.

2 Radionuclide measurement

The Comprehensive Nuclear-Test-Ban Treaty (CTBT) establishes the International Monitoring System (IMS) to ensure verification of compliance with the treaty. Prior to entry into force of the Treaty, the IMS is supervised and coordinated by the Provisional Technical Secretariat (PTS) and has been designed to provide, on a global scale, monitoring facilities capable of the detection and locating of nuclear explosions. For monitoring atmospheric radionuclides, a global network of radionuclide monitoring stations and radionuclide laboratories is established as part of the IMS. Kuwait has one radionuclide monitoring station. The station is operated by Kuwait Institute for Scientific Research (KISR). A Radionuclide Aerosol Sampler/Analyzer (RASA) [6] (Veridian System Division USA) is installed in the station.

The RASA samples and measures trace quantities of radionuclides in large atmospheric samples (PM10) and report the results to the central data center of CTBT. The RASA system equipment contains a gamma radiation detection system used to monitor the atmosphere for evidence of radionuclide activities. It also includes three mechanical subsystems consisting of a supply mechanism, a segmented sample head, and a multi-function T-bracket. The PM10 particles are collected for 24 hours, decayed for 24 hours, and measured for another 24 hours. The sampling rates are around 600m^3/hour.

3 Results and discussions

Many radionuclide elements such as Be-7, K-40, Pb-212, TL-208, Ac-228, Cs-137 etc. have been detected in Kuwait. But Cs-137 is especially interested since it is the key anthropogenic radionuclide indicative of nuclear debris. Due to Cs-137 has a half-life of 30.17 years, amounts of this radionuclide releases are still present in the soil and atmosphere as a result of past nuclear tests and reactor releases.

Figure 1 shows the Cs-137 concentrations detected from April 2004 to February 2005. There were 131 days when the Cs-137 was detected. The highest concentration was 270.70 µBq/m^3 (May 24-25, 2004) and the lowest was 1.40 µBq/m^3 (September 30-October 1, 2004). The average concentration of the study period was 10.54 µBq/m^3.

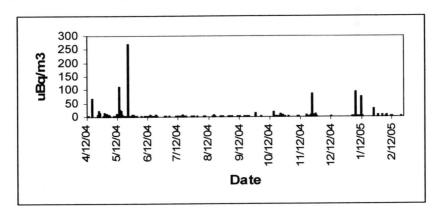

Figure 1:   Cs-137 concentration trend from April 2004 to February 2005 in Kuwait.

The monthly average Cs-137 concentrations and days detecting Cs-137 were shown in Figures 2 and 3. It can be seen that the higher concentrations were in May 2004 (22.3 µBq/m³) and January 2005 (22.9 µBq/m³) although the number of the days detecting Cs-137 were not varied a lot except May 2004 and December 2004. This discovery is partially agreed with previous measurements from 1995 to 1999 [5]. It still shows that the chance of detecting Cs-137 is in the spring and summer months; but that January 2005 had the highest concentration needs to be paid more attention. May 2004 had the highest number of days (25 days) with detecting Cs-137, but not the highest average concentration of Cs-137. Instead, January 2005 had the highest average Cs-137 concentration with only 10 days detecting Cs-137.

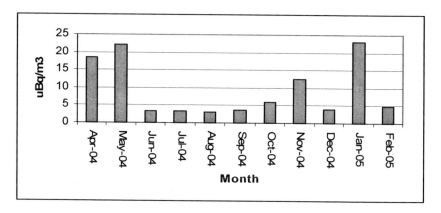

Figure 2:   Monthly average Cs-137 concentrations from April 2004 to February 2005 in Kuwait.

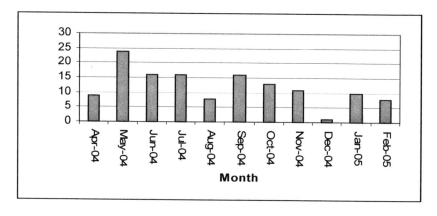

Figure 3:   Monthly days detecting Cs-137 from April 2004 to February 2005 in Kuwait.

3.1 Comparison of Cs-137 concentrations

Table 1 lists the Cs-137 concentrations obtained in Kuwait from 1995 – 1999 [5] and April 2004 – February 2005. It is obvious that the concentration of Cs-137 is almost the same level in the two study periods. Actually, it is not surprised to find that the two periods have the same concentration level since the half-life of Cs-137 is 30.1 years. If compared the Cs-137 concentrations obtained in Kuwait from April 2004 – February 2005 to those data obtained in other countries from 1995 – 1999 [5] and Germany from April 2004 to February 2005, the Kuwait Cs-137 concentration is still the highest (Table 1).

Table 1:   Cs-137 concentrations in different countries obtained from 1995 – 1999 and April 2004 – February 2005.

Time and Location	Ave. $\mu Bq/m^3$	Maximum	Minimum
1995 – 1999, Kuwait	10.60	107.84	1.44
1995-1999, Buenos Aires, Argentina	2.87	10.52	0.98
1995-1999, Schauinsland, Germany	0.75	17.34	0.12
April 2004 – February 2005, Sch. Ger.	2.19	21.47	0.80
April 2004 – February 2005, Kuwait	10.54	270.70	1.40

3.2 Health effect of Cs-137 in Kuwait

As discussed in reference 5, the human health effect of Cs-137 in Kuwait is not obvious. Bielgalski et al. [5] used a multi-compartment lung model [7] to assess the health effects. The model assumes that the particles deposition in the respiratory tract is governed by the size distribution of the inhaled aerosol, and that the clearance rate of the deposited particles is governed by the deposition of the particles. If using the same calculation method as discussed in reference 5, the calculated committed dose equivalent for airborne Cs-137 from May 24-25 is listed in Table 2. In this calculation, it still assumes Cs-137 aerosol median diameter of 1 μm with a geometric standard deviation of 4, standard inhalation rate of 20 $m^3/$ day, and exposure to this concentration for entire period. It can be seen that although a higher concentration of Cs-137 was detected in May 24-25, 2004 (270.70 $\mu Bq/m^3$), the committed dose equivalent to entire body was only 4.49E-11. This number is still less than the International Commission on Radiological Protection (ICRP) annual limit (5.00E-2).

3.3 Source apportionment of Cs-137 in Kuwait

Until now, we still cannot positive identified the sources of the Cs-137 in Kuwait. But the following wind-roses can prove very useful information.

Table 2: Committed dose equivalent for airborne Cs-137 in May 24-25, 2004 in Kuwait City, Kuwait.

Collection start	Collection stop	Atmospheric activity concentration, $\mu Bq/m^3$	Committed dose equivalent to entire body, Sv
May 24, 2004	May 25, 2004	270.70	4.49E-11
ICRP annual Limit (8)			5.00E-2

Figures 4–6 show the wind-roses of the days with higher Cs-137 in Kuwait. Those days were May 25-26 (270.70 $\mu Bq/m^3$), May 13-14 (114. .24 $\mu Bq/m^3$), and November 23-24 (84.81 $\mu Bq/m^3$). It can be seen from the wind-roses that the dominated wind directions were from southern-west. The wind-roses were created from meteorological data collected at a well calibrated meteorological station in KISR about 100 meters west of the RASA station.

Figure 7 shows the wind-rose for June 11-12, 2004 with the lower Cs-137 concentration. This figure also shows that the dominated wind direction was also from southern west, but had many other wind directions. Generally speaking, it seems that the Cs-137 sources in Kuwait City might be from the southern west directions.

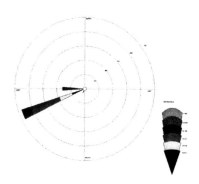

Figure 4: Wind-rose for Many 24-25, 2004.

The monthly wind-roses for May 2004 and August 2004 are shown in Figures 8 and 9. May 2004 had higher Cs-137 concentration compared to August 2004. From the wind-roses, it can be seen both months' dominated wind directions were from the same direction. Therefore, although the Cs-137 sources might be from the southern west, the Cs-137 concentrations can be depended on human and natural activities. For example, dust storms from the southern west directions can bring more PM10 in the atmosphere, and consequently more Cs-137.

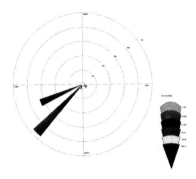

Figure 5: Wind-rose for May 13-14, 2004.

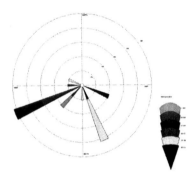

Figure 6: Wind-rose for November 23-24, 2004.

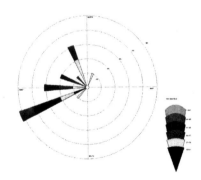

Figure 7: Wind-rose for June 11-12, 2004.

Table 3 lists Cs-137 concentration obtained in January of different years based on available information. We found that the highest average Cs-137 concentration was in January 2005 with 10 days' Cs-137 detections. It can be seen from Table 2 that it is not always the same trend. For example, there was no detection of Cs-137 in January in 1996 and 1997. This further indicates that many artificial and natural events can affect the concentration of Cs-137 in the atmosphere.

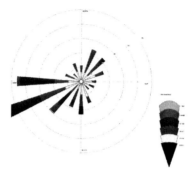

Figure 8:   Wind-rose for May 2004.

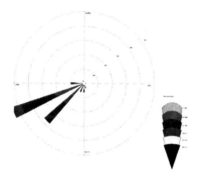

Figure 9:   Wind-rose for August 2004.

Table 3:   Comparison of detection days and concentrations of Cs-137 in January of different years.

Year	January Cs-137	
	Detection Days	Concentration $\mu Bq/m^3$
1996	0	0
1997	0	0
1999	2	2.77
2005	10	22.90

4 Conclusions

Many artificial and natural radionuclide elements have been measured in the Kuwait City RASA station. The average Cs-137 concentrations in the PM10 of the atmosphere in Kuwait City, Kuwait have been the highest for several years. This trend might be last for many more years. Although the Cs-137 concentrations in Kuwait will not affect human health, it is still worth to find the sources. This study indicates the higher chance to detect Cs-137 is not only in spring and summer, but winter is also included. The data collected from a nearby meteorological station indicates that the Cs-137 sources might from southern-west side. More attentions need to be paid to this direction.

Acknowledgements

The authors want to thank support from Kuwait Institute for Scientific Research (KISR), CTBTO and many individuals from Costal and Air Pollution Department, Environment and Urban Development Division of KISR.

References

[1] Holmes, C.W., Short-Lived Isotopic Chronometers- A Means of Measuring Decadal Sedimentary Dynamics, U.S. Geological Survey, Department of the Interior, Fact Sheet FS-073-98, 1998.

[2] Singhal, R.K., Estimation of Deposition Velocities for 85Sr, 131I, 137Cs on Spinach Radish and Beans Leaves in a Tropical Region under Simulated Fallout, Water, Air, & Soil Pollution, **158(1-4)**, pp181-193, 2004.

[3] Ebert, D., Hoerner, J., Kang, C., White, B., Biegalski, S. & Massari, J., Treansactions of American Nuclear Society 1990 Summer Meeting, San Diego, CA, June 1999.

[4] Eriksson, M., Distribution and Flux of 238Pu, 239, 240Pu, 241 Am, 137Cs and 210Pb to High Arctic Lakes in the Thule District (Greenland), Journal of Environmental Radioactivity, **75(3)**, pp285-300, 2004.

[5] Biegalski, S.R., Hosticka, B. and Mason, L.R., Cesium-137 concentrations, Trends, and Sources Observed in Kuwait City, Kuwait, Journal of Radioanalytical and Nuclear Chemistry, **248(3)**, pp643-649, 2001.

[6] General Dynamics, RASA Users Manual, Veridian Systems Division, USA, 2003.

[7] Cember, H., Introduction to Health Physics, Mc-Graw-Hill, Inc., New York, 1983.

[8] International Commission on Radiological Protection (ICRP), ICRP Publication 30, Part I, **5(1-6)**, 1981.

Environmental health risk by sly pollution: applied research on radon inside public buildings

S. Lo Nigro, F. Patania, A. Gagliano & F. Nocera
Energy and Environment Division of D.I.I.M.,
Engineering Faculty of University of Catania, Italy

Abstract

Radon (Rn) is a polluting gas coming from radioactive decays and it is not detectable by human senses as it is colourless, tasteless and odourless. Apart from the underground position of radioactive sources of such gas, it is able to cover very long paths through subsoil and to the surface at considerable distances from the underground starting points. Whenever it surfaces in the interior of buildings, passing through foundation structures, then it produces a sly pollution as its presence will be discovered only when it has harmed people. Owing to previous peculiarities, there is a considerable health risk in the case of such indoor air pollution and this risk can be mitigated only by precautionary measures as are used to periodically control Radon concentrations in indoor environments which are suspected to be polluted by Radon and then to set in action some techniques to reduce indoor radon concentration in polluted buildings. Beginning to face the Radon problem, the Province of Ragusa (Italy) set in action experimental research to discover the real concentrations of Radon in some public buildings in Ragusa town (ex IPAI building), Modica Town (technical Institute "Archimede") and Scicli Town (Civil Protection Agency Building). For reasons of space the aim of paper is to show results only for the IPAI building:
-   The techniques and the equipment used to survey the gas concentrations.
-   The analysis of results of the campaign of measurements that permit one to point out the reliability of methods as a function of the kinds of equipment.
-   The proposed techniques of mitigation of pollution.
Keywords: radon, indoor pollution, measurements and control.

1 Site of research, techniques and equipment for measurements

The whole of the research has been carried out in the towns shown by red spots in figure 1, that is the three towns of Sicily (Italy), but for reasons of space in this paper we will deal only with the part pertaining to the IPA building in Modica town where people attended a public school called "I.T.C. Archimede". In the campaign of measurement the following was carried out:

- Passive measures of Rn concentrations by method of gas absorption in active carcoil. The active carcoil was contained in canisters of metal, that is 70 gr. of carcoil for each canister with dimensions ϕ=10.2cm and h=2.9cm (figure 2). The measurements by canisters have been made with times of exposure of 48 hours for one week and repeated for four weeks. After exposure, carcoil has been analyzed in the laboratories of the Sicilian Centre of Nuclear Physic by sodium iodite spectrophotometer.
- Active measures of Rn concentration by Alphaguard - Genitron, that is a 3D ionisation chamber detector (figure 3) able to work both for "*gaseous natural diffusion*"(measurements of gas in the air) and "*gaseous pumping diffusion*" (measurements of gas in the subsoil)

Both kinds of measurements have been made in indoor rooms and in subsoil around the school. In the case of passive measurements in subsoil PVC tubes, appropriately punched, are positioned inside holes built in the ground (figures 4 and 5). The top of each tube has been closed with a special outlet plug able to house the canisters (figures 6 and 7) and all the holes in the top have been closed by a little inspection sump (figure 8). In the case of active measurement a probe has been positioned inside a PVC tube (figure 9) and connected to a 3D ionisation chamber by a very little tube in plastic material (figure 10). For outdoor measurement the equipment has been housed in a special metal container (figure 11).

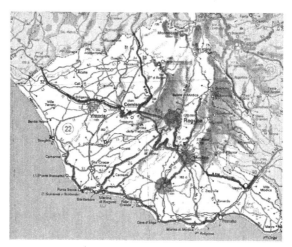

Figure 1:   Site of research.

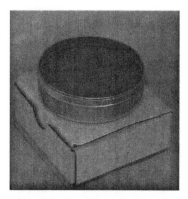

Figure 2: Carcoil container.

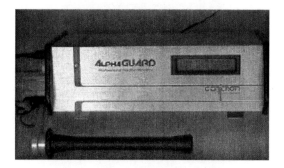

Figure 3: Ionisation chamber detector.

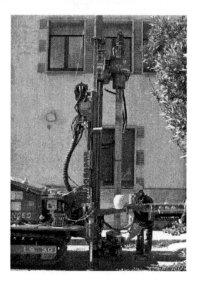

Figure 4: Hole preparation.

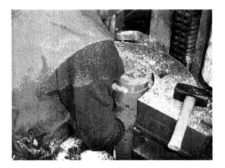

Figure 5: Tube positioning in the hole.

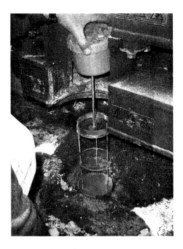

Figure 6: Outlet plug housing canister.

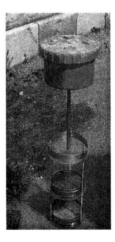

Figure 7: Plug with canisters.

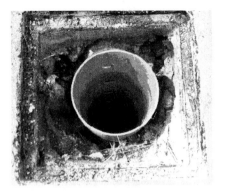

Figure 8:   Inspection sump.

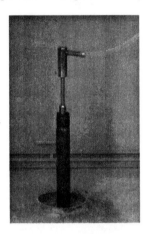

Figure 9:   Probe.

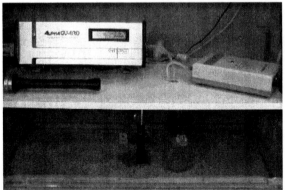

A: 3D Ionisation chamber
B:Probe
C:Pump
D:Filters

Figure 10:   Equipment for active measures.

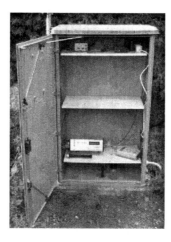

Figure 11:   Container for equipment used in outdoor measurements.

2   Factors favouring Rn pollution indoors

As is well known in technical literature [1–4], the factors are shortly summarised as follows:

- Intensity of gas flow coming from subsoil.
- Holes or breaks in trampling or in boundary walls that are in direct contact with the ground.
- Porosity and permeability of building surfaces in contact with the ground.
- Presence of doors and windows in the rooms.
- Presence of HVAC plants in the building.
- Ratio between the whole surface of the wrapper of the outside walls and that one in contact with the ground.
- Difference in air pressure between indoors and outdoors, independently from the producing causes.
- Presence of fine particulate matter (PM_{10}, $PM_{2.5}$, $PM_{1.0}$) in the air of indoor rooms.
- Climatic features in outdoor environments, especially referring to wind intensity and direction.
- Absence of air motions in the indoor environment.

3   Results of campaign of measurements

With reference to the maximum level of Rn concentration in the air, both Euratom 96/2000 directives and Italian law by decree n. 241/2000 fixed at 400 Bq/m^3 the alarm level for RN pollution. This value is estimated to be rather high by authors with particular reference to results carried out by ERRICCA European Project [5]. For reasons of space, some selected results are shown as follows:

- Figure 12 shows an example of the measured values of Rn given off from the subsoil of building.

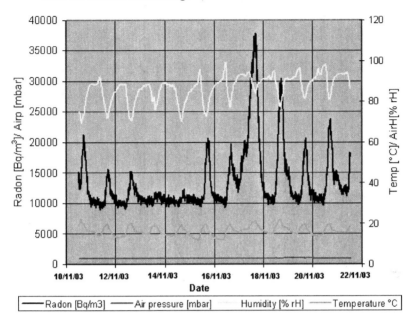

Figure 12:   RN given off from the subsoil of building.

- Figures 13 and 14 show examples of Rn measured values and indoor climatic features respectively for room n.1 and room n.4.

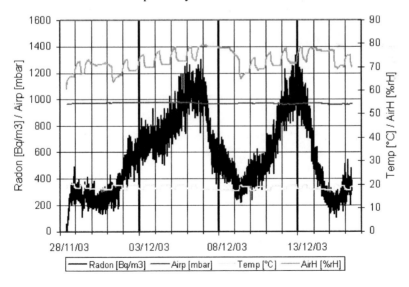

Figure 13:   Indoor climatic features and RN concentrations in room n.1.

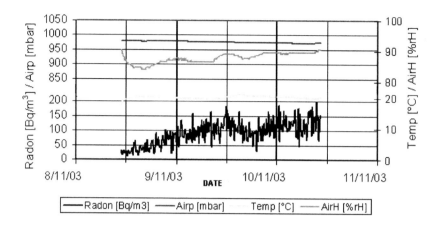

Figure 14: Indoor climatic features and RN concentrations in room n.4.

- Figure 15 shows the histogram of the average of RN concentrations for all rooms in the school.

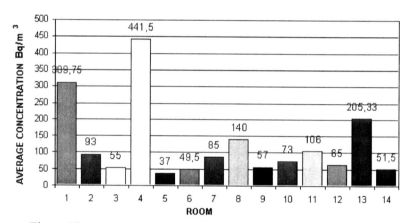

Figure 15: Average concentrations for each room of building.

- Table 1 shows an example of a comparison between data measured respectively by passive and active techniques.

Table 1: Data comparison between passive and active measurement techniques.

Exposure Period	Passive Method (canister)	Active Method (alphaguard mobile)	Factor
08–10 November 2003	85 Bq/m^3	92 Bq/m^3	1.08
9 November–01 December 2003	193 Bq/m^3	260 Bq/m^3	1.35
13–15 December 2003	245 Bq/m^3	586 Bq/m^3	2.39

For reasons of space it is not possible to show in this paper the peculiarities that caused the different values of Rn concentration in all of the investigated rooms, for this reason the authors prefer to draw the attention of readers to two particular cases, in fact a short analysis of the data in figure 15 to examine in detail rooms n.1 and n.4 that show a high average of Rn concentration and building peculiarities in accord with negative factors related in the previous paragraph n.2:

-   *Room n.1*: mean average 309,75 Bq/m^3, maximum value 586,00 Bq/m^3. The room is utilised as the larder of the school, it has no windows and the inlet door is the only aperture of the room which looks towards the outdoor environment. In this room about 11 m^2 of boundary surfaces are in direct contact with the soil, that is the floor made with marble slab upon a floor rough in concrete. Both the slab and the rough show evident cracks that permit the inlet of Rn from subsoil. The room is not frequently utilised and, in this way, there is no air motion or change of air: both factors favouring accumulation of Rn coming from subsoil into the room.

-   *Room n.4*: mean average 441,50 Bq/m^3, maximum value 637,00 Bq/m^3. The room is utilised as a service room to the hydraulic plant of the building, in fact it houses the pumps and the other related hydraulic equipment. A lot of holes or breaks are in the trampling that separates the room by a water tank staying in underground under the room. This room, as the n.1 room, is not frequently utilised, has no windows and has no motions or changes of air.

With reference to the different techniques to measure Rn pollution, the results shown in Table 1 allowed the claim to be made that the direct measurements by Alphaguard are more reliable than the ones obtained by the canisters. In fact the values of measurements obtained by the canisters have been undervalued by up to 40% in some cases. One supposes that the undervaluation is caused both by the manipulation suffered by the canisters on the way from the experiment site to the analysis laboratory and by the time spent during the transportation the experiment site to the laboratory.

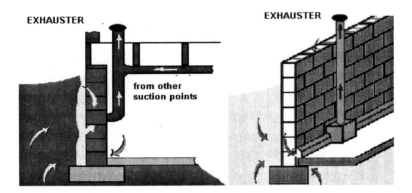

Figure 16:   Block Wall Depressurisation and Base Board Depressurisation.

4 Conclusions

The results of campaign of measurements and the investigations on situ permitted to focus on following remarks:
- the school is not very polluted by Rn gas, with a few exception: rooms nn.1, 4, 8 and 13
- to control and mitigate pollution in previous rooms the BBD (black Wall Depressurisation) or BWD (Based Board Depressurisation) (figure 16) techniques are suggested.
- Owing to very high emissions of Rn from subsoil (figure 12) people advise a continuous monitoring by active techniques in the class rooms
- The passive methods of measurement that do not offer a important reliability of measures could be used only for first general survey

Acknowledgement

The Authors wish to thank dott. Ing. Carlo Ricca for his precious contribution.

References

[1] ASTM Manual series: MNL 15- PCN 28-015094-17, "Radon, prevalence, measurements, health risk and control", Niren L. Nagda Editor, Philadelphia, June 1994.
[2] Patania F. and Gagliano A., Radon secret and detrimental effect on indoor health, II International Conference Cold Climate HVAC, Rowaniemy (Finland), March 1994.
[3] Patania F. and Gagliano A., Radon pollution dynamics in indoor environment: proposal about its control, International Conference Healthy Building, Budapest (Hungary), August 1994
[4] Patania F., Origini e controllo dell'inquinamento da radon parte I, Rivista Condizionamento dell'aria e refrigerazione n.11, pp. 1161-1168, Novembre 1995.
[5] Patania F. and Lo Nigro S., A new method to control health effect on radon indoor air pollution: final report", III International III International European Workshop (ERRICCA PROJECT FINAL REPORTED), Athens (Greece), March 1999.

Dioxin emission estimates and reduction options for Central and Eastern Europe

H. Kok[1], T. Pulles[1] & U. Quass[2]
[1]TNO Built Environment and Geosciences, Apeldoorn, Netherlands
[2]Müller-BBM GmbH, Gelsenkirchen, Germany

Abstract

The project "Dioxin Emissions in Candidate Countries" was commissioned by the European Commission to a consortium lead by TNO and was finished in the beginning of 2005. The project is part of the Commission's response to the Stockholm Convention on Persistent Organic Pollutants (POPs). The emissions have been estimated, using a method that is consistent for all countries in this study and the earlier EU Dioxin Inventory for the 15 "Old" EU Member States. The national inventory in this study has been discussed with national experts from each of the 13 countries. The results of the study show that the emissions of dioxins to air in the "New" EU Member States and the Candidate Countries are most probably comparable to those in the "Old" EU Member States. There is a small chance that the emissions are a factor 4 to 5 higher because of uncertainties in activity rates of dioxin emitting processes and emission per unit of activity. On the basis of the results we conclude that there is no reason to assume that the concentrations of dioxins in the air in the 13 countries are significantly higher than in the 15 "Old" EU Member States. This however does not exclude possible "hot spots", where relatively high concentrations could occur, due to for instance uncontrolled burning of chlorine containing wastes. Special attention must be given to prevent "illegal" activities in the field of waste combustion.

Keywords: dioxin emission, emission inventory, Central Europe, Eastern Europe, activity data, emission factors, waste incineration, primary metal industry, cement industry, residential heating, reduction measures.

1   Introduction

Dioxins and furans, more precisely polychlorinated dibenzo-p-dioxins (PCDD) and polychlorinated dibenzofurans (PCDF) have received wide attention both by scientists and by policy makers, developing international conventions and protocols aimed at protecting the environment from the so-called Persistent Organic Pollutants (POPs). Dioxins and furans (PCDD/F) are unintentionally formed in processes where chlorine containing organic material is heated to high temperatures. Such processes are combustion and incineration of wastes and fuels and certain manufacturing processes of chlorinated phenols and solvents, in pulp and paper industry (chlorine bleaching) and in the metallurgical industry.

As a starting point of any policy to decrease the environmental impact by POPs like dioxins and furans, a quantitative overview of the sources is absolutely essential. Dioxin and furan (PCDD/F) emission inventories have been compiled recently for continental scale [1; 2], for national scale [3] and for provincial / local scale [4; 5]. For the western European countries ('Old' Member States) a recent PCDD/F emission inventory is available [2]. For New EU Member States and Candidate Member Countries this was not the case. This was one of the reasons for the EU to commission the project "Dioxin Emissions in Candidate Countries". The 13 countries in Central and Eastern Europe, participating in this study are: Bulgaria, Cyprus, Czech Republic, Estonia, Hungary, Latvia, Lithuania, Malta, Poland, Romania, Slovak Republic, Slovenia and Turkey.

When the project was commissioned, these countries were referred to as EU Candidate Member Countries. Since June 2004, 10 of these countries are full members of the EU. Bulgaria, Romania and Turkey now are still candidate countries. In this paper we will continue to label these 13 countries as "New" Member States.

In the study the methods were developed to compile consistent and comparable inventories of PCDD/F for the 13 individual countries and to compare these with the inventories of the Old Member States.

This paper presents the results together with the differences in dioxin emissions from several industrial and non-industrial sectors in Old and New Member States. Recommendations are given for the reduction of dioxin load in populated areas.

2   Methods

A detailed description of the methods and data used in this study is available in the full report [6]. Below we summarise the main issues.

2.1 Procedure

The compilation of the dioxin emission inventory for the 13 countries in this study was a stepwise approach, aimed at making optimal use of both available expertise at the partners in the consortium and the knowledge and expertise in the countries.

2.2 Algorithm

The method applied in compiling the air emission inventory is the "top-down-approach", which is generally applied in almost all emission inventories. For each relevant sector and fuel, the emission is calculated by multiplying an activity rate with an appropriate emission factor:

$$Emissions_{sector,fuel} = Activity_{sector,fuel} \times Emission\ Factor_{sector,fuel}$$

Please note that only combustion processes will use the specification of "fuel". The total inventory then is simply the sum of these sector emissions for all sectors and fuels.

$$Emissions = \sum_{sectors,fuels} Emissions_{sectors,fuel}$$

In compiling the emission inventory for a country, for each relevant sector and fuel activity data and appropriate emission factors must be collected.

2.2.1 Sector and fuel definitions

Emission inventories in most countries are compiled using a set of sector definitions that has been developed under the work of IPCC to be applied in emission inventories for the Climate Change convention (UNFCCC). Recently, the Convention on Long Range Transboundary Air Pollution (LRTAP) also adopted a set of sector definitions that is fully consistent with these IPCC sector definitions.

2.2.2 Technologies

To calculate the emissions for each of the activities in the sectors emission factors are needed. These emission factors depend on the technology that is applied to perform the activity. Any activity could in principle be performed with different technologies in different countries representing the different technologies within one country. This is also reflected in available emission factors like the UNEP Chemicals Toolkit, in many cases differing by a factor of 10 between technologies [7].

2.2.3 Activity data

Activity data for the inventory were obtained from a series of publicly available data sources (e.g. IEA, EUROSTAT) and data used in the CEPMEIP-project [8]. Where updated data were provided by national experts, participating in the workshops, these replaced the data in the international data sets.

We assumed the uncertainties in the activity data, based on international statistics as +/- 30 % (95 % confidence interval), except for population sizes, which were assumed to be quite accurate (+/- 1 %).

2.2.4 Emission factors

The majority of emission factors are derived from the UNEP Chemicals Toolkit [7]. A number of countries have provided country specific emission factors based on dioxin emission measurements. If no information was available on the state of reduction technology used in principle we selected the highest one for that activity reflecting the idea that most of the industrial installations in Central and Eastern Europe will have limited abatement techniques.

For some activities (e.g. preservation of wood, cigarette smoking, fires), per capita emission factors were derived from the EU inventory [2].

Wherever the UNEP Chemicals toolkit provides emission factors for different technologies, these different emission factors were interpreted as the uncertainty range for these emission factors.

3   Results of emission inventory

3.1 Dioxin emission of 'new' EU member states

Taking the uncertainties as described above into account, the national total emissions in each of the 13 countries are estimated as presented in table 1.

Table 1:   Estimates for national total emissions to air in the 13 countries in grams for the year 2000.

Country Name	5 percentile	best estimate	95 percentile
Bulgaria	70	300	800
Cyprus	3	7	40
Czech Republic	85	320	990
Estonia	3	9	45
Hungary	45	120	450
Latvia	10	18	270
Lithuania	10	50	200
Malta	1	4	13
Poland	250	800	1900
Romania	120	500	1300
Slovak Republic	45	180	500
Slovenia	10	35	100
Turkey	200	1000	2800
Grand Total	**1300**	**3200**	**8000**

For each country, both the value as obtained from the inventory and the lower and upper limits of the 90 % confidence intervals are presented.

The total dioxin emission to air in the thirteen countries is estimated at 3.2 kg TE per year. The uncertainty range around this value is 1.3 to 8.0 kg TE per year (90 % confidence interval).

3.2 Sector contributions

Contributions by different sectors to the total emissions are given in Figure 1. Important sources are in the waste sector and industrial production (metals and minerals). Minor contributions are from product use and fuel combustion. The EU inventory for the "Old" EU member States shows a comparable distribution. Together these sources are responsible for over 60 % of the total dioxin emissions in the studied area.

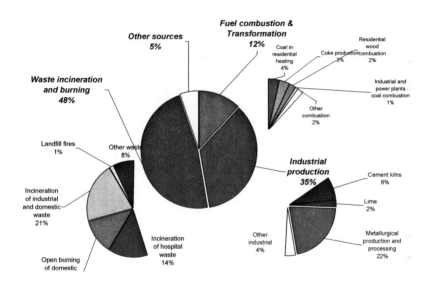

Figure 1:   Sector contribution to dioxin emissions to air in the 13 countries.

Major dioxin emission sources occur both in a limited number of larger industrial facilities and in numerous small residential sources (stoves, uncontrolled burning, fires etc.). Our best estimate of the contribution between these two source categories shows that 30 to 40 % of the emissions might arise from the small residential sources. This figure however is highly uncertain.

3.3 Dioxin concentration in populated areas and their potential health impacts

About one third of the emissions of dioxins to air are due to non-industrial (area) sources, where low level emission occurs in large numbers of small equipment (stoves, cars, open waste burning). These emissions obviously occur in the direct neighbourhood where people live and hence will give rise to elevated concentrations of dioxins in the direct surroundings of where people live. As an example, dioxin concentrations in ambient air of up to 8.000 fg TE/m³ (which is a factor of 200 above usual background concentrations) have been found in wintertime at Cracow, Poland [9]. Fugitive emissions from industrial activities carried out on industrial premises (e.g. dust resuspension by vehicles, dispersion from heaps) can have an impact on the adjacent areas. A recent screening of POPs concentrations in free-range chicken eggs frequently revealed elevated PCDD/F concentrations in the vicinity of industrial areas, proving direct impacts of industrial emissions on the food chain. In the area considered here such incidents were found in Slovakia, Czech Republic, Bulgaria and Turkey.

4 Reduction of dioxin emission

4.1 Emission reduction at waste incineration processes

Waste incineration comprises the incineration of municipal solid waste (MSW), hazardous waste, medical waste and sewage sludge. In the early 1990s flue gas concentrations of MSW incinerators in Germany were about 10 ng TE/m3 (TE = Toxicity Equivalent) [10]. According to the waste incineration directive incineration plants must comply with an emission limit value of 0.1 ng TE/m3 in the exhaust gas [11]. This means an emission reduction of about 99%. This reduction can be achieved by combining three types of measures:

- *Pre-incineration measures* e.g. removal of chlorinated compounds such as PVC). This however has shown little influence on the resulting concentration.
- *Incineration process control* to compensate for the natural variability in fuel quantity and the controlling factors that govern the rate of chemical reactions. Solid waste is not a homogeneous material and should be mixed very well before charging it to the furnace.
- *Post-combustion control* will remove unwanted contaminants from the waste gas stream.

Of these the third is the most important one. The three key aspects of such air pollution control systems are reagent addition, waste gas temperature control and particulate removal. First step in the removal of contaminants from the incinerator gases is the removal of particulates and acids by means of filters and chemical scrubbers. There are different possible additional techniques and their combinations that achieve a PCDD/F concentration of smaller than 0.1 ng TE/m3 in the cleaned gases. The systems are based on an activated coke bed filter or a flue gas injection system (injection of a mixture of lime and coke before a fabric filter). Annual costs for complete flue gas control systems for achieving all emission limit values (inclusive PCDD/F) stated in the waste incineration directive amounts to € 50 to € 100 per ton of domestic waste incinerated.

4.2 Emission reduction in industry

4.2.1 Emission reduction at sinter plants in primary metal industry
Sintering is the baking of moistened mixtures of small-particle iron ores with coke and lime to form lumps of a size which is suitable for the metallurgical process. In the sintering process dioxins are formed and adsorbed on dust particles in the waste gases from the sinter belt. The reduction measure usually used is dedusting of the exhaust air. The target value for the concentration of dioxin in the dedusted belt exhaust gases (< 0.5 ng TEQ/m3) can only be reached by an additional cleaning device (e.g. a second filtrating filter after cooling and adding an adsorbent like active carbon to the exhaust gases).

4.2.2 Emission reduction at cement kilns
Dioxins can be formed in/after the preheater and in the air pollution control device if chlorine and hydrocarbon precursors from the raw materials are available in sufficient quantities. The reformation of dioxins and furans is known to occur by de novo synthesis within the temperature window of cooling from 450 to 200 °C. Thus it is important that as the gases are leaving the kiln system they should be cooled rapidly through this range.

4.3 Emission reduction at residential heating

Residential heating in small-scale firing places takes place in the power range up to about 50 kW for cooking and heating purposes. Solid fuels like coal, coke and wood give relative high emissions of PCDD/F (10-100 ug TE/TJ). Oil fired stoves have a factor 10 lower and gas fired stoves a factor 100 lower emission per TJ energy input compared with solid fueled stoves [10].

Emission reduction can be achieved by reduction of energy demand, fuel-related measures and firing-place related measures. Reduction of energy demand is achieved by improved thermal insulation of houses. Fuel-related measures aim at the burning of standard dry and clean natural wood. However, in solid fuel firing places in households, illegal co-incineration of waste containing chlorine components and waste wood cannot be ruled out. Co-burning of wastes leads to a dramatic increase in the dioxin emission by solid fuel firing places [13].

According to the differences between the emission factors for solid, liquid and gaseous fuels replacement of solid fired stoves by oil fired stoves or preferably gas fired stoves would reduce the PCDD/F emissions to a great extent in populated areas.

5 Conclusions

Based on the inventory built for the 13 'New' EU Member States there is no significant difference in dioxin emissions between the thirteen countries in this study and the fifteen 'Old' EU Member States; hence no specific action to reduce dioxin emissions in these countries can be identified for the new EU Member States.

However, uncontrolled burning of domestic waste in backyards or co-incineration of waste in small stoves is a practice that should be paid attention to in view of the elevated PCDD/F concentrations in ambient air occasionally found. This would be also important for other reasons than for dioxin emissions (recovery of valuable materials; emissions of other pollutants as POPs, PAH, particulates, black smoke, etc.). The EU has already legislation in place that aims at improving waste management and waste treatment. The Commission could support programs to inform authorities and to educate the public to properly dispose of wastes via waste collection and waste treatment systems, using incineration in modern waste incinerators and land filling in modern well managed and well protected waste disposal sites.

Residential coal and wood combustion in small stoves also might be phased out because of other environmental problems like the emissions of particulates and PAHs. The emissions of dioxins from these sources add to the problems caused by the use of solid fuels for small residential heating systems.

Dioxin emissions from larger (industrial) facilities could be abated by technical measures. Implementation of the relevant EU Directives [11; 12] and Best Available Technologies (BAT) as described in the IPPC-BREF documents probably will significantly reduce the dioxin emissions from these larger industrial facilities. It should be monitored, however, if these improvements equally can be found also with respect to fugitive emissions from ground-near sources.

References

[1]   Berdowski, J.J.M., Baas, J., Bloos, J.P.J., Visschedijk, A.J.H., PYJ Zandveld, P.Y.J., *The European Emission Inventory of Heavy Metals and Persistent Organic Pollutants for 1990*. Forschungsbericht 104 02 672/03 des Bundesministers für Umwelt, Naturschutz und Reaktorsicherheit.

[2]   Quass, U., Fermann M. and Bröker G., The European Dioxin Air Emission Inventory Project--Final Results. *Chemosphere*, Volume 54, pp. 1319-1327, 2004.

[3]   Kakareka, S.V., Sources of persistent organic pollutants emission on the territory of Belarus, *Atmospheric Environment,* Vol 36, pp 1407-1419, 2002.

[4]   Caserini, S. and Monguzzi, A.M., PCDD/Fs emissions inventory in the Lombardy Region: results and uncertainties, *Chemosphere*, Volume 48, pp. 779-786, 2002.

[5]   Pulles, T., Kok H.J.G. and Pesik J., Dioxin emissions in the Haifa region, *TNO report* nr R 2004/016, TNO Apeldoorn, 2004.

[6]   http://www.envihaifa.org.il/heb/dioxins012004.pdf.

[7]   Pulles, T., Kok, H.J.G., Quass, U., Juery, C. and Mategovicova J., Dioxin emissions in Candidate Countries. *TNO report* R&I-A R 2005/054, 2005.

[8]   Standardized Toolkit for Identification and Quantification of Dioxin and Furan Releases, 1st edition, *UNEP Chemicals*, Geneva, 2003.

[9]   Pulles, T. and Visschedijk A.J.H., *Emission estimation methods for particulates: the CEPMEIP emission factor database.* http://www.air.sk/tno/cepmeip   http://www.dioksyny.pl/files/Results_ from_measurements_Poland_2002_Odense.pdf.

[10]   Detzel, A. et al., Investigation of emissions and abatement measures for persistent organic pollutants in the Federal Republic of Germany, *Research Report 295 44 365*, Federal Environmental Agency, Berlin, 1998.

[11]   Directive 2000/76/EC of the European Parliament and the Council of 4 December 2000 on the incineration of waste. *Official Journal of the European Communities*, L 332, pp. 91-111, 2000.

[12]   Best Available Techniques Reference Document on the Production of Iron and Steel. IPPC, Dec. 2001. http://eippcb.jrc.es/pages/FActivities.htm.

[13]   Launhardt, T., PCDD/F- und PAK-Emissionen aus Holzfeuerungsanlagen für den häuslichen Bereich. *Fach-seminar "Dioxin- und Gesamtemissiononsminimierungstechnieken mit Betriebserfahrungen".* VDI-Bildungswerk, 19 – 20 September 1996, München.

Atmospheric pollution and human health: the significance of a datable sedimentary archive from a small urban lake in Merseyside, UK

A. T. Worsley[1], C. A. Booth[2], A. L. Power[1], N. Richardson[1],
P. G. Appleby[3] & E. J. Wright[1]
[1]*Natural, Geographical & Applied Sciences,*
Edge Hill University College, UK
[2]*Environmental & Analytical Sciences Division,*
Research Institute in Advanced Technologies (RIATec),
The University of Wolverhampton, UK
[3]*Department of Mathematical Sciences, University of Liverpool, UK*

Abstract

Preliminary results from sediment cores taken at Speke Hall Lake, Merseyside (UK) are presented. They demonstrate the use of sediments from a small, man-made, urban lake to reconstruct the local environmental history from the last 250 years. The lake is set within the heart of the Merseyside region, which saw the instigation, and subsequent burgeoning of major industries, notably petro-chemicals during the nineteenth century and by the expansion of the use and manufacture of automobiles in the last century. Given the widely reported concerns over public health, the use of such datable environmental archives is promoted in order to examine the relationship between environment and human health.
Keywords: environmental pollution, palaeolimnology, mineral magnetism.

1 Introduction

There are considerable concerns about relationships between atmospheric quality and human health, particularly the links between lung disease and air quality, which are widely discussed [1, 2]. Many studies have investigated the possibility that atmospheric pollution is a direct cause of high mortality rates, increased hospital admission rates and many types of cancer [3]. Areas with the highest concentrations of atmospheric pollution are normally those with the highest density of industrial sites and major route ways [4]. Historically, the major sources of pollutants to the atmosphere were derived from the burning of fossil fuels, which released particulates and heavy metals [5]. Following legislation, in the 1950s, emissions have been controlled to some extent and the delivery of atmospheric particulates and heavy metals has been reduced [6]. However, the rapid rise of the automobile, over the last 50 years, has meant vehicle emissions are now a major component of atmospheric pollution [7].

Particulate materials, particularly <10 μm (known as PM10s), are acknowledged to contribute to serious human health problems [8, 9]. Indeed, it is now widely reported that particulates <2.5μm diameter (known as PM2.5) may be instrumental in contributing to a wide variety of diseases, most notably cancers [10, 11]. Similarly, high-density urbanisation and industrialisation goes hand-in-hand with serious concerns about human health, where high mortality rates, hospital admission and referrals are concentrated [12, 13].

2 Records of air pollution in urban sites

The majority of work reporting historical atmospheric pollution records come from relatively remote locations, either in peat deposits or lake sediments, well removed from the major sources of industrial output [14, 15]. A few studies [16, 17] have examined urban sites but the majority of work conducted within the urban setting has concentrated on contemporary monitoring of atmospheric pollution using road dusts, surface soils and filtration/capture equipment, and stations recording daily air quality [18]. While this contemporary monitoring yields significant spatial information about diurnal and seasonal changes, plus the relationship of air quality to weather patterns, there is a distinct need to generate information about the temporal patterns of atmospheric pollution. Lake sites within an urban setting, which will yield historical records, are rare and therefore hugely important, as they will allow the construction of datable, detailed historical archives of changes in atmospheric pollution, which may then be examined alongside the historical community health archives for the area in question.

3 The need for datable urban archives

To fully understand and appreciate the relationship between human health and atmospheric pollution, researchers must not only examine the contemporary situation but also the historic one, because both the nature of atmospheric pollution and the style of life in communities have changed considerably over time. This means that the physiological effects of changing types of atmospheric particulates upon humans may have altered. So there is a clear need to examine whether air quality has had an impact on local communities in the past. To do this, datable and detailed temporal records must be obtained. Until recently, the majority of historical environmental records have come from remote and rural locations and while this work clearly demonstrates that atmospheric pollution is widespread and ubiquitous [19], it does not allow for a very detailed examination of datable environmental archives (with records of disease) for *urban* communities. Public health archives become less reliable and lose clarity further back in time as they rely more on the recording of oral histories and increasingly scant documentation [20]. It is vital therefore, that sites from within the urban landscape are identified, tested for their suitability and then used for detailed investigation to produce a datable, accurate, temporal and high-resolution pollution history. Where that is possible, and when such records are generated, environmental and public health workers may test the relationship between them, in the hope that they will deepen our understanding of how community health has been affected by the changing nature of atmospheric pollution over time. It is from the sedimentary archives, rather than the local community histories, that reliable, accurate information about the nature and extent of atmospheric pollution may be obtained. Where that is achieved, medical health specialists may be able to determine the relative importance of local environment and lifestyle to the problems of community disease patterns, in particular, problems associated with lung disease and specific cancers.

The need then, is to identify and select urban sites that may be able to generate suitable sediment histories, and to submit them to a series of scientific techniques, to produce an environmental history for the site. Using historical maps, documents and archaeological records, lake sites found within modern conurbations and industrial centres can be subjected to rigorous investigations to determine their suitability. Sadly many such sites have either been in-filled, desilted or have totally disappeared under spreading urban developments. However, in South Merseyside, northwest England, a viable, small, anthropogenic lake site has been identified within an urban, industrial area, which has witnessed the birth and development of chemical industries. The lake has yielded a well-dated, high-resolution record of atmospheric pollution and land use change.

4   Lake sediments

Lake sediments have long been used as archives of environmental information since they act as natural repositories for atmospheric and catchment-based materials [21]. Many studies report their use in reconstructing environmental histories and lake sites of varying size, shape and situation around the world have been investigated documenting land-use change, lake acidification and erosion studies [22,23]. It is recognised that, if a lake has not been disturbed by drainage or desilting over the course of its history then as sediments accumulate they will capture a record of ecological change and anthropogenic impact at a range of resolutions. Both atmospheric deposition directly to the surface of the lake together with catchment input through inflowing streams or groundwater flow provides material, which becomes entrained within the deepening sediment column [24]. The lake and its catchment can then be seen as a 'trap' for local and regional environmental change. The sediments themselves may be subjected to a wide range of analytical techniques that allow the generation of information about atmospheric pollution and catchment (land-use) change.

5 Case study at the Speke Hall site

Surrounded by the urban areas of Speke, Halewood and Garston, in south Liverpool, the lake at Speke Hall is located in an area that includes the heavy industries of Widnes and Runcorn, East Wirral, the Stanlow oil refinery and the city centre and docklands of Liverpool (Figure 1). Major industries include coal and oil fired power stations, shipbuilding, chemical and petro-chemicals, pharmaceuticals and the burgeoning John Lennon International Airport immediately adjacent to the site. Urban communities and landscapes situated in and around these major sites receive the atmospheric pollution output generated by their industrial activity.

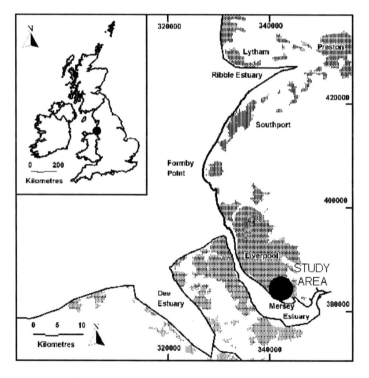

Figure 1: Location map of the study area.

The small lake at Speke Hall satisfies the requirements for the research programme, in that historical maps and documents attest to its anthropogenic origins, its maintenance, lack of disturbance and its longevity: in order to generate a suitable archive covering the rise of industrial development from the late seventeenth century onwards (the Industrial Revolution) the lake needed to be at least 300 years old. The site is approximately 11 km south of Liverpool

City Centre and lies close to the River Mersey (~20 m a.s.l.). At its deepest, the lake is 3-4m deep and it has a surface area of 30 m² derived from a modern–day catchment of approximately 620 m². There is no fluvial drainage either into or out from the lake at the present time.

5.1 Methodology

The lake was cored using a Gilsen hand operated piston corer and four cores were obtained from the deepest part of the lake. These were sampled at 0.5 cm intervals and the sediment dried at 35°C, packed into 10ml plastic pots [25] and subsequently subjected to mineral magnetic analyses (magnetic susceptibility measurements using a Bartington MS2 Magnetic Susceptibility Meter). Sediment chemistry was determined using an energy dispersive isotope source x-ray fluorescence (XRF) analyser [26]. Total concentrations of Aluminium (Al), Bromine (Br), Calcium (Ca), Iron (Fe), Lead (Pb), Manganese (Mn), Nickel (Ni), Potassium K), Silicon, Si), Sulphur (S), Titanium, (Ti), Zinc (Zn) and Zirconium (Zr) were obtained for Core 2. Of these Br, Cu, Ni, Pb and Zn are chiefly derived from atmospheric deposition [27] and Pb is used (Graph 1) for the purposes of this paper. Spheroidal carbonaceous particles (SCPs) were counted for the top 8 cm following procedures described by Rose [28]. Further SCP characterisation was conducted using a Scanning Electron Microscope (SEM), namely A Zeiss EVO-50 SEM, using an Oxford Instruments INCx-sight analyser, software V05.00.09 (21 Feb 2005), supplied by Carl Zeiss SMT Ltd. (Cambridge, U.K.), was employed. Work continues on the remaining samples.

Table 1: ^{210}Pb chronology for sediment core 2.

Depth		Chronology	
cm	G cm^{-2}	Date AD	Age (y)
0.5	0.03	1999	2
1.5	0.10	1994	7
3.5	0.28	1979	22
5.5	0.46	1963	38
7.5	0.65	1949	52
9.5	0.88	1932	69
11.5	1.15	1912	89
14.5	1.63	1881	120

5.2 ^{210}Pb dating

Dried sediment from core 2 was analysed for ^{210}Pb, ^{226}Ra, ^{137}Cs, ^{241}Am at Liverpool University's Environmental Radioactivity Laboratory. ^{210}Pb dates were calculated using the CRS dating model [29] and the 1963 depth was determined from the ^{137}Cs record, which places 1963 at a depth of 6.3 cm. The dating therefore suggests that sedimentation rates have been fairly uniform during the past century (0.013 g cm^{-2} y^{-1}). Table 1 shows the ^{210}Pb chronology of core 2; the dating results are discussed further in Worsley et al., [30]. But it is clear from Table 1 that 14.5 cm gives a date of 1881 and if the mean sedimentation rate is assumed for the lower core then at 24.5 cm it equates to a date of 1800. However, below this depth the sediment column is comprised of a thick clay layer (itself 24 cm deep), which represents the basal clay lining. Given that the lake (named the Higher Damme) was already in existence by the time that Addison's 1781 map was published and that detailed records from the Speke Hall Estate (1710-1719) clearly account for the "Higher Damme" [31], then the sedimentation rate for the core between 14.5 cm and 24.5 cm is notably lower, between 0.45 and 0.6 cm y^{-1}. This then includes the period of the Industrial Revolution and the start of the major industrialisation of the Mersey region.

(a)   (b)

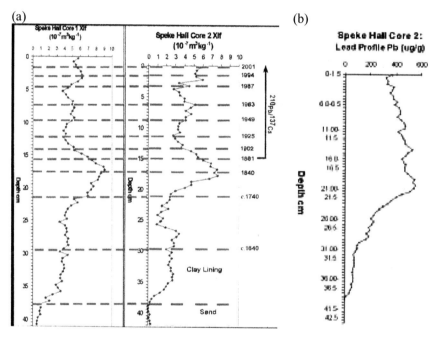

Figure 2:   Sediment profile data (a) χ_{LF} for cores 1 & 2, with radiometric datable horizons labelled and (b) Pb concentration profile for core 2.

5.3 Results and discussion

Low frequency magnetic susceptibility (χ_{LF}) for cores 1 and 2 and demonstrates the efficacy of χ_{LF} for correlation and any concerns of sediment disturbance in the past are dismissed (Figure 2). For reference, χ_{LF} (measured within a small magnetic field and is reversible, i.e. no remanence is induced) is roughly proportional to the concentration of ferrimagnetic minerals within the sample, although in materials with little or no ferrimagnetic component and a relatively large antiferromagnetic component, the latter may dominate the signal.

The profiles suggest three major phases:

Phase 3:	1970–2000 (4.5–0 cm)	Replacement of old industries, expansion of road and air traffic
Phase 2:	1881–1970 (14.5–4.5 cm)	Regional expansion of industrial Merseyside
Phase 1:	1700–1881 (24.5–14.5 cm)	Early industrialisation in the Speke area

The Pb profile (Figure 2b) is noteworthy because lead is important to the regional and local history, Lead was used extensively on the Speke Hall estate [31] and it was produced widely at Widnes as part of the manufacture of Sulphuric Acid [32, 33]. High values in the lower part of the core support the conclusion that the lower χLF values result from intensive local industrial activity. The values decline but still reflect the regional signal along with the magnetic measurements and the various peaks can be attributed to changes in the chemical industries along with the arrival of car and air transport [30].

SCP counts demonstrate that a major contribution of atmospheric pollution comes from combustion processes. The χLF peak at 3.5 cm (Figure 3) is therefore largely accounted for by these particulates. Implications for discussions about human health are paramount. Further results and discussion will be disseminated in future publications.

(a)   (b)

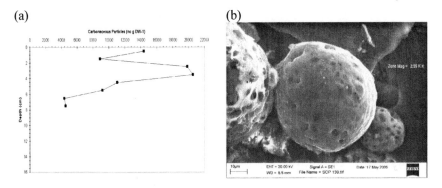

Figure 3:   (a) Spheroidal Carbonaceous Particle (SCP) counts for Core 1 and (b) SEM image of SCP grains.

6   Conclusions

A combination of sedimentary analytical techniques on sediment cores taken from Speke Hall Lake (Merseyside) demonstrate it is possible to reconstruct a datable archive of atmospheric pollution from within an urban area. Rather than relying on remote sites to produce such records, with care and detailed investigations into their history, small urban lakes and ponds can be used effectively. Records produced at Speke show the development of local and regional industry and its contribution to the atmosphere and they can therefore be used as a detailed record of atmospheric pollution. Public health and medical workers in turn can now use this information, as they strive to understand the contribution of the region's industrial legacy to community health problems.

Acknowledgements

This research forms part of the research development programme funded by Edge Hill University College. All authors would like to thank Mrs Barbara Hodson of the School of Applied Sciences at the University of Wolverhampton for her SEM technical support.

References

[1]   Brunekreef, B. & Holgate, S.T., Air pollution and health. The Lancet, 360, No. 9341, pp. 1233-1255, 2002.
[2]   Gulland, A., Air pollution responsible for 600 000 premature deaths worldwide. British Medical Journal, 325, pp. 1380-1381, 2002.
[3]   Parodi, S., Vercelli, M., Stella, A., Stagnaro, E. & Valerio, F., Lymphohaematopoietic system cancer incidence in an urban area near a coke oven plant: an ecological investigation. Occupational & Environmental Medicine, 60, pp. 187-195, 2003.
[4]   Department of Geography and Institute for Health Research Lancaster University. Understanding the factors affecting health in Halton: Final Report. August 2003.
[5]   Dugan, S., The Day the World Took Off: the Roots of the Industrial Revolution. Macmillan, London, 2000.
[6]   Blakemore, F.B., Davies, C. & Isaac, J.G., Effects of the changes in the UK energy demand and environmental legislation of atmospheric pollution by sulphur dioxide. Applied Energy, 62, pp. 283-295, 1999.
[7]   Williams, M., Atmospheric pollution: contribution of automobiles. Revue Francaise d'Allergologie et d'Immunologie Clinique, 327, pp. 219-221, 2000.
[8]   Etzel, R.A., How environmental exposures influence the development and exacerbation of asthma. Pediatrics, 112, pp. 233 – 230, 2003.
[9]   Le Tertre, A., Medina, S., Samoli, E., Forsberg, B., Michelozzi, P., Boumghar, A., Vonk, J.M., Bellini, A., Atkinson, R., Ayres. J.G., Sunyer, J., Schwartz, J. & Katsouyanni, K., Shot-term effects of particulate air pollution on cardio-vascular diseases in eight European cities. Journal of Epidemiology and Health, 56, pp. 773-780, 2002.
[10]   Lippmann, M., Winter air pollution and respiratory function. Occupational and Environmental Medicine, 60, pp 80-81, 2003.
[11]   Peters, A. & Pope, C.A., Cardiopulmonary mortality and air pollution. The Lancet, 360, pp. 1184-1185, 2002.
[12]   Fileul, L., Medina, S. & Cassadou, S., Atmospheric pollution and health: not patently obvious... and yet! Revue d'Epidemiologie et de Sante Publique, 50, pp. 325-327, 2002.

[13] Kelly, F., Oxidative stress: its role in air pollution and adverse health effects. Occupational & Environmental Medicine, 60, pp. 612-617, 2003.

[14] Lindstrom, M., Urban land uses influences on heavy metal fluxes and surface sediment concentrations of small lakes. Water, Air & Soil Pollution, 126, pp. 363-383, 2001.

[15] Dearing, J.A., Boyle, J.F., Appleby, P.G., Mackay, A. & Flower, R.J., Magnetic properties of recent lake sediments in Lake Baikal, Siberia. Journal of Palaeolimnology, 20, pp. 163-173, 1998.

[16] Merialinen, J.J., Hynynen. J. Palomaki, A., Mantykoski, K. & Witick, A., Environmental history of an urban lake: a palaeolimnological study of Lake Jyvasjarvi, Finland. Journal of Palaeolimnology, 18, pp. 75-85, 2003.

[17] Charlesworth, S.M. & Lees, J.A., The use of mineral magnetic measurements in polluted urban lakes and deposited dusts, Coventry, UK. The Physics & Chemistry of the Earth, 22, pp. 203-206, 1997.

[18] Shilton, V.F., Booth, C.A., Smith, J.P., Giess, P., Mitchell, D.J. & Williams C.D., Magnetic properties of urban street dusts and their relationship with organic matter content in the West Midlands, UK. Atmospheric Environment, (in press), 2005.

[19] Petrovsky, E. & Ellwood, B.B., Magnetic monitoring of air-, land- and water-pollution. In: Maher, B.A. & Thompson, R. (eds) Quaternary Climates, Environments and Magnetism. Cambridge University Press, 2000.

[20] Department of Geography and Institute for Health Research Lancaster University. Understanding the factors affecting health in Halton: Final Report. August 2003.

[21] Oldfield, F., Lakes and their drainage basins as units of sediment-based ecological study. Progress in Physical geography, 1, pp. 460-504, 1977.

[22] Dearing, J.A., Holocene environmental changes from magnetic proxies in lake sediments. In: Maher, B.A. & Thompson, R. (eds) Quaternary Climates, Environments and Magnetism. Cambridge University Press, 2000.

[23] Edwards, K.J. & Whittington, G., Lake sediments, erosion and landscape change during the Holocen in Britain and Ireland. Catena, 42, pp. 143-173, 2001

[24] Von Gunten, H.R., Sturm, M. & Moser, R.N., 200-year record of metals in lake sediments and natural background concentrations. Environmental Science & Technology, 31, pp. 2193-2198, 1997.

[25] Walden, J., Oldfield, F. & Smith, J. (eds) Environmental Magnetism: a practical guide. QRA technical Guide No 5. London, 1999.

[26] Boyle, J., Rapid element analysis of sediment samples by isotope source XRF. Journal of Palaeolimnology, 23, pp. 213-221, 2000.

[27] Galloway, J.N., Thornton, J.D., Norton, S.A., Volchok, H.L. & McLean, R.A., Trace metals in atmospheric deposition: a review and assessment. Atmospheric Environment, 16, pp. 1677-1700, 1982.

[28]   Rose, N.L., Characterisation of carbonaceous particles from lake sediments, Hydrobiologia, 274, pp.127-132, 1994.
[29]   Appleby, P.G. & Oldfield, F., The calculation of 210Pb dates assuming a constant rate of supply of unsupported 210Pb to the sediment. Catena, 5, pp. 228-233, 1978.
[30]   Worsley, A.T., Booth, C.A., Richardson, N. & Appleby, P.G., A record of recent environmental change from a small, man-made lake in urban Merseyside, UK. (in prep.), 2005.
[31]   Nicolson, S., Farming at Speke Hall 1066-1795. Liverpool, Mersyeside Archaeological Society, 1983.
[32]   Jones, A.D., Industry & Runcorn 1750 to 1960. Publicity & Information services Department, Halton Borough Council. January 1969.
[33]   Warren. K., Chemical Foundations: The Alkali Industry in Britain to 1926. Clarendon Press, Oxford, 1980.

Contamination by particulated material in blasts: analysis, application and adaptation of the existent calculation formulas and software

J. Toraño, R. Rodríguez, I. Diego & A. Pelegry
Mining and Mine Prospecting Department, University of Oviedo

Abstract

In the setting of a research project about the blasting negative effects granted with public funds coming from the Spanish Ministry for Development, several measurement campaigns were developed, in various locations and situations, where earth vibrations, aerial waves and dust in suspension simultaneously measured. Taking into account the dust negative effects (for human health, inhabited environment or plants) it is interesting to have available tools that allow the estimation of the particulated material quantities ejected in a blast (already studied by our research team in other cases). Here we show the application of the standardised computational methods for atmospheric contamination (developed for other applications) in the specific case of blasting in mining and civil works. To do so we have used the field data collected in blasts at a maritime port and at a limestone quarry. We will also show the advantages of using CFD when solving some of these problems, which is being studied in other research projects.
Keywords: particulated material, blast, atmospheric contamination, dust.

1 Dust generation in a blast

One of the main particle sources of the atmospheric contamination are the industrial activities. From their size and nature we can infer the affections that dust can induce in human beings. According to dust size we can categorize it in three groups: breathable dust (particles so small that go directly to lungs), inhaled dust (one part is retained by the upper part of the human breathing system, whit diameters around 10 μm) and total dust. Up to recent dates it was thought that the harmful action of those particles in people was limited to breathing system (National Institute for Silicosis Disease [4]) with the result of a first classification according to human beings affections: pneumoconiotic dust, toxic dust, inert dust and allergic dust.

Studies done "ad hoc" proof that during the last years there are more evidences of carcinogenic effects of dust containing free silica (International Agency for Cancer Research [5]) and the contribution of those particles to the cardiovascular pathologies (Ballester [6]). We must point out that the diseases produced by these contaminations have a special importance on children (World Health Organization Reports [7]). Blasting, or rock explosions, involves a high level of contamination by particulated material. This dust sources are intermittent, frequent, sporadic and very short in time. A cloud is produced, formed by the pulverized rock, the perforation debris and the projection of the dust previously settled in the blasting area.

2 Measurement campaigns to characterize the dust produced in a blast

The 4 measurement campaigns selected for this study were done in "El Musel" maritime port (blasts in concrete structures) and in "El Perejil" limestone quarry, both in Asturias, northern Spain. During the measurement campaigns we used dust collectors Met One (< 50 μ), which allow continuous measurement of PM-2.5, PM-10, total particles, atmospheric pressure and temperature, as well as meteorological stations (sensors E-sampler EX034 and HR-E Sampler EX593) in order to measure continuously air humidity and wind speed and direction.

2.1 Blasts in a maritime port

First blasts were done in 10th of April, 2004 at the dock of "La Osa" wharf (Figures 1 and 2), where a 100 meters long concrete dock wall was being demolished. The blasting characteristics are shown in Table 1. Meteorological conditions during the test were: temperature of 8°C, 1022 millibar atmospheric pressure, clouds, no rain, wind speed ranging 1-2 m/s and 40-60° of bearing in relation to the concrete wall, very small sunshine ratio (due to clouds) and relative humidity between 60-80%. We can say also that the ground was wet due to past days rain and the area was a suburban zone with wind flow obstacles in the back side of the dock and completely free from obstacles in the wind upcoming area.

Table 1:   Blasting characteristics.

Height, Burden and shots spacing(m)	3.80, 1.3 and 1.2
Length, diameter, slope, clay stopper	4 m, 54 mm, 5 (°) and 2.4 m
Main and Bottom Load	0.87 kg and 0.46 kg, dynamite
Number of shots and type of firing	80, non electric detonators

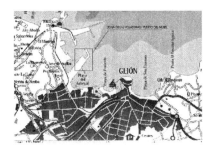

Figure 1: Port location.

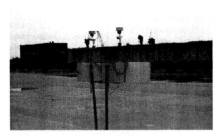

Figure 2: Dock wall and installed dust collectors.

In a first step the dust sensors were installed together 40 meters apart from the blast, one measuring PM-2.5 and another one PM-10; in a second step we brought one of the sensors close to the blast (12 m from it), measuring both of them total particles before and after the blast. Before the blast the PM-10 dust concentration ranged from 0.02 to 0.025 mg/m^3; PM-2.5 ranged again from 0.02 to 0.025 mg/m^3. Figures 3 and 4 show the concentration increase of total particles. Calculations done from the samples give values of: 40 m apart from the dock (C) = 0.220 mg/m^3 and 12 m from the dock (C) = 0.359 mg/m3. In 2 minutes, approximately, the particle concentration measurement gets stabilized again, as the dust cloud has already been displaced by the wind.

On 19th April, 2004 other two dock concrete pieces were blasted, as is shown in Figure 5. Meteorological conditions were: temperature of 11°C, 1007 millibar atmospheric pressure, clouds, no rain, wind speed ranging 4-5 m/s and 5-15° of bearing in relation to the concrete wall, very small sunshine ratio (due to clouds) and relative humidity between 60-80%. Again the ground was wet due to previous the day's rain and there were no obstacles to wind in the area. 2 dust collectors were installed 25 m and 50 m respectively apart and perpendicular to the dock. Table 2 and Table 3 show the blasts main characteristics. The sensor measured the particle concentration increase due to the 2 blasts in the same way as the previous blast. Dust concentration produced by blast in the points where the sensors were installed were: 25 m from the dock (C) = 1.069 mg/m^3, and 50 m from the dock (C) = 0.829 mg/m^3.

2.2 Blasts in a limestone quarry

The quarry is located in the core of the downfold geological structure and produces limestone (Figure 7). The meteorological conditions in the first measured blasts, 13th May 2004, were: temperature of 18°C, 1022.5 millibar atmospheric pressure, sunny day with no clouds, no rain, wind speed ranging 1-2 m/s and 90° of bearing in relation to the trench face, high sunshine ratio and relative humidity between 50-60%, upper part of bench wet. Country area. Blast characteristics are shown in Table 4 and Figure 8.

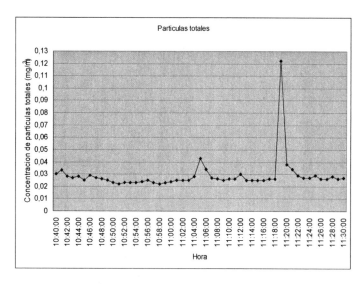

Figure 3:   Total particle sample @ 40m collector.

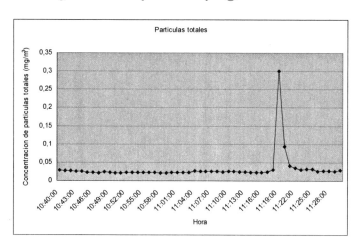

Figure 4:   Total particle sample @ 12m collector.

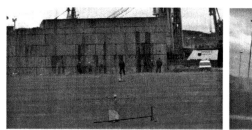
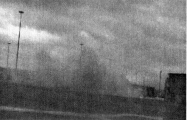

Figure 5: Initial time.   Figure 6: Dust dispersion.

Table 2:   Blast characteristics – First section of dock

Height, Burden and shots spacing(m)	3, 1,4 and 1,2
Length, diameter, slope, clay stopper	54 mm, vertical and 2,4 m
Main and Bottom Load	1,45 kg and 0.69 kg
Number of shots and type of firing	64 non electric detonators

Table 3:   Blast characteristics – Second section of dock

Height, Burden and shots spacing(m)	4.5, 1.4 and 1.2
Length, diameter, slope, clay stopper	54 mm, vertical + horizontal, 2.4 m
Main and Bottom Load	1.74 kg, 0.69 kg and 1.71 kg
Number of shots and type of firing	44, non electric detonators

Two dust collector were installed 125 meters apart from the bench in the covering area, measuring PM-2.5 and PM-10 before blasting; further on total particles were measured before and after the blasting (Figures 9 and 10).

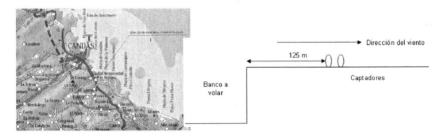

Figure 7:   "El Perecil" quarry map.   Figure 8:   Sensors location.

Table 4:   Characteristics of the bench blasting (UEE explosives).

Height, Burden and shot spacing (m)	18, 4 and 5
Length, diameter, slope, clay stopper	120 mm, 15°, horizontal, 3 m
Total Load (dynamite), Nr of shots	1175 kg and 13
Bottom and Head firing, Detonating cord type and firing	EZDET (25/350 ms) and Ms N° 16 (450 ms)
Firing and detonating cord	Electrical Nr 0 and EZTL (17ms);20m

The particle PM-2.5 concentration ranged between 0.03 and 0.05 mg/m^3 and PM-10 concentration ranged between 0.035 and 0.06 mg/m^3. Total particle concentration alter the blast were similar, with values of 0.156 mg/m^3 and 0.199 mg/m^3 , which means a mean value of 0.177 mg/m^3. Figures 11 and 12 show the dust formation and dispersion phases, as well as the position of the dust collectors. Although the blast boost down and straight the dust cloud it then follows the wind direction, slides over the bench face, overpass it and then were dispersed.

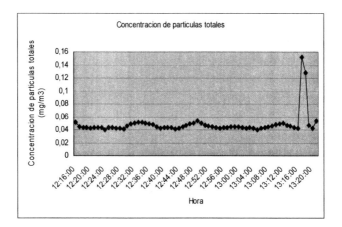

Figure 9:   Total particules sample – collector 1.

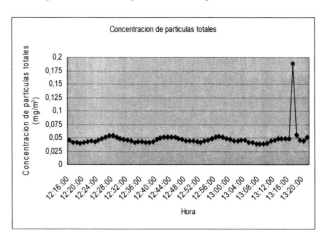

Figure 10:   Total particules sample – collector 2.

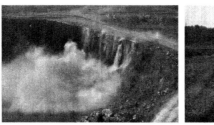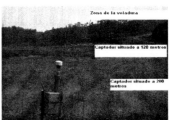

Figure 11: Dust creation.   Figure 12: Samplers detail.

21st May 2004 blasts and its main characteristics are shown in Table 5. Dust concentration produced by the blast was, where the dust collectors were installed, 0.406 mg/m^3 200 m apart from the bench and 0.733 mg/m^3 120 m apart. In the same way as in the previous cases, dust was boosted down and straight and then back following wind direction.

Table 5:   Characteristics of the blasting (UEE explosives). 21-04-04.

Height, Burden and shot spacing (m)	16,2, 4 and 5
Length, diameter, slope, clay stopper	120 mm; 15° and horizontal; 2,83 m
Total Load (dynamite) and shot Nr	1300 kg ; 12
Bottom and Head firing	EZDET(25/350ms);Ms Nr16 (450ms)
Firing and detonating cord	Electrical Nr0;EZTL (17ms); 19 m

3   Blast simulation using isc3 software

3.1 Maritimal port blast

We will use ISC3 software [8] and [9] in order to simulate the blasts measured. Meteorological field data are introduced in the ISC3, obtaining Table 6 as the meteorological values output. Figure 13 shows the inferred wind rose. Dust sources are introduced defining the size of the blasted dock, its emission height and the amount of emitted pollutant. Source used will be polygonal type, as it allows us to define the irregular shape of the dock, using UTM coordinate systems in order to maintain portability with software Aermod. We will also define in the software the particle nature, its size distribution and its density, s well as the source coordinates and the measuring point's coordinates in order to simulate the same configuration as we had in the blast measuring campaigns.

Starting from the coordinates assigned to the source we establish two receptors types. The first is a discrete network made by 2 node receptors that simulate the position of the samplers in the field tests and that will allow us to check the modelization against the field measurements. The second one is a regular Cartesian mesh of receptors, located in the wind downstream that will show us the pollution level where we do not have samplers. So once we have checked with the first type of receptors that the software is doing right by comparing measured values with the simulated ones, we can rely on the simulated values that are given by the second type of receptors.

Table 6:   Meteorological calculated values.

Random Flow Vector	Wind Speed (m/s)	Ambient Temperature (K)	Stability Category	Rural Mixing Height (m)	Urban Mixing Height (m)	Friction Velocity at the Application Site (m/s)	Monin-Obukhov Length at the Application Site (m)	Roughness Length at the Application Site (m)	Global Horizontal Radiation (W/m2)	Relative Humidity (%)
141,0000	1,5433	280,9	4	398,2	613,8	0,3179	-56,3	1,0000	0	70

The emission rate by area unit is the parameter that will be modified, tuned, until we get the adjustment of the simulation to the field data. Once all the parameters are introduced we obtain results shown in Figure 14 and Table 7, where we are showing respectively concentration isosurfaces and the values obtained by the software simulation in the sampled points. We can clearly see how the dust is dispersed in the wind direction in an opening cone shape (figure 15). If we proceed in the same way with the second blasting measurements we obtain analogue outputs shown in Figures 16, 17 and Table 8. This time the source has to be double, as the dock is made by two different areas (one point source and another polygonal source).

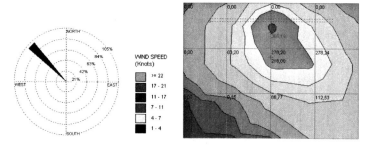

Figure 13: Wind rose.   Figure 14.

Table 7.

Dust concentration	
Field measures	ISCT3 Simulation
359 μg/m³	366 μg/m³
220 μg/m³	218 μg/m³

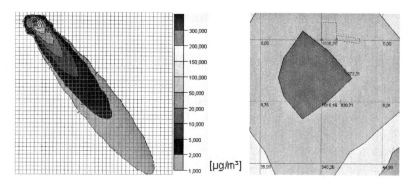

Figure 15.   Figure 16.

Table 8.

Dust concentration	
Field measures	ISCT3 Simulation
1069 μg/m³	1072 μg/m³
829 μg/m³	820 μg/m³

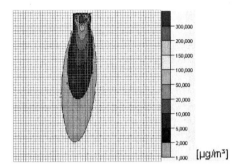

Figure 17.

3.2 Limestone quarry blasting

Following the methodology described in the previous case the results for the first group of samples are shown in Table 9 and in figure 18. Figure 19 shows the cone dispersion (concentration) of the particulated material as was obtained from the simulation.

Table 9.

Dust concentration	
Field measures	ISCT3 Simulation
177 μg/m³	177 μg/m³

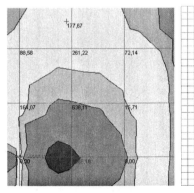

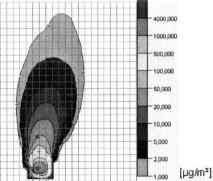

Figure 18.   Figure 19.

Proceeding again in the same way the second group of blasts calculations are shown in Table 10, Figure 20 and Figure 21.

Table 10.

Dust concentration	
Field measures	ISCT3 Simulation
733 μg/m^3	825 μg/m^3
406 μg/m^3	400 μg/m^3

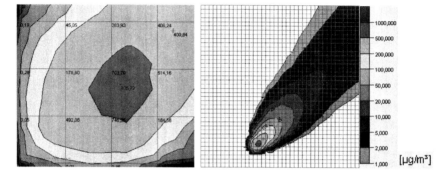

Figure 20.   Figure 21.

4 Conclusions

In mining and civil works blasts is possible to establish prediction models that simulate with enough accuracy and simplicity the behaviour of the emission and propagation of the particulated material using easy-to-use software as ISC3, [8] and [9]. This is done through the adjustment of the software using a simple measurement campaign deploying dust collectors and meteorological sensors. In case of complex blasting geometries or highly irregular terrain is necessary to use other modelization tools as numerical codes (CFD).

References

[1] J. Toraño et al. (2003) Oviedo University-Ministry for Development Contract FOM 1540/2002 (within the Priority Action Framework "New Technologies and Constructive Systems", of the Sectorial Area "Building and Cultural Heritage Conservation" National R&D&I Plan 2000-2003).
[2] J. Toraño, R. Rodríguez, J.M. Rivas, A. Pelegry (2004) Diminishing of the dust quantity during the management of granular material in an underground space. XII International Conference on Modelling Monitoring and management of Air Pollution (Air Pollution 2004).
[3] J. Toraño et al. (2004) Oviedo University, Carbonar Company and FICYT (R&D Foundation) Contract IE 03-86

[4] Several studies at "Instituto Nacional de Silicosis" (National Institute for Silicosis), Spain.
[5] Annual Report of the International Agency for Cancer Research. 1997.
[6] Ferrán Ballester (2003): Estudio multicéntrico español sobre la relación entre contaminación atmosférica y mortalidad. EMECAM-EMECAS. Medicina Clínica. Madrid.
[7] Environmental Contamination and Global Climate Change. The future for our children. Fourth Ministerial Conference on Environment and Health, WHO. Budapest, 2004.
[8] ISCST3 and AERMOD of software ISC-AERMOD View 4.6.2b from Lakes Environmental Software.
[9] ISCST3, (1999): U.S. EPA, 1999. Addendum - Users Guide for the Industrial Source Complex (ISC3) Dispersion Models, Volume 1. Office of Air Quality Planning and Standards, Research Triangle Park, NC. RAMMET, U.S. EPA - 454 / B-96-001 (Revised June 1999)

Population exposure to urban highway traffic emissions

N. Barros, T. Fontes, C. Brás & L. M. Cunha
*Center of Environmental Modelling and Systems Analysis,
Fernando Pessoa University, Portugal*

Abstract

In this paper is presented firstly the traffic and emission characterization of Via de Cintura Interna (VCI), an urban highway at Oporto city, Portugal, with more than 4 000 vehicles/hour during rush hours. Emission estimates were carried through on the basis of emission factors to road transport published in the Atmospheric Emission Inventory Guidebook. A weighed emission factor has been calculated for nitrogen oxides (NO_x) and vehicle class, according to the Portuguese fleet composition (vehicles age, type of engine and average speed). Furthermore, during a three-week period, an outdoor nitrogen dioxide (NO_2) monitoring campaign was carried out in a domain around the VCI (100 m for each side), in particular near residential buildings. The results demonstrate that higher NO_2 concentrations are seen in the sub-domain with higher circulation of heavy-duty vehicles and where buildings are adjacent to VCI hindering pollutant dispersion. Meteorological conditions, such as wind intensity and direction, temperature and solar radiation were monitorized too. The NO_2 concentrations obtained by the monitoring campaign have been used to create scenarios of population exposure to NO_2, having taken into account the time-activity patterns of residents. It was verified that higher exposures occur when the population lives in Boavista, in contrast with the favourable scenario that corresponds to life in Prelada and those working in Espinho city. The work and results presented in this paper are a part of the methodology used in the scope of the ImpactAir Project. This project, started in 2003 in Oporto city, has the main objective of evaluating the impact of urban highway (VCI) traffic emissions on air quality and the health of the local population.
Keywords: air pollution, traffic, population exposure, health risk.

1 Introduction

Health effects of pollution are continuously under study. In 1999 it remained unknown whether the absolute concentration of pollution or the rate of change of concentrations had the greatest effect on different health end-points [1]. Epidemiological studies have confirmed the impact of air pollution on different respiratory health parameters and mortality. The effects of air pollution in population health depend directly from pollutants concentrations and exposure time and may be sharp or chronic. The knowledge of population health before the occurrence of harmful effects is important in the establishment of prevention programs [2]. Depending on the effects related to each substance, atmospheric pollutants are regulated with respect to different exposure times.

In urban environments and especially in those areas where population and traffic density are relatively high, human exposure to hazardous substances is expected to be significantly increased. This is often the case near busy traffic axis in city centers, where urban topography and microclimate may contribute to the creation of poor air dispersion conditions giving rise to contamination hotspots. High pollution levels have been observed in street canyons. Within these streets, pedestrians, cyclists, drivers and residents are likely to be exposed to pollutant concentrations exceeding current air quality standards [3]. Vehicular exhaust emission has gradually become the major air pollution source in modern cities and traffic related exposure is found to contribute significantly to total human exposure level [4]. Although technological improvements and more stringent emission standards have led to a remarkable reduction in emission levels for new vehicles over the last 25 years, these reductions are being counteracted by the continuing increase in traffic volumes [5]. There are studies focused on the association between road proximity and respiratory disease, lung cancer and stroke mortality. Some of these studies were conducted in countries across Europe [6, 7, 8] in United States [9, 10], in Hamilton, Canada [11], etc.

This paper focused on the study of population exposure to traffic emissions of VCI, in the scope of ImpactAir Project. VCI is an urban highway that crosses the city of Oporto, making the linking between Arrábida and Freixo bridges over Douro River. It serves not only the urban traffic, but also the long-range traffic between the main cities of the Peninsular Northeastern. As urban highway, VCI presents proper characteristics that distinguishes it from other arteries of Oporto city and the remaining highways of the country, provoking inevitably diverse environmental, socio-economic and health impacts.

2 The ImpactAir project

The main objective of the ImpactAir project (Urban Large Traffic Lines Impact on Health and Air Quality; The VCI Case) is to evaluate the emission impact of VCI on air quality and health of the local population. Additionally, a numerical model will be implemented and evaluated in order to predict the outdoor and indoor air quality near VCI and other Large Traffic Lines (LTL's). The numerical model should be a tool for people involved in urban planning and air quality management.

The project is divided in four tasks that consist of: indoor and outdoor air quality campaigns to measure traffic related pollutants; application of epidemiological questionnaires to sensitive and control groups; development, application and evaluation of a numerical model to predict emission impacts from traffic of VCI and other LTL's in air quality and health; and finally, the elaboration of a good practice manual to reduce those impacts and support politic decision maker.

3 Methodology and results

The methodology presented in this paper is a part of the work done in the scope of ImpactAir project. Firstly NO_x emissions estimates were calculated on the basis of emission factors to road transport published in Atmospheric Emission Inventory Guidebook [12] and traffic counts in VCI during April 2004. At the same time, during a three-week period, an outdoor NO_2 diffusive sampler monitoring campaign was carried out. Meteorological conditions, such as wind intensity and direction, temperature and solar radiation were also monitorized and have been taken in account. Finally, the results of this campaign and time-activity patterns have been used to create scenarios of population exposure to NO_2.

3.1 Traffic analysis and emission estimates

In this study 4 sub-domains of VCI were selected: Boavista, Prelada, Amial and Antas (Figure 1). In these sub-domains, strategic access points to center city with high traffic flow and sensitive zones (hospitals, schools, sport and residential zones) are placed.

3.1.1 Traffic analysis
The images recorded on video cameras located in the study sub-domains (Figure 1), have been used to do the traffic countings for vehicle category between 30/03/2004 and 05/04/2004. The differentiation of 5 vehicle categories was carried through having in account the definitions adopted by the Emission Inventory Guidebook [12], the Insurance Portuguese Institute [13] and the characteristic of VCI: passengers cars (PC), light duty vehicles (LDV), buses (B), heavy duty vehicles (HDV) and motorcycles (M) with more than 50 c.c. The countings have been done throughout 24 hours, in alternating periods of 15 minutes, in each felt of VCI, in a total of 8 days: 1 day in Amial (Wednesday), 2 in Antas (Tuesday and Saturday) and Boavista (Thursday and Monday) and 3 in Prelada (Saturday, Sunday and Monday).

The variation of daily average of traffic in VCI (Figure 2) evidences that minimum values of traffic happen during the night, between 04H00 and 05H00, while maximums between 08H00 and 19H00. In average, in VCI circulate about 107.000 vehicles/day in both directions, of which 82.6% are PC; 11.3% LDV;

5.4% HDV; 0.3% B and 0.4% M. This average distribution floats relatively little in each direction (Arrábida/Freixo or Freixo/Arrábida), but in the opposite, a significant difference is verified when weekend and workdays are compared, in particular for the categories of PC and HDV on Sundays, as expected, given the legislation in limiting the circulation of HDV in these days. The highest percentage of PC and M is verified in Prelada and Amial sub-domains (Figure 3), LDV and B in Antas and HDV in Boavista. Prelada is the sub-domain where the total flow of traffic is biggest and Antas the calmest sub-domain.

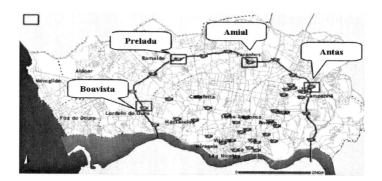

Figure 1: Locations of the video cameras in VCI sub-domains.

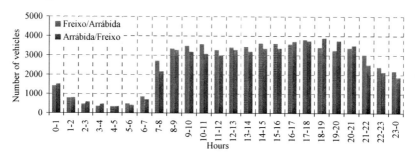

Figure 2: Daily average variation of traffic in VCI.

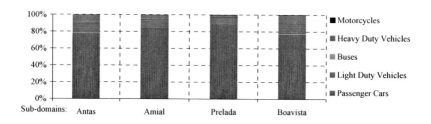

Figure 3: Average (%) of vehicle categories in the 4 sub-domains.

3.1.2 Emission estimates

For estimate traffic emissions, emission factors of road transport were used. These emission factors were selected by those published in the Atmospheric Emission Inventory Guidebook [12], and weighed in accordance with the Portuguese vehicle fleet composition in terms of certain parameters, as the average age of the vehicles, fuel, type of engine, tare and driving patterns in VCI [14]. The average speed of 20 km.h^{-1} was consider for rush hours with slow traffic movement and 75 km.h^{-1} for normal circulation. In this way, the weighed emission factors were calculated and applied to the traffic countings, getting hourly emissions, for NOx - Model LTE (Line Traffic Emissions) [14]. The higher emissions of NOx were seen in Boavista sub-domain while that less raised emissions were located in Antas sub-domain. The direction of traffic with bigger emissions was the Freixo/Arrábida.

3.2 Outdoor NO$_2$ diffuse sampler monitoring campaign

To have a first idea of the most exposed and sensible zones to air pollution from traffic in the VCI area, a preliminary outdoor NO$_2$ diffuse sampler campaign was carried out in April of 2004, in the 4 sub-domains: Antas, Amial, Prelada e Boavista. In each sub-domain have been defined 2 sampling lines of NO$_2$ measurements, with intervals of 150 meters. Parallel to these, with a distance of 100 meters, another 2 lines for each one of the sides of the VCI was defined (Figure 4). The samplers (with an expanded uncertainty of 17,8% at concentration levels of 20-40 μg.m^{-3}), in a total of 46, had been placed between 3 and 10 meters of height to verify vertical concentration dispersion.

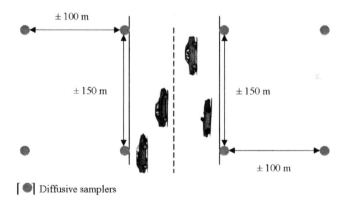

[⬤] Diffusive samplers

Figure 4:   Scheme of the diffuse samplers location in VCI.

The results of the preliminary campaign showed that in all the sub-domains the NO$_2$ concentrations are, in average, higher than 40 μg.m^{-3}, and that Boavista and Amial have the highest average values, 76,6 and 62,6 μg.m^{-3}, respectively. Prelada and Antas are the sub-domains that present a lower average concentrations with, 49,1 μg.m^{-3} and 52,5 μg.m^{-3}, respectively. Comparing these results with the European Union Directive 1999/30/EC [15], it can be verified that Boavista, Amial and Antas sub-domains exceed the annual limit value for human health protection (52 $\mu g.m^{-3}$ for year 2004). The locals with higher concentrations of NO_2 are the closest to VCI, where average concentration reach values two times higher than ones located away from the VCI, about 100 meters. In most of the sampling points, the NO_2 concentration diminishes with height, being exception locals surrounded by buildings, where the dispersion of pollutants becomes less efficient and, eventually, recirculation takes place. The influence of some closest streets and avenues with high flow traffic in the concentrations of the NO_2 is remarkable, as it is on case of Amial Street, in the Amial sub-domain, and Boavista Avenue in the Boavista sub-domain (Figure 5).

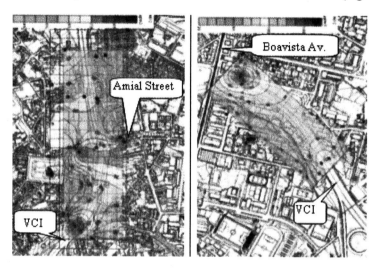

Figure 5: Results of the preliminary outdoor NO2 monitoring campaign in Amial and Boavista sub-domains (different scales).

3.3 Meteorological parameters

Meteorological factors influence the dynamics of the atmosphere, and the dispersion of the emitted pollutants. In the scope of the ImpactAir project, wind direction and speed, solar radiation and temperature were measured. The results obtained for the period of the preliminary outdoor campaign show that the average temperature value is 13,1°C. Lowest values of temperature correspond to the sunrise and highest to the period of the afternoon between 12H00 and 17H00 UTC. As expected, solar radiation is null in the period of the night and in the daylight it reaches a maximum value at 13H00 UTC. Wind speed increases gradually during the day, reaching maximum values of between 14H00 and 16H00 UTC. With the end of the afternoon, wind speed starts to reduce, until reaching minimum values over night period. The analysis of the wind direction (Figure 6) demonstrates a North/Northwest and Southeast predominance. Having in account that in Boavista sub-domain the tracing of VCI is perpendicular to the direction of the predominant wind, the transport and dispersion of atmospheric pollutants emitted by traffic is strongly conditioned/limited by the existing buildings. This interpretation is consistent with the results of the preliminary campaign, where high values of NO_2 were observed in this sub-domain and relatively lower values were observed in Prelada and the Antas sub-domains, which ones are more exposed to wind, facilitating the transport and dispersion of the emitted pollutants.

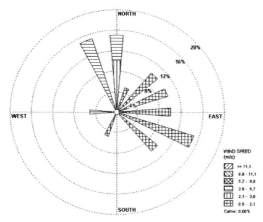

Figure 6:   Wind direction and speed rose in the study area.

3.4 Population exposure

Several methods of measuring/estimating individual exposure have been used. This methods include passive portable monitoring equipment, which have the advantage that they can be used to determine individual exposures but also for establishing large-scale databases with indoor and outdoor data [16]. If the concentration of a pollutant to which a person is exposed can be measured or modelled and the time spent in contact with the pollutant is known, exposure is determined from concentration and time. It is often assumed that the concentration is constant within a given microenvironment j for some finite interval, Δt_j. Thus, any particular exposure e_j within a given microenvironment j is given by:

$$e_j = \overline{C}_j \Delta t_j, \tag{1}$$

which means that a person stays within the microenvironment with average concentration $\overline{C}_j$ for the interval Δt_j [17].

In this study, having in account the hour average concentrations of NO_2 measured in the preliminary campaign and, for the same period, hour average concentrations of NO_2 monitorized by the monitoring stations located in Oporto Metropolitan Area, exposition scenarios were defined. In a first stage it was evaluated in which cities of the Oporto Metropolitan Area (Figure 7) work the residents of Oporto city, using an origin/destination data matrix work trips [18].

The highest number of trips was verified for Oporto and Matosinhos cities, while the lowest was verified for Espinho. Assuming that an individual lives in the VCI domain (Boavista, Prelada, Amial or Antas), staying at home or around of it during 15 hours and works in Oporto, Matosinhos or Espinho city during a period of 9 hours a day, 12 exposure scenarios have been made. Examples of these scenarios are: the individual lives in Amial sub-domain (15 hours) and works in Espinho (9 hours).

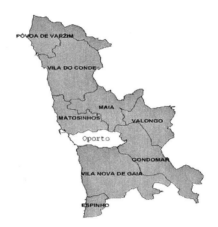

Figure 7:   Map of Oporto Metropolitan Area.

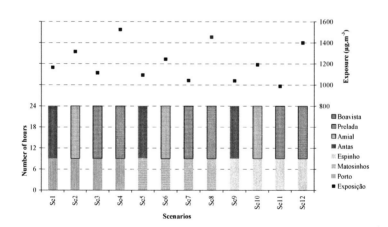

Figure 8:   Exposure scenarios for NO_2.

As it is observed in Figure 8, the worst scenario (with higher exposition of an individual to NO_2) is that where population lives in Boavista and works in Oporto city center, followed by those scenarios where the individual lives in Boavista and works in Matosinhos and/or Espinho. The favourable scenario is that one the population lives in Prelada and works in Espinho.

4 Conclusions

The analysis of daily traffic variation in VCI sub-domains allowed to evidence that the biggest flow of traffic is verified in Prelada, in contrast with Antas, the calmest sub-domain. Although traffic flow in Boavista is not so intensive as in Prelada, NO_2 measurements showed higher concentrations. This can be explain by the fact that in Antas and Prelada sub-domains there are few constructions in height and some agricultural fields, what having in account that the predominant wind is of the North/Northwest, with some frequency of Southeast, results in one better dispersion of pollutants, less loaded atmospheres. On the other hand, in Boavista sub-domain the number of HDV (diesel vehicles) in circulation is bigger than in the other sub-domains, what leads to an increase of the NO_2 concentrations.

Atmospheric NO_x emission estimations were in accordance with the results of the preliminary outdoor monitoring campaign, indicating that the higher NO_2 emissions are verified in Boavista sub-domain.

According to the results of the preliminary outdoor campaign, the most problematic zones in terms of pollutants concentrations are those near VCI and at 3 meters of height. The concentrations tend to diminish in height, being exception, points involved by buildings, where the dispersion of pollutants becomes less efficient. It is still notable that in Boavista and Amial sub-domains, densely populated areas, NO_2 average concentrations are above the established limit values [15], and, as such, preoccupying in terms of public health impact.

Relatively to the NO_2 exposition scenarios, it was verified that higher exposure occurs when people lives in Boavista, in contrast with the favourable scenario that corresponds to live in Prelada and work in Espinho.

Acknowledgments

The authors wish to acknowledge the Science and Technology Foundation for financing the ImpactAir project (Ref. POCTI/ESP/47806/2002), and for the grant of Tânia Fontes (Ref. SFRH/BD/19027/2004). Special thanks go to City Council of Oporto, for traffic counts data provision.

References

[1]   Guerreiro, C., Clench-Aas, J. & Bartonova A., Air pollution exposure monitoring and estimating. Part III. Development of new types of air quality indicators. *Journal of Environmental Monitoring*, **1**, pp. 327-332, 1999.

[2]   Regional Administration of Health – Center of Portugal. Air quality and public health – Occurrence of respiratory diseases. October 2001-March 2002.

[3]   Vardoulakis, S., Fisher, B.E.A., Pericleous, K. & Flesca, N.G., Modelling air quality in street canyons: a review. *Atmospheric Environment*, **37**, pp. 155-182, 2003.

[4]   Chan, L.Y., Chan, C.Y. & Qin, Y., The effect of commuting microenvironment on commuter exposures to vehicular emission in Hong Kong. *Atmospheric Environment*, **33**, pp. 1777-1787, 1999.

[5]   11th International Symposium, Transport and Air Pollution. Graz, Austria 19-21 June 2002. *Atmospheric Environment*, **37**, pp. 5135-5136, 2003.

[6]   Wyler, C., Fahrlander, C. B., Kunzli, N., Schindler, C., Liebrich, U. A., Perruchoud, A., Leuenberger, P. & Wuthrich, B.; the Swiss Study on Air Pollution and Lung Diseases in Adults (SAPALDIA Team), Exposure to motor vehicle traffic and allergic sensitisation. *Epidemiology*, **11**, pp. 450-456, 2000.

[7]   Hoek, G., Brunekreef, B., Goldbohm, S., Fischer, P. & van den Brandt, P. A., Association between mortality and indicators of traffic-related air pollution in the Netherlands: a cohort study. *The Lancet*, **360**, pp. 1203, 2002.

[8]   Maheswaran, R. & Elliot, P., Stroke mortality associated with living near main roads in England and Wales. *Stroke*, **34**, pp. 2776–2780, 2003.

[9]   English, P., Neutra, R., Scalf, R., Sullivan, M., Waller, L. & Zhu, L., Examining associations between childhood asthma and traffic flow using a geographic information system. *Environmental Health Perspectives*, **107**, pp. 761–767, 1999.

[10]   Langholz, B., Ebi, K. L., Thomas, D. C., Peters, J. M. & London, S. J., Traffic density and the risk of childhood leukaemia in Los Angeles case–control study. *Annuals of Epidemiology*, **12**, pp. 482–487, 2002.

[11]   Jerrett, M., Arain, A., Kanaroglou, P., Beckerman, B., Potoglou, D., Sahsuvaroglu, T., Morrison, J. & Giovis, C., A review and evaluation of intraurban air pollution exposure models. *Journal of Exposure Analysis and Environmental Epidemiology*, **15**, pp. 185–204, 2005.

[12]   EMEP (2002) Emission Inventory Guidebook - Technical report n° 30, 3° Edition, *European Environment Agency*, Copenhagen.

[13]   Insurance Portuguese Institute. Parque Automóvel Seguro 2000-2001, Portugal.

[14]   Barros, N., Fontes, T. & Brás, C., Comparação das Emissões do Tráfego Rodoviário por Análise dos Factores de Emissão, *Department of Science and Technology Magazine, Fernando Pessoa University*, **1**, pp. 29, 2004.

[15]   Council Directive 1999/30/EC of the 22 April 1999 relating to limit values for sulphur dioxide, nitrogen dioxide and oxides of nitrogen, particulate matter and lead in ambient air.

[16]   Committee on Advances in Assessing Human Exposure to Airborne Pollutants, Human exposure assessment for airborne pollutants: advances and opportunities. U.S. *National Academy of Sciences*, 1991.

[17]   Committee on Risk Assessment of Hazardous Air Pollutants – National Research Council Science and judgment in risk assessment. *The National Academies* Press, 672 pages, 1994.

[18]   National Institute of Statistics. Inquérito à Mobilidade da População Residente, Portugal, 2000.

Purification characteristics of golden pothos for emitting air-pollutants from plywood using a gas sensor

T. Oyabu[1], T. Onodera[2], A. Sawada[1] & M. Tani[1]
[1]Graduate School of Regional Economic Systems,
Kanazawa Seiryo University, Japan
[2]Graduate School of Information Science and Electrical Engineering,
Kyushu University, Japan

Abstract

Sick-house syndrome widely occurs in general domiciles. Its cause is from various types of chemical substances generated from building materials. The airtight structure is also one of the main causes for the syndrome. The most prevalent chemicals are formaldehyde, toluene and xylene. It is well known that plants have purification capabilities for these chemicals in an indoor environment. It is strongly desired to reduce the pollution level for multiple chemical sensitivity in domiciles and buildings. Foliage plants are very effective in reducing the pollution concentration. In this study, the purification characteristics of golden pothos for polluting chemicals emitting from a piece of building board are examined using a tin oxide gas sensor. The experiments are carried out in an airtight chamber of 200 liters. The number of plant pots were also changed from 0 to 3 in the experiments. As for the results, pothos had high purification capabilities for those chemicals and the capabilities increased as the number of pots were added. The purification rate reached almost 100% at over three pots in the chamber experiment. The approximate function of the purification characteristic is derived using an exponential function. The system can introduce the pollution level in an indoor environment using this expression. It is felt that this model can be effective in estimating the pollution level and the design of an indoor environment.
Keywords: foliage plant, air-pollutant, purification, formaldehyde, gas sensor.

1   Introduction

Various kinds of chemical substances are used in an indoor environment and these chemicals have occurred in human surroundings. Therefore, some residents fall into multiple chemical sensitivity (MCS) and sick-house syndrome, and they can not be fit for their daily life due to these diseases. The Ministry of Land, Infrastructure and Transport of Japan suggested that housing companies should measure the pollution levels of formaldehyde, toluene, xylene, ethyl-benzene and styrene in a built residence and publish the results officially. It has been reported that plants have a capability to remove atmospheric pollution [1-4]. In these studies, it was reported that a potted plant was put in an experimental chamber and a polluting chemical was injected into the chamber and the concentration of the chemical decreased with the passage of time. Various kinds of plants have capabilities to purify many kinds of atmospheric pollutants[5][6]. In a real domicile, the pollutants, however, generate continuously, and the generating volume increases as the atmospheric concentration of the pollutant decreases. We looked at how much the purification capability of the plants in those environments and measured the purification characteristics of the plants using a tin oxide gas sensor.

In this study, a piece of plywood was put in the chamber together with potted plants and the characteristics of polluting level were measured. The number of potted plants required to obtain a clean environment, was derived by a computer simulation. It became obvious that over three potted plants are required in the experimental environment of this study. The results can be practicable in domiciles and buildings.

2   Experimental

Experiments were carried out in a thermo-hygrostat room (Tabai: TBR 5HA2G3A). An experimental chamber of 200 liters was installed in the room. A piece of plywood (JAS (Japanese Agricultural Standard): F2, 300×300×9mm) and potted pothos were put in the chamber. The temperature and humidity in the thermo-hygrostat room were controlled at 22 degree centigrade and 60%RH. The sunlight was isolated in the experimental room and the light intensity was controlled at 730 lux using fluorescent lights. The temperature in the chamber was about 22 degree centigrade and the humidity was over 75%RH. The humidity was strongly influenced by plant-biorhythm. The experimental system is shown in Fig.1. It was always agitated in the chamber by a fan. The plywood and potted plants were put together in the chamber. The number of pots was increased to three. These pots were the same size (15cm in diameter and 17cm in height) and the plants were also about same size. A photograph of these pots is shown in Fig.2. The formaldehyde concentration in the chamber was measured using a tin oxide gas sensor (Figaro TGS#860). The sensor is named AMS in this paper. The real concentration was derived using a measuring instrument (RIKEN CO., FR-85) and the data were corrected using the relationships.

This type of gas sensor has been used to detect various types of atmospheric pollutants [7,8]. The tin oxide gas sensor is one of the more popular sensors and is available on the market now. The sensor has a high reliability and cost-performance. The sensor, which was used in this experiment, was developed to detect ammonia gas selectively. It does not have high gas-selectivity. The sensor and a load resister (R_L) were connected in series and dc voltage (V_c) was applied to the circuit. The voltage of both the ends of the load resistance was introduced as the sensor output (V_{out}). $V_{out} = R_L V_c / (R_s + R_L)$, where R_s means sensor resistance. The surface of the sensor element is usually covered with oxygen and hydroxide molecules. The molecules cover the sensor surface with binding free electrons inside sensor bulk. For example, when methyl alcohol gas comes near the sensor surface, the following reactions (eq.(1) and (2)) occurred, and aldehyde (CH_3CHO) or ethoxy (C_2H_5O) were generated. As for the results, conduction electrons return into the sensor-bulk, and the sensor resistance R_s decreases and V_{out} increases. Namely, when the concentration of a reducing gas in the atmosphere increases, R_s decreases and output V_{out} increases, and V_{out} come up to V_c level. A photograph of the sensor used in this experiment is shown in Fig.3. The output voltage was inputted every minute through an A/D converter.

$$C_2H_5OH + O^- \rightarrow CH_3CHO + H_2O + e \qquad (1)$$

$$C_2H_5OH + O^- \rightarrow C_2H_5O + OH + e \qquad (2)$$

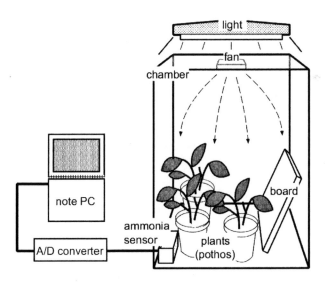

Figure 1:   Measurement system.

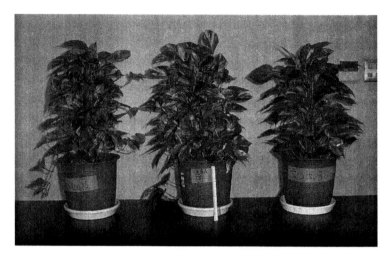

Figure 2:   Photograph of three potted plants used in this study.

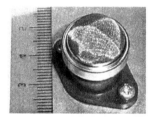

Figure 3:   Photograph of the sensor adapted in this study.

3 Results

3.1 Plant purification-characteristics

The correlation between the gas sensor output (V) and formaldehyde concentration (C) can be expressed using the following equation.

$$C = \exp[(V - 2.61)/0.474] \quad (3)$$

The purification characteristics of potted pothos are shown in Fig.4. The concentration is indicated using the unit of (mg/m^3) in the figure. The characteristic (a) was measured when only plywood was put in the chamber. The (b) means the characteristic when plywood and one potted pothos were installed. It reaches a maximum value after about eight hours from the beginning of the experiment and the concentration is about $0.3mg/m^3$ after 24 hours. The level in (a) is $0.67mg/m^3$. The maximum value of (b) is 0.34 mg/m^3. The characteristic (c) means the case when two pothos pots were inserted with the plywood. The maximum concentration (C_{max}), the time (t_{max}) at which the characteristic reached

C_{max} and C_{24} which means the concentration after 24 hours are also examined. In (c), C_{max} is 0.217mg/m^3, t_{max} is 3 hours and C_{24} is 0.15 mg/m^3. In characteristic (d), C_{max} is 0.18 mg/m^3, t_{max} is 2 hours and C_{24} is 0.1153mg/m^3. These values are shown in Fig.5. C_{24}, t_{max} and C_{max} decrease as the number of pot (n) increases. The relationship between C_{24} and n can be expressed using the eq. (4). The C_{24} does not decrease largely if the number of pots increases over 4. The concentration (C_0) in the thermo-hygrostat room was about 0.108 mg/m^3. When n is greater than 4, the concentration can be controlled below C_0 which is considered the outside concentration of the chamber.

$$C_{24} = 0.59 \exp(-n) + 0.08 \qquad (4)$$

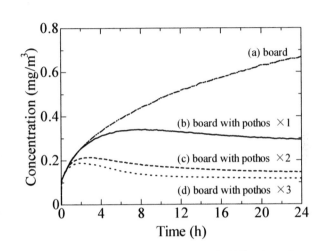

Figure 4:   Sensor outputs for a building board.

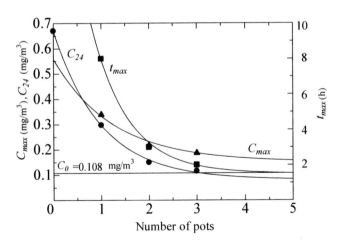

Figure 5:   The characteristics of C_{max}, C_{24} and t_{max} as a function of the number of pots.

3.2   Simulation for plant purification-capability

It is possible to derive the relationship between the formaldehyde concentration ($C(t)$(mg/m^3)) in the chamber and the emission volume per hour $E(t)$(mg/m^3) from the characteristic (a) in Fig.4. It is indicated in eq.(5). In the equation, t means time (h) and $\Delta C(t)$ means the variation concentration for Δt. V_0(m^3) means the cubic volume of the chamber which is 200 liters.

$$E(t) = \Delta C(t) \times V_0 / \Delta t \qquad (5)$$

The result when eq.(5) is applied to the characteristic (a), is shown in Fig.6. It is obvious that the emission volume of formaldehyde from the plywood decreases as the concentration in the chamber increases. The approximate function of $E(t)$ and $C(t)$ which is introduced in Fig.6, is expressed in eq.(6).

$$E(t) = 0.0418 \exp\left[-6.53 C(t)\right] + 0.0019 \qquad (6)$$

First, the concentrations in each plot of the characteristics (b), (c) and (d) in Fig.4 are derived, the values are substituted for the eq.(6). The $E(t)$s for (b), (c) and (d) can be obtained. The $E(t)$ can be also expressed as eq.(7) using the plant purification volume $P(t)$(mg) and the formaldehyde concentration change $C_v(t)$(mg/h).

$$P(t) = E(t) - C_v(t) \qquad (7)$$

$E(t)$, $P(t)$ and $C_v(t)$ characteristics for three pothos pots are shown in Fig.7. $P(t)$ increases with the passage of time. $E(t)$ decreases at a time and increases after that. The difference between $E(t)$ and $P(t)$ is $C_v(t)$. $E(t)$ and $P(t)$ take almost same value after 12 hours, namely emission volume and purification volume by plant are nearly equal. Therefore, $C_v(t)$ is nearly zero after 12 hours.

Total purification volume of three pothos pots for a day is about 0.46mg/day according to the $P(t)$ characteristic in Fig.7. Similarly, the values for two pots and one pot are 0.37 mg/day and 0.16 mg/day. Mean plant purification volume for a day and a pot is about 0.165 mg/(day $\times$ pot). The purification volume $P(t)$ for the number of pots (n) is derived and the relationship can be expressed using the eq.(8). We can simulate the $P(t)$ for n using eq.(8).

$$P(t) = \alpha\left(1 - \exp(-\beta t)\right) \qquad (8)$$

where

$$\alpha = 0.0031\left(1 - \exp(-0.344n)\right)$$
$$\beta = 0.886\left(1 - \exp(-0.534n)\right)$$

We can also estimate the concentration variation of formaldehyde as a function of time using the derived equations. Namely, the emission volume $E(t)$

can be introduced using the formaldehyde concentration at $t(h)$. The initial concentration (C_0) was in the thermo-hygrostat room. $C_0 = 0.108\text{mg/m}^3$. The $C_v(t)$ can be also introduced using the values of $E(t)$ and $P(t)$ in eq.(7). This $C_v(t)$ is added in every $t(h)$ successively and the concentration-variation as a function of time can be estimated accurately. The estimated results are shown in Fig.8. The number of pots (n) is adopted as a parameter in the figure. The figure is very similar to Fig.4. The estimated concentrations for $n=4$ and 5 become lower than the value of outside (C_0) after 24 hours. This result is almost equal to the result of Fig.5.

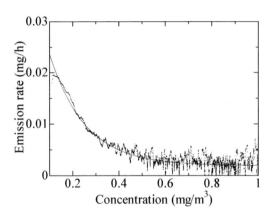

Figure 6: Formaldehyde emission rate vs. concentration in the chamber.

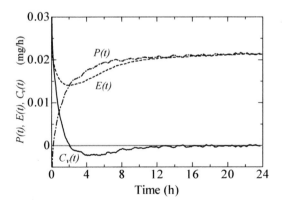

Figure 7: $P(t)$, $E(t)$, $C_v(t)$ as a function of time.

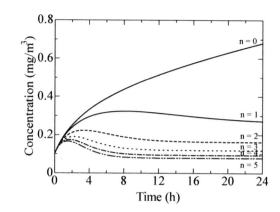

Figure 8:   Estimation of formaldehyde concentration as a function of time.

4   Conclusions

The purification processes of plants for formaldehyde, which generates from a piece of plywood, are examined. The potted pothos is adopted as a subject. It is shown quantitatively that the emission volume from the plywood decreases as the atmospheric concentration increases. It also became obvious that the formaldehyde concentration decreased by increasing the number of pots. The total purification volume could not increase by a simulation even if the number of pots exceeded a threshold value. The value was four in this experiment. The optimum number of pots in various types of indoor environment can be derived on the basis of these results.

The influence of ventilation must be also considered in the future.

References

[1] Oyabu, T., Onodera, T., & Takenaka, K., Purification Capability of Potted Plants for Removing Atmospheric Formaldehyde. *Proc. of 5th Int. Conf. on Engineering Design and Automation*, Las Vegas, USA, pp.1080-1085, 2001.
[2] Oyabu, T., Onodera, T., Kimura, H., & Sadaoka, Y., Purification Ability of Interior Plant for Removing of Indoor-Air Polluting Chemicals Using a Tin Oxide Gas Sensor. *J. Jpn. Soc. Atmos. Environ.*, 36(6), pp.319-325, 2001.
[3] Oyabu, T., Takenaka, K., Onodera, T., & Nanto H., Purification Ability of a Potted Plant and Soil for Atmospheric Gasoline. *Proc. of 1st Int. Congress on Petroleum Contaminated Soils, Sediments, and Water*, London, UK, p.117, 2001.
[4] Oyabu, T., Sawada, A., Onodera, T., Takenaka, K. & Wolverton B. C., Characteristics of Potted Plant for Removing Offensive Odors. *Sensors and Actuators* B, 89, pp.131-136, 2003.
[5] Wolverton, B. C., *How to grow fresh air*, Penguin Books: New York, 1996.

[6] Wolverton, B. C. & Wolverton, J. D., Plants and Soil Microorganism: Removal of Formaldehyde, Xylene, and Ammonia from the Indoor Environment. *J. Missil. Acad. Sci.*, 38(2), pp.11-15, 1993.

[7] Oyabu, T., Sensing characteristics of SnO2 thin film gas sensor. *J. Appl. Phys.*, 53(4), pp.2785-2787, 1982.

[8] Oyabu, T., Osawa, T., & Kurobe, T., Sensing characteristics of tin oxide thick film gas sensor. *J. Appl. Phys.*, 53(11), pp.7125-7130, 1982.

Ventilation improvement in fire smoke control

L. Santarpia, F. Gugliermetti & G. Zori
Department of "Fisica Tecnica", Rome University "La Sapienza", Italy

Abstract

Thermal gradients, wind pressure and mechanical ventilation systems determine a natural airflow travelling the two atmospheres. A fire ignition in a confined space increases thermal gradients and determines a growing smoke flux towards adjacent atmospheres. A free air jet from an air curtain system reduces the exchange airflow and improves fire and smoke compartimentation. Two theoretical analyses are used for the air curtain device dimensioning in emergency conditions. The results provide guidelines to improve the project quality.
Keywords: air curtain, confined fire, smoke control, ventilation device.

1 Introduction

Smoke management methods can modify smoke movement to protect occupants and fire fighters, and to reduce property damage. Barriers and smoke vents, supplying and exhausting big air quantities (purging dilution) of air in fire space, are traditionally used. Doors coupled with mechanical fans are a very common system in smoke control, while as the single smoke purging is unable to provided the needed air flow attracted through the open door by pressure differences. In many practical applications escape routes towards refuge areas are not equipped with doors, especially in large common-space. In this case the use of air curtains, with the barrier function, could be useful reducing or delaying smoke infiltration towards escape ways. Atria in commercial multi-stories buildings, exhibition halls, sports arenas, railway stations are typical examples of large commonplaces where is suggested to apply an air curtain system.

There are a lot of works and guidelines (NFPA 1995 [1], Klote and Milke 1992 [2], Tamura 1995 [3], Yamana and Tanaka 1985 [4], Hansell and Morgan 1994 [5]), standards and codes devoted to the design of smoke controls, but few papers regards on air curtain system used as a smoke barriers. Preliminary studies about air flow rates and pressure field analyses produced by air curtain systems can be find in Gugliermetti and Santarpia [6, 7, 8]

This paper presents a practical application of smoke control by an air curtain systems focused to the emergency ventilation system controlling smoke diffusion in an underground subway station.

2 Background

Smoke diffusion in a burning confined space can be analysed in function of the fire dynamic and the exhaust ventilation efficiency [9].

A possible approach for an air curtain device project and to achieve the fire smoke control in a railway deep subway station is to consider a steady fire with an upper layer exhaust [10, 11]. The stationary fire condition determines a constant smoke production rate. This choice involves a security condition, assuming a constant heat release rate and a well fire oxygenation (maximum heat release rate). In this case the air curtain system can operates protecting emergency exits and reducing evacuation time.

The high temperature fire floats toward the ceiling smoke, making a smoke layer whose thickness is z_f. The outlet airflow, G_{out}, stabilizes the smoke layer thickness; its value is carried out by a mass balance in the smoke layer control volume (Fig. 1).

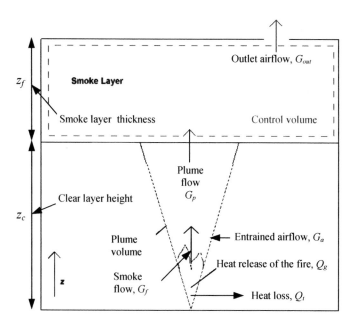

Figure 1:   Smoke layer mass balance.

The smoke layer thickness, z_f, (and consequently the height of lower clear layer, z_c,) is constant in the time when: $G_{out} = G_p$. The G_p flow, coming from the plume towards the smoke layer, is a mixture of entrained air, G_a, and smoke, G_f. This plume flow generated, G_p, can be estimated as:

$$G_p = C_1 \left(Q_g - Q_t \right)^{\frac{1}{3}} (z - z_0)^{\frac{5}{3}} + C_2 \left(Q_g - Q_t \right) \qquad (1)$$

where:

G_p	= mass flow in plume at height z, kg/s;
Q_g	= heat release rate of fire (HRR), kW;
Q_t	= fire heat radiative loss (RHRR), kW;
z	= height above top of the fuel, m;
z_0	= plume virtual origin, m;
C_1	= 0.071;
C_2	= 0.026.

The amount $\left(Q_g - Q_t \right)$ symbolizes the convective heat release rate, Q_c, of the plume (CHRR). The virtual origin, z_0, is a function of the fire surface and acts shifting the plume origin above the top of the fuel ($z_0 > 0$) or below the top of the fuel ($z_0 < 0$). The Heskestad's relationship for the virtual origin is:

$$z_0 = C_3 Q_g^{\frac{2}{5}} - 1.02 D_f \qquad (2)$$

where:

D_f	= diameter of fire, m;
C_3	= 0.083.

The effective diameter of a fire, when the surface is rectangular, can be expressed by:

$$D_f = 2 \sqrt{\frac{S}{\pi}} \qquad (3)$$

where:

S	= surface of fire, m².

When the fire is starting and developing, before reaching steady conditions (Fig. 1), the low smoke temperature not allows the defined upper and lowers layer creation. In this case the outlet airflow, G_{out}, is calculated supposing a perfect smoke mixing in the confined space where the fire is developed.

The smoke mass balance in the confined volume, V, is:

$$V \cdot dC = G_f \cdot dt - G_{out} \cdot C(t) \cdot dt \qquad (4)$$

where:

dt	= infinitesimal time interval, s;
G_f	= smoke mass production, kg/s;
$C(t)$	= time dependent smoke mass concentration, kg_{smoke}/kg_{total};

Separating the variables:

$$dt = -\frac{V \cdot dC}{G_{out} \cdot C(t) - G_f} = -\frac{V}{G_{out}} \cdot \frac{d(C(t) - G_f / G_{out})}{(C(t) - G_f / G_{out})} \tag{5}$$

Integrating and setting $C = C_0$ when t = 0, we can obtain:

$$C(t) = \frac{(G_{out} \cdot C_0 - G_f) \cdot e^{-\frac{G_{out}}{V}t} + G_f}{G_{out}} \tag{6}$$

The outlet airflow, G_{out}, can be properly estimated if maximum smoke concentration is lower than security alert level, C_s, during the evacuation from the subway station.

3 Ventilation system project

3.1 Description

The depth subway stations are characterized by tunnels (for train transit), central docks and ascending scales. The emergency ventilation system consists in a metallic duct installed at the ceiling connected to the airshaft. The ventilation duct intakes the air and the smoke from several longitudinal grilles disposed with step of 2.5 m.

The surface subway stations are characterized by a rectangular section. In this case the exhaust ventilation system intakes the air and the smoke from two localized airshafts (Fig. 2).

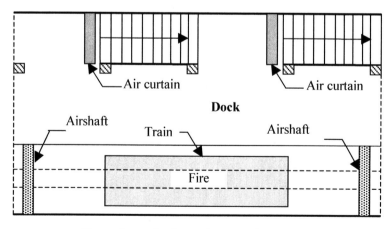

Figure 2:   Surface subway station layout.

An air curtain system is installed at the start of each ascending scale (emergency exit). This ventilation device starts to operate when the fire is beginning, and the emergency conditions are announced by alert signal, to improve the exit practicability in smoke presence.

Two different operating settings are used to carry out the inlet and outlet ventilation both in normal and emergency conditions.

3.2 Evacuation time

Experimental results, published in the scientific literature, [12] shown a temperature value above the fire surface lower than 200 °C. A sprinkler plant (the activation temperature is set to 68°C) assure an effective temperature value lower 200 °C in the first five minutes (during the evacuation phase). Past 5 minutes, the developing fire becomes uncontrollable and determines not acceptable risks, and the evacuation phase must be completed before this period. The emergency action sequences when a fire starts are shown in Tab. 1.

Table 1:   Event-action sequence.

Time	Event	Action	Temperature
0 sec.	Start fire	Start evacuation	25°C
30 sec.	Fire detection	Start emergency ventilation system	50°C
1 min.	Sprinkler head breaking	Emergency ventilation full operative	80°C
3 min.	Developing fire	75% of occupants evacuated	150°C
4 min.	Smoke concentration growth	Evacuation complete	200°C

3.3 Project design procedure

3.3.1 Outlet ventilation system
The minimum outlet airflow is determined from the number of the air changes per hour (ACH), parameter fixed by technical provisions, both for normal as for emergency operational conditions (Tab. 2).

Table 2:   Air changes per hour (ACH).

	ACH (h^{-1})
Normal	2
Emergency	8

The correct outlet airflow must be determined to avoid danger caused by the high indoor pollution level (smoke, CO, CO_2, …) and by the temperature.

3.3.1.1 Developing fire A smoke mass balance in the subway station premise can be used to determine the smoke concentration vs. time during the evacuation phase, $C(t)$. Setting the maximum smoke concentration level, $C_s = 25\%$, and the smoke production rate, $G_f = 16$ kg/s (that corresponds to HRR = 3 MW), the smoke concentration, $C(t)$, is calculated with eqn. (5).

The operating phase, shown in tab. 3, are considered to compute the smoke concentration.

Table 3:   Operating phase.

Phase	Time	Description
1 - initial phase	$0 < t < 1$ min.	time gap between normal and emergency operating state (normal outlet airflow and maximum smoke release rate)
2 - dilution phase	$1 < t < 10$ min.	outlet airflow set to emergency state and maximum smoke release rate.
3 - final phase	$t > 10$ min.	outlet airflow set to emergency state and zero smoke release rate.

The smoke concentration vs. time are synthesized in tab. 4 and shown in fig. 3.

The emergency outlet airflow, G_{out}, during the fire developing is 155.000 m³/h for a depth station and 200.000 m³/h for a surface station.

Such disproportion (about 30% of airflow) is due, for the surface stations, to the directly air extraction from the airshaft, in this case air mixed to smoke outlet airflow is induced from the adjacent tunnel.

Table 4:   Concentration vs. time.

Phase	Time (min)	Depth station (V = 8000 m³)		Surface station (V = 7000 m³)	
		Ventilation (m^3/h)	Smoke concentration (%)	Ventilation (m^3/h)	Smoke concentration (%)
1	0.0		0.0		0.0
	0.5	64000	5.8	100000	6.4
	1.0		11.1		11.9
2	1.5		14.6		14.9
	2.0		17.5		17.2
	2.5		19.9		18.9
	3.0		21.8		20.2
	3.5		23.4		21.1
	4.0		24.8		21.8
	4.5		25.8		22.4
	5.0		26.7		22.8
	5.5	155000	27.5	200000	23.1
	6.0		28.1		23.3
	6.5		28.6		23.5
	7.0		29.0		23.6
	7.5		29.4		23.7
	8.0		29.6		23.8
	8.5		29.9		23.8
	9.0		30.1		23.9
	9.5		30.2		23.9
3	10.0		24.9		18.0
	10.5		20.5		13.5
	11.0	155000	16.9	200000	10.1
	11.5		13.9		7.6
	12.0		11.5		5.7

3.3.1.2 Steady fire When steady conditions are reached the dimensioning the extraction system can be carried out by the model of the plume illustrated (§ 2). The dimensioning is obtained directly through the esteem of the HRR and it leads to the same result obtained following the methodology illustrated in § 3.3.1.1.

Assuming the following values for the calculations:

- HRR = 3MW
- Convective heat fraction $(Q_c/Q_t) = 0,7$
- Fire surface = 30 m²

A value for virtual origin, z_0 = -4,26 m, and an outlet airflow G_{out} = 40 m³/s (144000 m³/h), are obtained. Such values are sufficient to determine a free height from smoke, zc, constant in the time, of approximately 5 m above the dock.

Therefore the outlet airflow (155000 m³/h) is consistent in order to guarantee the ventilation emergency to complete the evacuation of the premises (about 5 min.). For the surface stations the outlet grille airflow must be 30% greater to compensate the air-smoke entrained from the tunnels.

The air changes per hour carried out with the present model are 19, approximately 60% greater than the provision values suggested as minimum value (Tab. 2).

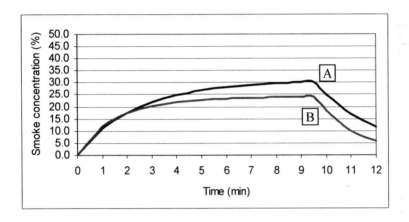

Figure 3:   Depth (A) and Surface (B) stations smoke concentration vs. time.

3.3.2 Inlet airflow

The outlet airflow going out to the premises captures external renewal air through the galleries and the exodus way. This airflow, flowing in opposite exodus versus, contrasts the premise evacuation (the difference of pressure in correspondence of the emergency exits could interfere with the opening of the fire doors). A solution at this problem is the inlet airflow system.

To avoid the smoke diffusion in exodus way a localized inlet grille is installed on the exit proximity. The vertical inlet airflow width creates a pressure gradient contrasting the air jet flowing on the communicating doorway. The air jet can be considered as a linear vertical air curtain system operating with not recirculated airflow [13].

The project design can be guided by ASHRAE procedure, therefore, in emergency operating conditions, it can be useful applied the procedure presented in Tab. 5 by Santarpia et al. [14]. The procedure is based on a momentum ratio, $r_M = M/M_0$, where M is the airflow momentum on the exodus way when the air curtain is OFF and M_0 is the air curtain jet momentum.

Table 5: Design procedure.

Setting:	Width of push grille	m	d
	Door height	m	H_d
	Outdoor temperature	°C	t_e
	Indoor temperature	°C	t_a
	Velocity coefficient	–	$\phi = 0.7$
	Width of opening	m	L
	Momentum ratio	-	$r_M = \dfrac{M}{M_0}$
Carrying out:	Pressure gradient (ρ_e outdoor air density ρ_a indoor air density)	Pa	$\Delta p_{max} = (\rho_e - \rho_a) \cdot g \cdot \dfrac{H_d}{2}$
	The average speed of the air flow through the opening when the air curtain is OFF	m/s	$v_m = \dfrac{2}{3}\phi \cdot \sqrt{\dfrac{2 \cdot \Delta p_{max}}{\rho_m}}$
	Air curtain vertical discharge velocity	m/s	$v_{in} = \sqrt{\dfrac{r_M v_m^2 \cdot \dfrac{H_d}{2} \cdot \rho_m}{d \cdot \rho_{in}}}$
	Air curtain airflow	m³/h	$G_{in,tot} = 3600 \cdot d \cdot L \cdot v_{in}$

The principal technical dimensioning parameter is the momentum ratio; in normal operating condition r_M can be set to 10, while in emergency operating condition r_M can be set to 32.

In Tab. 6 are shown the dimensioning data carried out both with ASHRAE method and with the Tab. 5 procedure.

On the Authors procedure (tab. 5), the air curtain airflow, $G_{in,tot}$, can be carried out in function of the indoor steady temperature T_a, door height H_d, and air curtain grille d, with:

$$G_{in,tot} = G_{in} \cdot L = 3600 \cdot H_d \cdot \sqrt{r_M} \cdot \sqrt{\frac{2}{9}g\phi^2} \cdot \sqrt{d} \cdot \sqrt{\frac{\theta_a}{\theta_e} - 1} \cdot L \quad (7)$$

g is the gravity acceleration, θ_a and θ_e are the indoor and outdoor Kelvin temperature.

4   Remarks

The Authors air curtain airflow dimensioning procedure is more precautionary than ASHRAE method in emergency condition (airflow 20-30% greater).

Moreover the inlet airflow balances the outlet airflow and improves security in exodus ways.

Table 6:   Design results.

Setting:		ASHRAE		Authors model		
		Depth	Surface	Depth	Surface	Unit
	E =	0.3	0.3	-	-	
	f =	10	10	-	-	
	d =	-	-	0.6	0.6	m
	r_M =	-	-	32	32	
	H =	3.2	2.7	3.2	2.7	m
	Te =	25	25	25	25	°C
	Ta =	200	200	200	200	°C
	Tem =	200	200	200	200	°C
Carrying out:						
	$d = \dfrac{H_d}{f} =$	0.32	0.27	-	-	m
	ρ_e =	1.18	1.18	1.18	1.18	kg/m³
	$\rho_a = \rho_{in}$ =	0.75	0.75	0.75	0.75	kg/m³
	ρ_m =	0.968	0.968	0.968	0.968	kg/m³
	Δp_{max} =	6.74	5.7	6.74	5.7	Pa
	$v_{in} = \sqrt{\dfrac{2 \cdot \Delta p \cdot f}{\beta_0 \cdot \rho_{in} \cdot E}} =$	23.4	21.5	-	-	m/s
	$v_m = \dfrac{2}{3} v_{max} =$	-	-	1.74	1.60	m/s
	$v_{in} = \sqrt{\dfrac{r_M v_m^2 \cdot \dfrac{H_d}{2} \cdot \rho_m}{d \cdot \rho_{in}}} =$	-	-	22.4	18.9	m/s
	$G_{in} = 3600 \cdot v_{in} \cdot d =$	26944	20883	32256	27216	m³/h x m
	L =	4	7,2	4	7,2	m
	$G_{in, tot} \approx$	108000	150000	129000	196000	m³/h
	$G_{out} \approx$	155000	20000	155000	20000	m³/h
	$\Delta G = G_{out} - G_{in, tot} =$	47000	50000	26000	4000	m³/h

Acknowledgement

This work has been supported with the economical contribute of the "Fondazione Cassa di Risparmio di Roma" in the frame of a national program devoted to the human health protection.

References

[1]   NFPA, 1995. NFPA 92 B. Guide for smoke management systems in malls, atria and large areas. Quincy, Mass: National Fire Protection Association

[2]   Klote J.H. and J.A. Milke, 1992. Design of smoke management systems. Atlanta, ASHRAE: American Society of heating, Refrigerating and Air-Conditioning Engineers Inc.

[3]   Tamura G.T., 1995. Smoke movement and control in high-rise buildings. Quincy, Mass, NFPA: National Fire Protection Association.

[4]   Yamana T. and T. Tanaka, 1985. Smoke control in large spaces. Fire science 5: 41-54

[5]   Hansell G.O. and H.P. Morgan, 1994. Design approaches for smoke control in atrium buildings. BR-258. Garston, U.K., BRE: Building Research Establishment.

[6]   Santarpia L., Gugliermetti F., 2002. Smoke movement and management in larges spaces. Heat and Technology (Vol.1). - International Journal of heat and technology.

[7]   Santarpia L, Gugliermetti F., 2000. Air curtains to reduce outdoor pollutants infiltration through buildings aperture. Proc of Intren Conf. HB2000, Helsinki, August 5-10.

[8]   Santarpia L. Gugliermetti F., 1999. A phenomenological approach to the performance of shutter type air curtains Proc. Of Air pollution 99, 27-29 July, San Francisco.

[9]   Klote J.H., 1994. Method of predicting smoke movement in atria with application to smoke management. NIST- 5516. Gaithersburg, NIST: National Institute of Standards and Technology.

[10]   Klote J.H., 1997/1. Prediction of smoke movement in Atria: Part I-Physical concepts. Ashrae Transactions: 103(2).

[11]   Klote J.H., 1997/2. Prediction of smoke movement in Atria: Part II-Application to smoke management. Ashrae Transactions: 103(2).

[12]   Heskestad G., 1988. Fire Plumes- Handbook of fire protection engineering. Boston, Mass, SFPE: Society of Fire Protection Engineers

[13]   ASHRAE HVAC Application Handbook, 1999. Handbook Editor, ASHRAE, 1791. Tullie Circle, Atlanta.

[14]   Santarpia L., Gugliermetti F., Zori G. Dynamic efficiency of air curtain systems. HEFAT2005, 4th International Conference on Heat Transfer, Fluid Mechanics and Thermodynamics. 19-23 September 2005, Cairo, Egypt.

Section 3
Food contamination

Mercury in Amazonian fish from Madeira River basin, Rondônia State, Brazil

P. A. S. Gali[1], D. M. Bonotto[1], E. G. da Silveira[2] & W. R. Bastos[2]
[1]Departamento de Petrologia e Metalogenia,
Instituto de Geociências e Ciências Exatas-UNESP, Rio Claro, Brazil
[2]Departamento de Geografia,
Fundação Universidade Federal de Rondônia-UNIR, Porto Velho, Brazil

Abstract

This investigation was carried out at the Madeira River basin, located in the state of Rondônia, Brazilian Amazon. Fish from Madeira, Jaciparaná, and Jamari rivers between 7 and 11° parallels south and between 62 and 65° meridians west in Rondônia state, Brazil, were sampled and chemically analyzed for mercury in order to evaluate if the inputs of this metal into the food-chain is occurring in levels reaching values above those recommended by the World Health Organization. This is because such an element is very dangerous when ingested by humans and its presence was extensively identified some years ago in the area, since it was utilized as an amalgam in processes for recovering alluvial gold.
Keywords: mercury, fish, statistical distribution, Madeira River basin, health hazard.

1 Introduction

In aquatic systems, heavy metals (including mercury) and other elements are mainly transported in the solid phase, either sorbed onto particle surfaces and coatings, or incorporated into mineral grains. Thus, 90-99 percent of the total metal load in rivers is transported in the particulate phase, depending on the geochemical behavior of the metal and the nature of the physical and chemical environment [1]. Upon discharge to river waters, metal speciation or complexation, and other physical-chemical parameters such as pH, redox conditions, and nature of the solid-metal species interaction, determine the partitioning of the metal between solid and liquid phases, controlling its dispersion throughout the aquatic environment, where adsorption on fine particles has been recognized as a key process in its transport [2-4].

The sources of trace metals in aquatic systems determine their distribution ratio between the aqueous and solid phases, when the metal contents of river solids depend significantly on allochthonous influences. Mining activities involve the extraction, processing, and disposal of large quantities of rock, being responsible, very often, by the release of metals that are introduced either directly or indirectly to rivers and streams [5]. The major problem affecting mercury during mining activities is related to the fact that it is widely utilized as an amalgam in processing alluvial gold ores, mainly in rainforest areas [6, 7].

The gold exploitation in several areas of the Brazilian Amazon has caused environmental problems due to the presence of mercury in the biosphere, whether in liquid, ionic or vapour form. Special attention has been given to mercury inputs at the Madeira River in the Amazon area by numerous investigators [6, 8-13] since is one of the largest tributary of Amazon River and the gold mining was officially allowed and practiced since the Andean headwaters, causing the release of metallic mercury to the atmosphere and waterways [14].

The gold mining activities on the Madeira River extended from the Bolivian headwaters, on the Beni River, down to the city of Porto Velho, capital of Rondônia State, and, despite to be practically absent in the present days, mercury has been evaluated in the aquatic system by local authorities and environmentalists due to the possibility of occurring contamination in people [15]. Contamination of the aquatic food-chain of the Madeira River tributaries has been demonstrated [20], being reported that 86% of the piscivorous fish collected in the Beni River exhibited high mercury concentrations, i.e. values exceeding by almost four times the WHO safety limit [16].

This investigation focused the mercury presence in fish of the Madeira River basin, Brazilian Amazon, following the previous interest in the area due to possible intoxication on animal and human population due to the ingestion of this metal in food.

2   Material and methods

The Madeira River is one of the largest tributaries of the Amazon River, extending from Bolívia and crossing the city of Porto Velho, capital of Rondônia State in Brazil, which is the most populated site (population approximately 300,000, according to the 1999 census) along it. The Aw-tropical rainy climate (Köppen classification) characterizes Rondônia State, i.e. the relative air humidity ranges from 74.2 up to 90.8% and air temperature from 20.7 up to 32.2°C [17]. The wet season (average rainfall = 250 mm/month) occurs between October and April, whereas the dry season (average rainfall = 20 mm/month) between May and September [17]. Such rain regime influences directly the water level height of the Madeira River (Fig. 1).

This study provided Hg distribution data for 419 samples of fish from Madeira, Jaciparaná, and Jamari rivers in the Madeira River basin between 7 and

11° parallels south and between 62 and 65° meridians west in Rondônia state, Brazil (Fig. 2). The samples were obtained between April 1994 and January 1998 in the central market located at the city of Porto Velho, as well collected directly from the rivers after using roads and small boats, because the selected area is not suitable for navigation. The specimens were identified according to their popular name during the fieldwork. Afterwards, they were stored in polyethylene bags that were kept in iceboxes and transported up to the laboratory.

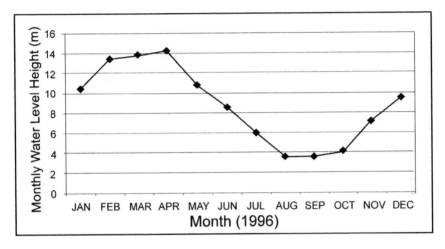

Figure 1: The average monthly water level height of the Madeira River during 1996 [17].

The weight and length of the specimens were recorded at the laboratory according to standard procedures [18]. It was also indicated if their skin contains scales or not, as well their possible scientific name based on criteria applied to Amazonian fish [18]. Then, a fillet was cut from the back of the specimen and maintained under freeze (-5 °C) up to the time of analysis.

Digestion and extraction procedures were used for Hg analysis in the samples. About 0.5 g of each sample was weighed in Teflon beakers/tubes, 1 mL of 30% H_2O_2 was added plus 2 mL of a 1:1 H_2SO_4-HNO_3 mixture and 5 mL of 5% $KMnO_4$. This material was inserted in a 630 W microwave oven and maintained there (temperature~55°C) during about 35 minutes. Alternatively, digestion was also performed in an opened system. Afterwards, the solution was brought to room temperature (~25°C) and the excess $KMnO_4$ was neutralized with some drops of 12% hydroxylamine hydrochlorate. The volume was raised up to 10 mL with ultra pure water prepared on a Milli Q system that uses ion exchange resin and Millipore 0.22 μm filter.

The analyses of total Hg concentrations were done using atomic absorption spectrophotometers with cold vapor generation. The equipment utilized is a Perkin Elmer model FIMS-400 atomic absorption spectrophotometer, containing a cylindrical cell with quartz window, an Hg lamp (253.7 nm), a specific detector for absorption on the Hg wavelength, a system of flow injection analysis, and a cold vapor generator system. The parameters of calibration utilized in this equipment consisted on an Ar flow of 50 mL.min^{-1}, a 3% HCl flow of 9-11 mL.min^{-1}, and a 0.2-0.5% NaBH$_4$+NaOH flow of 5-7 mL.min^{-1}. The concentrations of the analytical solutions for obtaining the calibration curve of the equipment varied between 2 and 40 µg.L^{-1}, and were prepared from a 2 µg.mL^{-1} stock solution preserved with 5% HNO$_3$ + 0.01% K$_2$Cr$_2$O$_7$. Each aliquot representing the sample (0.5 g) was divided in three sub-aliquots. All analytical determinations were made in triplicate for each sub-aliquot, yielding, therefore, nine measurements for each sample. The final result for each sample (Table 1) corresponded to the mean value of the nine readings.

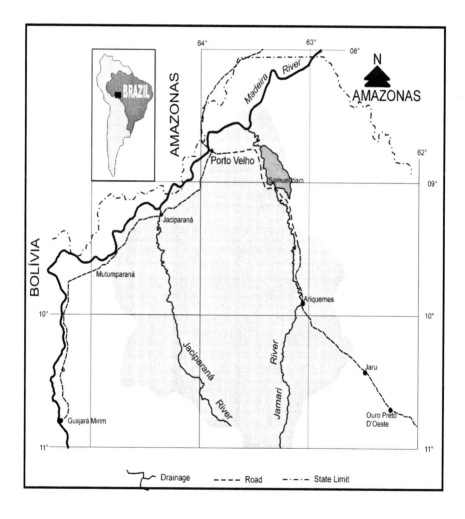

Figure 2:   Location of the area for sampling fish in Rondônia State, Brazil.

Table 1:   Average Hg content in fish from the Madeira River basin, Brazil.

Popular name	Scientific name	N*	Hg (ppm)
Acará	*Geophagus* sp.	10	0.09
Acari Bodó	*Lipsarcus pardalis*	1	0.04
Apapá	*Pellona* sp.	1	0.81
Aruanã	*Osteoglossum bicirrhossum*	2	0.68
Bacu	*Pterodoras granulosus*	1	0.01
Bico de Pato	*Hemisorubim platyrhynchos*	3	0.53
Bicudo	*Boulengerella ocellata*	4	0.90
Branquinha	*Potamorhina latior*	16	0.09
Cará	*Cichlasoma spectabile*	3	0.29
Caratinga	Not identified	1	0.04
Cascudinho	*Pareiorhapis duseni*	7	0.04
Cascudo	*Plecostomus* sp.	3	0.04
Croatá	*Platynematichthys notatus*	2	1.86
Curimatã	*Prochilodus* sp.	38	0.12
Curimba	Not identified	1	0.08
Dourado	*Brachyplathystoma flavicans*	4	0.43
Filhote	*Brachyplathystoma filamentosum*	7	0.96
Jacundá	*Crenicichla reticulata*	5	0.37
Jaraqui	*Semaprochilodus taeniurus*	7	0.18
Jatuarana	*Hemiodus notatus*	9	0.10
Jaú	*Paulicea leutkeni*	2	0.52
Lírio Braço de Moça	*Platystomatichthys sturio*	4	0.46
Mandi	*Pimelodus* sp.	6	0.34
Mandubé	*Ageneiosus brevifilis*	3	0.95
Mapará	*Hypophtalmus edentatus*	18	0.56
Matrinchã	*Brycon* sp.	1	0.05
Pacu	*Mylossoma* sp.	21	0.07
Peixe Cachorro	*Hydrolycus scomberoides*	9	0.97
Pescada	*Plagioscion squamosissimus*	14	0.33
Piau	*Laemiyta* sp.	4	0.07
Piau Apará	Not identified	3	0.21
Piau Aracu	*Laemolyta* sp.	6	0.16
Piau Botafogo	*Shizodon vittatum*	3	0.04
Piau Cabeça Gorda	*Leporinus friderici*	5	0.20
Piau Cabeça de Meia	*Schizodon fasciatum*	14	0.14
Pintado	*Pseudoplatystoma* sp.	22	0.92
Piramutaba	*Brachyplathystoma vaillanti*	1	0.09
Piranha	*Serrasalmus* sp.	46	0.80
Pirapitinga	*Colossoma bidens*	3	0.08
Pirarucu	*Arapaima gigas*	4	0.26
Sardinha	*Triportheus elongatus*	11	0.26
Surubim	*Pseudoplatystoma fasciatus*	1	0.38
Tambaqui	*Colossoma macropomum*	8	0.15
Traíra	*Hoplias malabaricus*	34	0.46
Tucunaré	*Cichla ocellaris*	49	0.36
Tucunaré açu	*Cichla* sp.	2	0.30

* N = number of samples.

3 Hg content in selected fish

The average values of the Hg content in the analyzed fish are greatly variable, ranging from 0.01 to 1.86 ppm (Table 1). The species sampled are widely spread over the area, being commonly consumed by the population. However, considering the number of specimens sampled per specie, the economic importance and the use in alimentation, four types were selected for initial evaluation of the data obtained. They are: *Prochilodus* sp., *Serrasalmus* sp., *Hoplias malabaricus*, and *Cichla ocellaris*. A summary of the parameters obtained for these fish is shown in Table 2.

The WHO safety limit [16] for ingestion of mercury in fish is 0.5 ppm and considering the range of values reported in Table 2, only the specimens of *Prochilodus* sp. do not reach the maximum allowable limit in any analyzed sample. These fish ingest organic matter and microorganisms associated to mudstone at the bottom of lakes and margins of rivers, realizing long migration for reproduction. *Serrasalmus* sp., *Hoplias malabaricus*, and *Cichla ocellaris* are classified as carnivorous fish, and among them the average Hg content is higher in *Serrasalmus* sp. (0.8 ppm) that exceeds the WHO safety limit of 0.5 ppm.

However, such contamination level is lower than that found in other piscivorous fish in the Amazon area, since values exceeding by almost four times the WHO safety limit have been reported [8]. The same relationship between the Hg content and the alimentation pattern of the specie had been identified in previous studies developed in Brazil, with the higher Hg contents occurring in individuals of higher trophic levels [10-13].

Table 2:   Weight, length, and Hg content in fish from the Madeira River basin, Rondônia State Brazil.

	Serrasalmus sp.	*Prochilodus* sp.	*Hoplias malabaricus*	*Cichla ocellaris*
Number of samples	46	38	34	49
Weight (g)				
Minimum value	500	200	250	100
Maximum value	2100	2000	1200	2000
Average value	884	556	533	560
Length (cm)				
Minimum value	14	22	20.5	21
Maximum value	36.5	42.5	46	44
Average value	27	28	31	29
Hg (ppm)				
Minimum value	0.1908	0.0029	0.1018	0.0627
Maximum value	2.1681	0.3380	1.1876	0.8432
Average value	0.8051	0.1203	0.4628	0.3551

4 Statistical analysis of the data

The Hg content data obtained for *Prochilodus* sp., *Serrasalmus* sp., *Hoplias malabaricus*, and *Cichla ocellaris* were submitted to statistical analysis, as reported in Table 3. All data adjust to a normal distribution (Fig. 3), inclusive those obtained for *Cichla ocellaris* that indicate a bi-modal normal distribution.

Table 3: Statistical distribution of the mercury content in fish from the Madeira River basin, Rondônia State, Brazil.

Hg content range (ppm)	Average Hg content (ppm)	Frequency	Frequency percentage	Cumulative percentage
Serrasalmus sp. (N = 46)				
0.1908 - 0.2861	0.2400	4	8.7	8.7
0.2861 - 0.4289	0.3600	3	6.5	15.2
0.4289 - 0.6430	0.5400	12	26.1	41.3
0.6430 - 0.9641	0.8000	15	32.6	73.9
0.9641 - 1.4456	1.2000	8	17.4	91.3
1.4456 - 2.1675	1.8100	3	6.5	97.8
2.1675 - 3.2499	2.7100	1	2.2	100.0
Prochilodus sp. (N = 38)				
0.0018 - 0.0040	0.0029	1	2.6	2.6
0.0040 - 0.0088	0.0064	0	0	2.6
0.0088 - 0.0194	0.0141	0	0	2.6
0.0194 - 0.0429	0.0312	1	2.6	5.2
0.0429 - 0.0948	0.0689	8	21	26.2
0.0948 - 0.2095	0.1523	26	68.5	94.7
0.2095 - 0.4630	0.3366	2	5.3	100
Hoplias malabaricus (N = 34)				
0.1000 - 0.1506	0.1253	2	5.9	5.9
0.1506 - 0.2268	0.1887	2	5.9	11.8
0.2268 - 0.3416	0.2842	11	32.3	44.1
0.3416 - 0.5144	0.4280	9	26.5	70.6
0.5144 - 0.7747	0.6445	4	11.8	82.4
0.7747 - 1.1667	0.9707	5	14.7	97.1
1.1667 - 1.7570	1.4618	1	2.9	100
Cichla ocellaris (N = 49)				
0.0500 - 0.0771	0.0636	1	2	2
0.0771 - 0.1189	0.0980	1	2	4
0.1189 - 0.1833	0.1511	9	18.5	22.5
0.1833 - 0.2827	0.2331	14	28.6	51.1
0.2827 - 0.4359	0.3594	6	12.2	63.3
0.4359 - 0.6722	0.5542	15	30.6	93.9
0.6722 - 1,0366	0.8547	3	6.1	100

Statistical tests of correlation were performed between weight and length and between the Hg content and weight for the data obtained for *Prochilodus* sp., *Serrasalmus* sp., *Hoplias malabaricus*, and *Cichla ocellaris*. Fig. 4 plots all relationships found among these parameters, where it is possible to see that the weight of the specimens is directly related to their length, as expected. The Hg content raises in accordance with the weight of the carnivorous fish *Serrasalmus* sp., *Hoplias malabaricus*, and *Cichla ocellaris* (Fig. 4), evidencing the cumulative effect of mercury in tissues, i.e. the increase in weight is normally related to the age of the specimen, that causes a longer assimilation of Hg present in food, not in the metallic form, but bio-available in the ionized (organic) form. Beyond the Hg content values in the non-piscivorous fish *Prochilodus* sp. not exceed the WHO safety limit of 0.5 ppm, the Hg content and weight in these fish are not related (Fig. 4), reinforcing the importance of the alimentation habit on the Hg bioaccumulation.

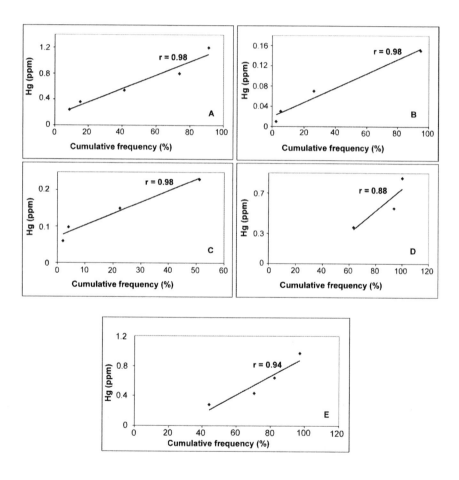

Figure 3: The average Hg content in a) *Serrasalmus* sp., b) *Prochilodus* sp., c) *Cichla ocellaris* (N=25), d) *Cichla ocellaris* (N=24), and e) *Hoplias malabaricus* plotted on a probability graph.

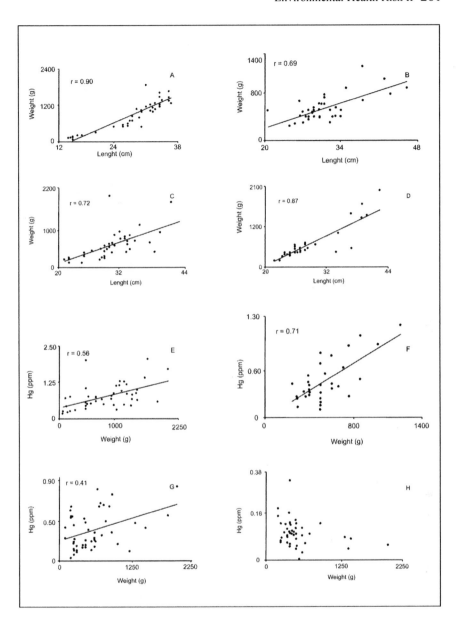

Figure 4:   The relationship between weight and length in a) *Serrasalmus* sp., b) *Hoplias malabaricus*, c) *Cichla ocellaris*, d) *Prochilodus* sp., and the relationship between the Hg content and weight in e) *Serrasalmus* sp., f) *Hoplias malabaricus*, g) *Cichla ocellaris*, and h) *Prochilodus* sp.

References

[1]   Miller, J.R., The role of fluvial geomorphic processes in the dispersal of heavy metals from mine sites. J. Geochem. Explor., 58, pp.101-118, 1997.

[2]   Lockwood, R.A. & Chen, K.Y., Adsorption of Hg (II) by hydrous manganese oxides. Environ. Sci. Technol., 7, pp. 1028-1034, 1973.

[3]   Gambrel, R.P., Khalid, R.A. & Patrick Jr., W.H., Chemical availability of Hg, Pb, and Zn in mobile bay sediment suspensions as affected by pH and oxidation-reduction conditions. Environ. Sci. Technol.,14,.431-436, 1980.

[4]   Luoma, S.N., Bioavailability of trace metals to aquatic organisms – a review. Sci. Total Environ., 28, pp. 1-22, 1983.

[5]   Salomons, W. & Förstner, U., Metals in the hydrocycle, Springer-Verlag: Berlin, 353 p., 1984.

[6]   Pfeiffer, W.C., Lacerda, L.D., Malm, O., Souza, C.M.M., Silveira, E.G. & Bastos, W.R., Mercury concentrations in inland waters of gold-mining areas in Rondônia, Brazil. Sci. Total Environ., 87, pp. 233-240, 1989.

[7]   Cramer, S.W., Problems facing the Philippines. Int. Min., pp. 29-30, 1990.

[8]   Maurice-Bourgoin, L.,Quiroga, I.,Chincheros, J.&Courau, P.Mercury distribution in waters and fish of the upper Madeira rivers and mercury exposure in riparian Amazonian populations.Sci.Total Environ,260, 73-86, 2000.

[9]   Lacerda, L.D., Amazon mercury emissions. Nature, 374, pp. 21-22, 1995.

[10] Malm, O., Pfeiffer, W.C., Souza, C.M.M., & Reuter, R., Mercury pollution due to gold mining in the Madeira River basin. Ambio, 19, pp. 11-15, 1990.

[11] Malm, O., Contaminação ambiental e humana por mercúrio na região garimpeira de ouro do Rio Madeira, PhD Thesis, Universidade Federal do Rio de Janeiro: Rio de Janeiro, 1991.

[12] Lacerda, L.D., Pfeiffer, W.C., Ott, A.T. & Silveira, E.G., Mercury contamination in the Madeira River, Amazon: mercury inputs to the environment. Biotropica, 21, pp. 91-93, 1989.

[13] Pfeiffer, W.C. & Lacerda, L.D., Mercury inputs into the Amazon region, Brazil. Environm. Technol. Lett., 9, pp. 325-330, 1988.

[14] Azcue, J.M., Guimarães, J.R.D., Mudroch, A, Mudroch, P., & Malm, O., Bottom and suspended sediment sampling for studies on the behavior of mercury and other heavy metals in southwestern Amazon rivers and a reservoir, Brazil. Handbook of techniques for aquatic sediments sampling, eds. A. Mudroch, & S.D. MacKnight, CRC Press: Boca Raton, pp. 203-228, 1994.

[15] Cleary, D., Thornton, I.L., Brown, N., Kazantzis, G., Delves, T. & Worthington, S, Mercury in Brazil. Nature, 369, pp. 613-614, 1994.

[16] WHO (World Health Organization), Environmental Health Criteria - I. Mercury. Geneva, pp. 1-131, 1976.

[17] Nunes, D.D., Hidrovia do rio Madeira. Research Report PIBIC-UNIR/CNPq, Universidade Federal de Rondônia: Porto Velho, 1999.

[18] Santos, G.M., Pesca e ecologia dos peixes de Rondônia, PhD Thesis, Instituto Nacional de Pesquisas da Amazônia: Manaus, 213 p., 1991.

Human exposure of methyl mercury through fish consumption: a Lake Ontario case study

G. K. Luk

Department of Civil Engineering, Ryerson University, Canada

Abstract

The consumption of fish accounts for the most significant source of MeHg accumulation in human. The rate of mercury accumulation depends on many factors, including the amount, size, type and frequency of fish consumed, as well as the contamination levels of the aquatic habitat. The ability to accurately predict the human exposure of mercury through fish consumption is very critical for drawing public consumption guidelines. This paper describes the development of an innovative method for the estimation of human exposure of mercury through mathematical modelling. The paper provides a practicable mathematical tool for estimating the human mercury exposure through fish consumption, by a combination of fish mercury bioaccumulation models with surveyed information of fish-eating habit. The efficacy of the model is demonstrated through application to some common Lake Ontario fish species.

Keywords: methyl mercury, human exposure, fish, bioaccumulation, diet, concentration, fish consumption, mathematical models.

1 Introduction

Mercury and its compounds are widely distributed in the environment. Mercury occurs naturally in the environment as mercuric sulphide, from the degassing of the earth's crust through volcanic gases and the weathering of rock in mountains [17]. It has desirable properties such as the ability to alloy with most metals, liquidity at room temperature, electrical conductivity, and the ease of vaporizing and freezing, making mercury an important industrial metal. As a result, mercury has over 3,000 industrial applications, including gold-mining, electrical equipment, chloralkali, paint, fungicide, military, medicine, and dentistry [16].

When mercury is discharged into water bodies, it is first oxidized to the divalent mercuric ion (Hg^{2+}), and then transformed by bacteria action into a highly toxic, poisonous form called methyl mercury (MeHg) [2]. The MeHg in the water and sediments is almost 100% absorbed and stored by bottom fauna and plankton. This toxin gradually works its way up the food chain, causing an increased MeHg concentration in the upper trophic level fish, an effect known as bioaccumulation. It is commonly accepted that longer food chains result in greater bioaccumulation [14]. Once inside the body of a fish, MeHg is tightly bound to the protein of the fish tissues including muscles, and it is slowly metabolized or eliminated from the fish. Eventually, MeHg enters into human who consume the upper level top-predatory fish.

Fish is an important component of the human diet in the Canadian Food Guideline, since it provides dietary protein and many other nutrient benefits. The U.S. EPA estimates that approximately 85% of people consume fish or shellfish over the course of a month, while 60% consume fish four or more times a month, or, on average, at least once a week. As a result, the consumption of fish accounts for the most significant source of MeHg accumulation in human. Unfortunately, there is no known method of cooking or cleaning that is capable of removing MeHg in seafood. Therefore, human has a potentially high health risk when they consume contaminated fish. Mahaffey [10] estimated that the aquatic food web provides more than 95% of human MeHg intake, suggesting that fish is the predominant source of MeHg for most people.

Once MeHg enters into the body of human, it accumulates in the liver, kidneys, brain or blood, and causes a multitude of acute and chronic health effects. It also affects the central nervous system, and in severe cases irreversibly damages areas of the brain [15]. Adverse effects such as impairment of vision and speech, loss of motor coordination, neuropathy and death, and psychological symptoms such as memory loss, weakness and fatigue, anxiety and flight of ideas have been reported [7]. According to Health Canada [6], the maximum tolerable daily intake of mercury for the general population is 0.47 µg/kg of body weight, but the limit for women of childbearing age and children under 15 are more severe, at 0.20 µg/kg, since mercury can seriously damage the fast-growing brain and nervous system of a child or fetus. Since most of the MeHg is absorbed by humans through fish consumption, another guideline to protect the human health from mercury is through fish consumption advisories. As an example, the province of Ontario recommends that women of childbearing age and children eat no more than four meals of fish per month from what is called the "clear fish category", and none at all from any other categories shown in its Guide to Eating Ontario Sport Fish [12].

In spite of the high official and public concern over the mercury pollution problem, a review of the scientific literature indicates that no commonly-accepted methodology is available for the estimation of human exposure of MeHg through the consumption of fish. This is because the rate of mercury accumulation depends on many factors, including the amount, size, type and frequency of fish consumed, as well as the contamination levels of the aquatic habitat and hence individual fish species. It has been observed that even for fish occupying similar trophic levels of the food chain, their choice of habitat and physiological profile can result in very different patterns of bioaccumulation [8]. The objective of this paper is to develop an innovative method for the estimation of human exposure of mercury through the predominant pathway of diet with the use of mathematical modelling. It is envisaged that the model will provide a highly practicable tool from which useful consumption guidelines for the public may be drawn, while remaining flexible enough to accommodate specific studies of localized populations.

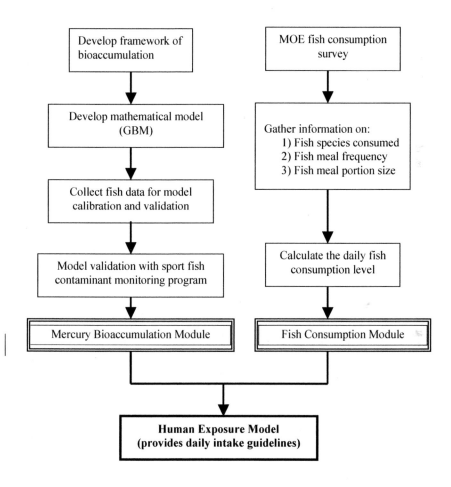

Figure 1:   Organization chart for estimating MeHg dietary exposure.

2 Materials and methods

2.1 Study methodology

The wealth of information and research performed on past fish bioaccumulation models may serve as a framework for modeling the mercury exposure of human. The paper will demonstrate how localized surveyed information of fish consumption may be used to construct a scientifically-based estimation of the average daily exposure of mercury from the fish diet. Figure 1 is an organization chart describing the major components of the study methodology. The human exposure model is developed from two important components: the bioaccumulation module and the fish consumption module. The effectiveness of the developed model is demonstrated through application to two popular Lake Ontario fish species, Chinook Salmon (*Oncorhynchus tshawytscha*) and Lake Trout (*Salvelinus namaycush*).

2.2 Mercury bioaccumulation module

Numerous examples are available on the mathematical models of mercury bioaccumulation in fish [3, 5, 8, 9, 13]. These existing models may be classified into two main categories: the first type is based on regression analysis of collected fish data [3], and the second type is based on the concept of fish bioenergetics [8, 9, 13]. The bioenergetics-based modeling framework is gaining popularity because it incorporates a direct correlation between the energy requirement, the diet, and the pollutant bioaccumulation of the fish. In addition, it allows for a detailed mechanistic representation of all the major pathways of accumulation, whereby model parameters can be related to the physiochemical properties of the fish. For the demonstration of this study, a generic bioaccumulation model (GBM) [9] is chosen to describe the bioaccumulation of MeHg in Lake Ontario's fish. The model has a clear representation for the pathways of mercury intake and excretion, and has been validated to effectively predict the mercury concentrations in many species of fish [1]. It is based on the concept of bioenergetics, derived from an energy balance of fish from food source to support normal activities and growth. Fish needs energy for various life functions such as swimming and foraging activities. To satisfy these requirements, they feed on zooplankton, crustacean and small fish from their diet. In addition, they take in water through the gills for oxygen exchange. When the water and diet items are contaminated with MeHg, mercury will enter the fish's body along with these intake pathways. Therefore, a direct correlation can usually be observed between the metabolic activity level of the fish, the diet requirements, and the pollutant accumulation. The model is based on a mass-balance of the MeHg that enters into the fish body through the pathways of water and food, and leaves through excretion, as follows:

$$\left[\frac{dP}{dt}\right]_{body} = \left[\frac{dP}{dt}\right]_{food} + \left[\frac{dP}{dt}\right]_{water} - \left[\frac{dP}{dt}\right]_{clearance} \qquad (1)$$

where P is the total body burden of mercury in the fish per unit wet weight (ppm); and t is the time (weeks). When the bioenergetics expressions are incorporated into the equation, the final mass-balance equation is given by:

$$\left[\frac{dP}{dt}\right] = \left[\frac{E_{pf}\ C_{pf}}{q_{fd}\ E_{fd}}\right]\left[\alpha_{lr}\ W^{\tau}+\ q_f(\beta+1)\ \left(\frac{dW}{dt}\right)\right]+$$
$$\left[\frac{E_{pw}\ C_{pw}}{E_{ox}\ C_{ox}\ q_{ox}}\right]\left[\alpha_{lr}\ W^{\tau}\ +\ q_f\ \beta\ \left(\frac{dW}{dt}\right)\right]\ -\ k_{cl}\ P \qquad (2)$$

In the equation, E is the efficiency of assimilation; C is the concentration of mercury (ppm); q is the energy equivalence (kcal/(g-wk)); α_{lr} is the low routine metabolism (kcal/(wk-g$^{\tau}$)); W is the wet weight of the fish (g); τ is the body weight exponent for metabolism; β is the proportion of growth rate that represents the energy for food conversion; and k_{cl} is the clearance rate combining waste egestion and growth dilution (wk^{-1}). The subscripts 'pf' and 'pw' represent pollutant from food and water respectively, 'fd' is the value of the food or prey, 'f' is the value of the fish, and 'ox' represents values of oxygen.

A computer program was developed in Visual Basic 5.0 [9] to provide weekly simulation with graphical display of the mercury bioaccumulation patterns in different fish species. One of the most important input for the model is the composition and the level of contamination of the diet of individual fish, which is age and species-specific. An attempt is made to re-construct the diet pattern, based on food web information and data collected from past studies on fish stomach's contents, as demonstrated in Table 1 [1, 3].

2.3 Fish consumption module

Since 1978, the Ontario Ministry of Environment (MOE) has periodically surveyed the fishing habit and fish consumption by the Lake Ontario population. The survey is carried out once every few years, in which questionnaires on fishing habit and consumption are randomly sent to residents of Ontario. Based on the results, the MOE publishes consumption advice to people in the province in the form of a bi-annual edition of "Guide to Eating Ontario Sportfish" [12]. The survey is made up of 19 questions, ranging from the respondent's personal information, knowledge of the Fish Guide, to fishing frequency, fishing locations, and fish consumption habits (on both sport and commercial fish). For this paper, the latest-published survey data set collected in 1995 [11] is selected to represent the fish consumption habit by Ontarians of different age groups. From the results of the survey, information on the distribution of the fish species consumed, fish meal frequency, and the meal portion size may be obtained.

Table 1:   Re-constructed diet composition.

Fish species	Age group (age group)	% Diet items	MeHg conc. (ppm)
Chinook Salmon	Juvenile (0 – 1)	Terrestrial insects 100%	0.0040
	Mature (1 – 7)	8% Small invertebrates	0.0500
		11% Medium rainbow smelt	0.0355
		82% Medium alewife	0.0300
Lake Trout	Juvenile (0 – 2)	45% Small slimy sculpin	0.0240
		35% Small rainbow smelt	0.0215
		20% Small alewife	0.0165
	Young (2 – 4)	18% Medium slimy sculpin	0.0315
		45% Medium rainbow smelt	0.0285
		38% Medium alewife	0.0300
	Mature (4 – 8)	30% Medium rainbow smelt	0.0355
		70% Large alewife	0.0430

3   Model results

3.1 Tolerable daily intake

Health Canada recommends a maximum tolerable daily intake (TDI) of mercury for the general population as 0.47 µg/kg, and for children and women of childbearing age as 0.20 µg/kg. Since the acceptable mercury intake is highly dependent on body weight, some estimation of the human weight distribution would be required to calculate the tolerable intake for different spectrum of the population, and the data by Halls and Hanson [4] is adopted. For the demonstration in this study, five major groups of the population are identified: Children, women of childbearing age, young adults, mature adults, and seniors. The maximum daily tolerable mercury uptakes for these groups are calculated in Table 2.

3.2 Factor of safety

Fish is not the only source of mercury for human, since appreciable amounts of mercury may be absorbed by human from breathing contaminated air, from consuming other contaminated food sources, and from other unknown sources. As such, a safety factor of 2 is considered appropriate to apply to the acceptable intake of mercury from fish for the general population. Applying this safety factor, the tolerable levels of mercury intake for the four identified groups are re-established and included with the original levels in Table 2. In general, males can accept 10% higher daily mercury consumption than can females.

Table 2:   Maximum daily tolerable mercury uptakes for 5 study groups.

Study groups	Age range	TDI (µg)
Children	10 – 15	4.5
Women of Childbearing age	20 – 35	6.1
Young adults	20 – 25	15.1
Mature adults	40 – 55	16.5
Seniors	≥ 65	10.3

3.3 Actual mercury uptake from fish consumption

The amount of fish consumed on a daily basis may be estimated from the survey data, based on the information collected on fish consumption habits. With this, the actual mercury uptake from fish consumption may then be estimated for the two study species as summarized in Figure 2. Calculations are performed for people eating anywhere between one to four meals of fish per week. The symbol curves represent the total amount of mercury consumption of different diet habits, and the horizontal lines are the suggested TDI levels for various groups of population. Whenever the curves are higher than the TDI, there is a health concern. Therefore, the intersection point of the curves and TDI may be used to estimate the size restriction of fish consumption.

4 Discussion

A lot of useful recommendations may be drawn from Figure 2. For example, the results show that there is practically no risk for the general population who regularly eat 1 meal or less of Chinook Salmon per week. This, however, does not apply to children under 15 and women of childbearing age, because a part of the 1-week curve is above the TDI for these groups.

The results can also give some recommendations on the selection of fish size to be consumed. As an example, for a senior who eats 2 meals of normal serving portion (of around 220 g) of Chinook Salmon per week, the results show that he should limit the consumption to a maximum fish size of 10 kg total weight. Obviously, the more frequent is the fish consumption, the more stringent is this size restriction. Therefore, the same group eating Chinook Salmon three times a week should consume a fish less than 3.5 kg to be on the safe side. If this size happens to be much less than the typical size available for that fish, then three meals a week is simply too much for the study group, and consumption frequency should be reduced.

Another important result from the analysis is the level of contamination of the different species. Of the two fish species, Lake Trout has a higher risk than Chinook Salmon. Therefore, a person who is concerned about MeHg exposure should make a point of selecting a less contaminated fish species habitually. As demonstrated from this research, a lot of highly useful recommendations on the choice of fish may be provided if a multiple-species analysis of commonly available fish is carried out.

WIT Transactions on Biomedicine and Health, Vol 9, © 2005 WIT Press
www.witpress.com, ISSN 1743-3525 (on-line)

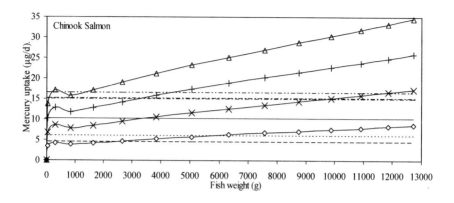

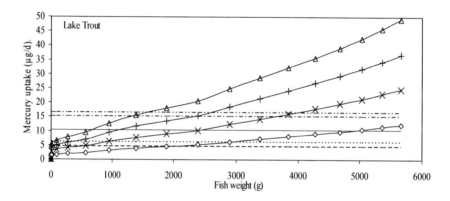

Legend

Frequency of fish per Week	Once ◊	Twice x	3 Times +	4 Times Δ	
Study Group	Children	Women of c/b age	Young adults	Mature adults	Seniors
	--------	....	---·---·--	---··---··--	_____

Figure 2: Results of the MeHg human exposure model.

Results from this research also reveal two very important guidelines for the consumers. Firstly, moderate fish consumption of less than twice a week should pose no major risk to the general population in terms of MeHg exposure. On the other hand, a person eating four fish meals a week should be very vigilant over the type and size of the fish consumed. Secondly, even though most consumers prefer a bigger fish because of the ease of preparation and absence of fine bones, results from this analysis clearly indicates that the choice may not be a healthy one. This is especially significant considering that no amount of cooking or cleaning will remove the accumulated mercury of the fish. In addition, unlike other types of fat-soluble contaminants such as PCBs which can be avoided if the skin, intestines, and head of the fish are removed, mercury is protein-bound and tends to accumulate in the tissues or meat of the fish quite uniformly.

Another factor to consider is the highly cumulative effect of mercury in human. While the tolerable daily intake of mercury provides some guidelines on daily fish consumption, the bioaccumulation effect of mercury over the life span should not be neglected. Results from this and other studies have clearly confirmed that mercury is bioaccumulated in human and animals over time and it is only eliminated from the body at a very slow rate. Therefore, while it may be acceptable to exceed the tolerable daily limit occasionally, a fish-lover who consumes fish consistently as a regular part of the diet should be more cautious about the possible cumulative effect.

5   Conclusions

Fish is an important dietary component of human, containing a good source of proteins, omega-3 fatty acids, and many other nutrient benefits. However, consumption of fish on a regular basis may also lead to an increased risk of MeHg exposure. This paper describes the development of an innovative method for the estimation of human exposure of mercury through mathematical modelling. By a judicious combination of fish mercury bioaccumulation models with surveyed information of fish-eating habit, it was found that the method provided a scientifically-based estimation of the average daily exposure of mercury from fish consumption. It provides a highly practicable tool from which useful consumption guidelines for the public may be drawn, while remaining flexible enough to accommodate specific studies of some localized individual populations. To reduce the potential mercury exposure in the human body, people should choose smaller fish within a species, because they are typically younger and haven't been exposed to mercury for as long as the older, bigger fish. It is also better to eat a variety of fish, especially the less contaminated species, to avoid high exposure to mercury.

Acknowledgements

This study is made possible through a Natural Science and Engineering Research Council (NSERC) grant to the author. The assistance of staff at the Ministry of Environment in providing fish surveillance data is highly appreciated.

References

[1]   Au-Yeung, W.C., 2002. Methylmercury bioaccumulation in sport fish and the relation to human exposure. M.A.Sc. Thesis, Ryerson University, Canada.

[2]   Boening, D.W., 2000. Ecological effects, transport, and fate of mercury: a general review. Chemospere 40, 1335-1351.

[3]   Borgmann, U., Whittle, D.M., 1992. Bioenergetics and PCB, DDE, and mercury dynamics in Lake Ontario lake trout (*Salvelinus namaycush*): a

model based on surveillance data. Canadian Journal of Fisheries and Aquatic Sciences 49, 1086-1096.

[4]   Halls, S.B. and Hanson, 2002. Adults Height and Weight Charts. Available in web page http://www.halls.md/chart/child-growth/height-weight.htm

[5]   Harris, R.C., Snodgrass, W.J., 1993. Bioenergetic simulations of mercury uptake and retention in walleye (*Stizostedion vitreum*) and yellow perch (*Perca flavescens*). Walter Pollution Research Canada 28 (1), 217-236.

[6]   Health Canada, 2003. Warning/Advisories – Information on mercury levels in fish. Publications Health Canada, Ottawa.

[7]   Huggins, H.A., 1988. Mercury & other toxic metals in humans. Proceedings of the International Conference on Biocompatibility of Materials. Life Sciences Press, Tacoma.

[8]   Luk, G.K., Brockway, F., 1997. Application of a PCBs bioaccumulation model to Lake Ontario lake trout. Journal of Ecological Modelling 101(1997), 97-111.

[9]   Luk, G.K., 2001. Ecotoxicology modeling of methylmercury bioaccumulation. In: Villacampa, Y., Brebbia, C.A., Uso, J.L. (Eds.), Ecosystems and Sustainable Development III. WIT Press, Boston.

[10]   Mahaffey, K.R., 1999. Methylmercury: a new look at the risk. Public Health Reports 114, 396-415.

[11]   Ministry of Environment (MOE), 1998. The results of the 1995 – 1998 survey for "Guide to Eating Ontario Sport Fish" questionnaire. Ministry of Environment, Ontario.

[12]   Ministry of Environment (MOE), 2003. 2003 - 2004 Guide to eating Ontario sport fish. Queen's Printer, Ontario.

[13]   Norstrom, R.J., McKinnon, A.E., DeFreitas, A.S.W., 1976. A bioenergetics-based model for pollutant accumulation by fish. Journal Fish Resources Board Canada 33, 248-267.

[14]   Rasmussen, J.B., Rowan, D.J., Lean, D., Carey, J.H., 1990. Food chain structure in Ontario lakes determines PCB levels in lake trout and other pelagic fish. Canadian Journal of Fisheries and Aquatic Science 47, 2030-2038.

[15]   Thompson, P. 2000. Mercury:a fact sheet for health professionals. Missouri State University, available in

[16]   http: //www.orcbs.msu.edu/AWARE/pamphlets/hazeaste/mercuryfacts.html

[17]   World Health Organization (WHO), 1989. Mercury environmental aspects. WHO, Geneva, Switzerland.

[18]   Zelikoff, J.T., Thomas, P.T., 1998. Immunotoxicology of environmental and occupational Metals. Taylor and Francis Ltd, Lon

Section 4
Occupational health

Microbiological risk in operating rooms: new strategies for infections surveillance

A. Frabetti[1], A. Vandini[1], S. Pantoja Rodriguez[1], F. Margelli[1],
M. Cavicchioli[4], M. Migliori[3], D. Arujo Azevedo[1],
P. Balboni[2] & S. Mazzacane[1]
[1]CERTECA Laboratory, Air Technology Research Center,
Department of Architecture, University of Ferrara, Italy
[2]Department of Diagnostic and Experimental Medicine,
University of Ferrara, Italy
[3]Hospital Manager, Emilia Romagna Region, Italy
[4]CENTO HOSPITAL Manager, Italy

Abstract

In this paper the authors describe the program of epidemiological overseeing of the surgical site infections activated in the operating department of the Cento Hospital (Ferrara).

The purpose of the program is to systematically collect the data related to the frequency and distribution of the infections contracted during a surgical intervention and to analyze the environmental factors correlated to them, the concentration of particles and of UFC, the characteristics of the ventilation system, the number of people in the room, the type of clothing, the systems of cleaning and disinfection, the type of intervention etc.

The objective of the research consists of identifying the actions for prevention of the infections and to get an indicator of the quality of the surgical activities.

Since the greatest obstacle to this kind of activity is related to the man-hour cost for the information collection, researchers of the University of Ferrara and the Cento hospital have setup an electronic system of automatic acquisition of the field data using computer technologies of different types (RFID-Radio Frequency IDentification sensor, PC pocket, net computer and programs).

The management of continuous relief of the pollution level established in the operating rooms during every intervention, the automatic acquisitions of the main environmental parameters (temperature, relative humidity, instant air flow rate of climatization plant, state of the doors, level of pressurization of the room, level of stoppage of the absolute filters etc.) and of the clinical overview of the patient allow detailed knowledge of the conditions in which every surgical intervention is developed. Particular attention is paid to the state of hypothermia of the patient that is monitored in continuously before, during and after the operation, since according to some authors this determines an increase in the probability of contamination of the wound. The surgical wound is controlled daily in the hospital up to the moment of patient release and every three months for one year from the intervention, so as to record possible complication.

This adopted strategy allows to verification in the respect of the behavioral protocols of the medical and nursing personnel.

Keywords: surveillance, infection rate, microbiological and physical pollution.

1   Introduction

Nosocomial infections (NI) are acquired during hospital care which are not present or incubating at admission. Infections occuring more than 48 hours after admission are usually considered nosocomial. Definitions to identify NI have been developed for specific infection sites and they derived from those published by CDC of Atlanta [1-3].

Studies throughout the world document that nosocomial infections are a major cause of morbidity and mortality [4-11]. A high frequency of nosocomial infections is evidence of a poor quality of health service delivery, and leads to avoidable costs. SSIs represent the second most common type of nosocomial infection at a rate between 20% and 30% of the total events [13,14]. SSIs develop in 2% to 5% of patients undergoing surgical procedures each year in the United States, resulting in at least 500,000 infections (100,000 in Italy), and high costs extra hospital charges [12,13]. In Europe the SSI rate varied widely from 1.5-20% of patients undergoing surgical procedures often unspecified in consequence of inconsistencies in data collection methods, surveillance criteria and wide variations in the surgical procedures; the SSI's healthcare cost estimated range from € 1.47-19.1 billion. The development of a surveillance process to monitor this rate is an essential first step to identify local problems and priorities, and evaluate the effectiveness of infection control activity. Surveillance, by itself, is an effective process to decrease the frequency of hospital-acquired infections [16-18] and their costs.

Since 1970s CDC's National Nosocomial Infection Surveillance (NNIS) system has been serving as an aggregating medium to collect data of NI in USA and in the North of Europe. NNIS system is a voluntary, hospital-based reporting system established to monitor HAI and guide the prevention efforts of infection control practitioners. NNIS establishes a national risk-adjusted benchmark for NI rates and invasive device-use ratios [19,20] by using uniform case definitions and data collection methods and computerized data entry and analysis.

For a long time in Italy the problem of hospital-acquired infection was to be an interesting object of investigation for SSN and other national and international institutions.

In 1984 OMS had just indicated the priority to control the developing of nosocomial infections (NI) within year the 2000; successively were produced two national Ministerial Circulars (n° 52-20/12/85, n° 8-30/01/88) with the same aims.

Finally were emanated Ministerial Acts (PSN 1998-2000; PSR 1999-2001) that declared the necessity to reduce the incidence of NI of 25%; these acts were addressed to characterize systems for prevention and surveillance of NI.

Following these formatives, Azienda USL of Ferrara (Delibera n° 58-13/01/2000), had instituted the "Prevention and Infection Control Committee" with the aim to characterize, organize and verify the strategy to pull down NI in any kind of health-care environment.

Considering that the responsible health authority should develop a national (or regional) programme to support hospitals in reducing the risk of NI.

At this aim, we are monitoring the internal conditions "at rest" and "in activity" of the 4 operating rooms of Cento Hospital under different profiles:
-   physical pollution (particulate concentration in the air) by KANOMAX GEO-α instrument;
-   air, material surfaces and wound microbiological pollution (active and passive monitoring using Surface Air System (SAS), Contact plate dishes, tampons);
-   characteristics of ventilation system (supply and extraction air flow rates, pressurization level, type of filters, air distribution and velocity on the wound field, air temperature and relative humidity and so on);
-   hypothermia phenomena for the patient, sweatiness index and comfort degree of medical staff (Dallas Semiconductors I-BUTTONs and BABUC/A system LSI Lastem);
-   morbosity of the patient, antibiotic profilaxis and anaesthetic infusion;
-   environmental contest (number of persons, clothing and drapes, state of the doors, if opened or closed, operating protocols and so on).

Until now all data were collected in a writing-papers, but in the future they will collect into a central server by a supervision system and electronic devices utilizing RFID sensors (Radio Frequency IDentification) and bar code readers (Figure 1).

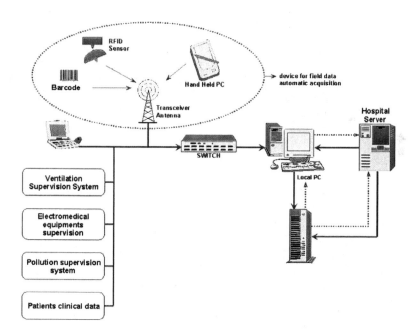

Figure 1.

2 Materials and methods

2.1 Period and setting

The results reporting in this paper were collected in a period of two month (February and March 2005) but the study is yet in progress and it will continuing for a period of three years.

The study was carried out in the operating room (OR) of Orthopaedic Department in Santa Annunziata Hospital in Cento (Ferrara-Italy), which has a turbulent air flow circulation system (22 air changes/h) that includes two HEPA filters (1 on every air terminal and 1 on central unit).

2.2 Microbiological monitoring

2.2.1 Air monitoring

Nowadays the evaluation of the level of air microbial contamination in places at risk is considered to be a basic step toward prevention [21-27]. However, there are still problems to be solved relating to methodology, monitoring, data interpretation and maximum acceptable levels of contamination.

At the moment, the only effective means of quantifying airborne microbes is limited to the count of cfu. The cfu count is the most important parameter, as it measures the live micro-organisms which can multiply. Air samples can be collected in two ways: by active air samplers or by passive air sampling (the settle plates). Both methods are widely used.

Passive air sampling is performed using settle plates at frequency of one sampling for 1 hour during every orthopaedic surgery. Microbes carried by inert particles fall onto the surface of the nutrient, with an average deposition rate of 0.46 cm/s being reported [29]. Followings the CDC's guidelines (8Ascca), we evaluated microbial sedimentation with Contact plate dishes "Agar Clean Room Contact FDA" of 55 mm diameter containing plate count agar TSA (Tryptone Soia Agar) with the addition of Tween-Lecitine. The dishes were left open to air according to the 1/1/1 standard (for 1 h, 1 m from the floor and about 1 m from the patient) over three operating tables [26].

Sampling started in correspondence of the surgical incision. The plates were sent to the bacteriology laboratory at the end of the operation and incubated at 37°C for 48 h and at 25°C for another 24 h before bacterial counts were counted. The number of CFU is measured in cfu/plate. Only the total aerobic bacterial count was evaluated; identification and speciation of bacteria isolated were not performed. The results were compared with index of microbiological contamination of air (IMA index). IMA index was devised in 1978 [31] with the aim of unifying and standardizing the technique of air sampling by settle plates. The IMA classes and the maximum acceptable IMA levels for each environment at risk were empirically defined by performing a large number of tests in different environments [28,30,31,32].

In this study we have selected the Petri dishes of 55 mm diameter because they are useful both for passive and active monitoring and for the control of surfaces (contact plates). Moreover a triple cover of these plates assures a high grade of sterility that is requisite for their use in an operating theater. However in view to uniform our study to international standards, we'll be going to do a comparison between the results obtained by the utilization both Petri dishes 55mm in diameter and 90mm in diameter.

The microbial air contamination can be measured by counting the number of cfu per cubic metre (cfu/m^3) of air. For this purpose active air samplers are used, which collect a known volume of air, blown on to a nutrient medium by different techniques. There are many different types of active samplers, in this study we used Surface Air System sampler (SAS; "SAS SUPER 100" PBI International). SAS was placed nearest the site of surgical incision in according to standard [34].

SAS was programmed to introduce 6000 l of air in one hour and to blow the air on to contact plates of 55 mm in diameters containing plate count agar TSA (Tryptone Soia Agar) with the addition of Tween-Lecitine. After 1 h the plates were incubated at 37°C for 48 h and at 25°C for another 24 h; finally the counts of CFU was performed and compared with the IMA index [32].

2.2.2 Material surfaces monitoring

OR surfaces (walls, floor and electomedical instruments) were monitored by the use of Contact plate dishes at the frequency of 1 hour every 15 days. Then the plate is incubated at 37°C for 48 h and at 25°C for another 24 h before bacterial counts were taken. The number of CFU is measured in cfu/plate.

2.2.3 Wound microbiological pollution monitoring

The rates of wound microbiological pollution were monitored by the application over the surgery wound of a sterile tampon. These tampons were passed by on a contact plate dishes and then incubated at 37°C for 48 h and at 25°C for another 24 h before bacterial counts were counted. This sampling was carried out for 1 month for each orthopaedic surgery at sutured wound before its disinfection.

2.3 Particulates concentration monitoring of air

Particulates concentration monitoring of air (0,3 μm , 0,5 μm, 1 μm, 3 μm e 5 μm) was performed with Kanomax Geo-α instrument (Pollution) according to ISO 14644 norm for a period of one week. In the operating theatre at *rest* measurements were carried out, in 6 points (140cm high) every 2 minutes to define optimum monitoring time(τ) which was resulted to be $\tau = 30$ min. Instead, in active operating theatre this instrument was located only in one place over a bracket 170cm high near operating table and acquired measurements every 2 minutes during all the days' surgeries.

2.4 Ventilation of system data

The collection of ventilation system data was performed by a central supervision system linked to the local equipment which was able to register every state function in real time.

2.5 Hypothermia phenomena monitoring

Hypothermia that develops in patients undergoing operating surgery; hypothermia is join to inhibition of thermoregulator system due to both anaesthetic treatment and low temperature of operating room; for this reason, hypothermia could increase the morbidity and mortality after operating surgery [35]. The sampling was performed by use I-BUTTONs (Dallas Semiconductors) that are small instruments like a buttons to which is possible both capturing and registering the temperature and the humidity of the skin of the patient and medical staff.

Two model of buttons are using:
- DS1921H model that measure the temperature
- DS1923-F5 model that measure the humidity

These buttons are able to register until 4096 data in different moments. Many application forms for the button are codified in literature, but we decided to utilize Olesen's application form [36], where three buttons on the body (chess, arms and legs) are considered. Moreover I-button for humidity was positioned on the epigastric zone.

2.6 Microclimatic monitoring: Babuc

Following ISPESL Italian guidelines (D.P.R. 14.01.97) and UNI EN ISO 7730 norm we performed the microclimatic sampling with the use of BABUC/A system (LSI-Lastem), formed by two parts: one that acquire and elaborate data and the other that its constituted by a group of sensors:
- a psychometric probe for measuring both dry (Td) and wet (Tw) temperatures,
- a globe thermometric probe for measuring mean radiant temperature (Tr),
- an anemometer for air velocity (Va) measuring.
BABUC/A was placed at 1,5 m high from the floor (area: 36 m^2) in OR. The first measurements were collected in operating room at rest in different points.

The verification of microclimatic conditions during orthopedic surgery is going under study.

2.7 Active surveillance of SSI

Patients undergoing total joint knee and hip replacement surgery, hemi-artroplasty were monitored as part of the hospital's overall surveillance programme during February 2005. We used a standardized data collection form to obtain statistic data. Details collected included demographic data, the date and type of procedure, morbidity, American Society of Anesthesiology (ASA) pre-operative assessment score, peri-operative antibiotic prophylaxis, pre e post-operative blood transfusion and type of anaesthesia.

After orthopaedic surgery were reviewed inpatients for postoperative SSIs. Notifications of possible infections were also requested from us to nursing staff, surgical team, and staff in the care intensive unit; they was informed when patients have suspected SSIs. In addition patients undergoing hip and knee arthroplasty were followed up at one, three, six and 12 months after surgery and notifications of suspected infections were collected.

If a SSIs was suspected by the nursing or medical staff, they discussed the case to classify the infections according to the CDC (The Center for Disease Control and Prevention) definitions of surgical site infections (the organ/space and deep incisional categories were combined in this survey).

2.8 RFID technology

RFID system are used in a wide variety of industry applications, including automatic fare collection on bridges, toll roads, and public transit; wireless pay-at-the-pump payment programs, and hands-free access control security systems in offices and factories.

RFID tags consist of an integrated circuit (IC) attached to an antenna; data is stored on the IC and transmitted trough the antenna. Tags can be smaller than a grain of rice or as large as a brick. RFID tags are either passive (not battery) or active (self-powered by a battery). Data transmission speed and range depend on the frequency used, antenna size, power output and interference. Tags can be read-only, read-write, or a combination, in which some data (such as a serial number) is permanently stored, while other memory is left available for later encoding or to be updated during utilization. Information is sent to and is read from RFID tags over RF signals.

RFID tags can be read through packaging, shipping containers, and most materials except metal. An important characteristic of them is that dozens of tags can be read effectively by the same reader simultaneously. Because tags are reusable, they can improve efficiency in many operations by reducing labor and materials costs.

The aim of our study is to reduce the medical staff working time (collecting all data and information, actually hand-taken, with tagging wireless technology), to realize a hands-free control security system for pre/post-operating nursing (medicine administration, disposable control, etc.) and operating (anaesthesia, clinical information, prosthetic components and others) activities and finally to reach a higher information technology level in the clinical managemant to look up the services quality reducing the double-entry and permitting a faster information finding.

3 Results

During two month (February and March 2005) we monitored 104 orthopaedic surgeries of which only 62 were election surgeries interesting for us to use for developing a new method for SSIs survillance. These election orthopaedic surgeries were composed by 29 total hip replacement (ATA), 8 total knee replacement (PTG), 19 shoulder artroscopy (SPALLA) and 6 reconstruction of knee ligament (LCA).

Microbiological data, collected with passive method, was compared with IMA index; OR was placed in IMA1 class because the UFC counts ranged between 0 to 6 CFU/dm^2/h. Only 4 surgeries (3 ATA, 1 LCA) were resulted more contaminate than other with a range between 5-10 CFU/dm^2/h placing OR in IMA2 class (Figure 2).

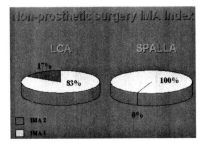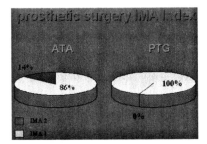

Figure 2: IMA Index values related with different orthopaedic surgery.

For a period of one month we monitored and collected data of 40 surgeries with the active air sampling (SAS) and the same results, as passive air sampling were obtained. Moreover we had monitored all 104 surgeries with passive air sampling to determinate the daily total microbial charge; we had registered that microbial charge didn't growth at the end of the day but was maintained constant between first operation and last one. We reported in this text the results of two days (Figure 3). The other results are completely similar.

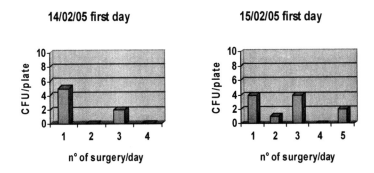

Figure 3: 5 graphic that show the daily total microbiological charge.

During the two months of observation and collection of data we didn't reveal any case of SSIs not even at 30th day after surgery, but is necessary to going on with the monitoring of wound for a much longer period of time especially for election prosthetic surgery that required one year of observation after surgery. The wound tampons results are all negative as the results of surfaces monitoring.

Through the results of particulates concentration in OR *at rest* we had calculated ISO class and as shown in table 1 the values obtained placing room in ISO5 class.

Table 1:   ISO classification results

C_n	particle / m^3			
D	Particle diamteter			
N	$N = \log(C_n) - 2{,}08 \cdot \log(0.1/D)$			
diameter	0.3 μm	0.5 μm	1 μm	5 μm
CLASS	4.2	3.9	4.1	5.0

In activity OR the values collected maintaining the room in ISO6 class. We had noticed that while trend of the particulates concentration curve was the same for every dimensions of particulate, the differences between the values are sensitive to particulates diameter, to different kinds of operations and to different events during the same operation.

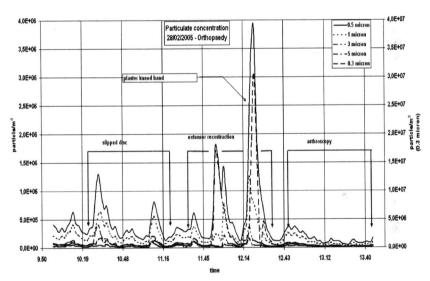

Figure 4:   Particulates concentration *in activity* OR.

Regarding the results of termic stress monitoring, their elaboration and analysis are in progress, as the developing and the definition of RFID technology that is in progress too.

4 Discussion

Providing feedback to the use of conventional surveillance methods requires a significant amount of time for the collection, analysis and feedback of data by the operating staff.

One of the aims of our studies is to create and offer another methodology to collect data for surveillance, to identify the actions for prevention of the infections and to get indicator of quality for the surgical activities.

During two month were collected many data of election orthopaedic surgery in the Cento Hospital, about microbiological and physical monitoring of air and active monitoring SSIs surveillance.

Regarding the microbiological monitoring it can be demonstrated that turbulent airflow with absolute HEPA filter is very efficiently.

Regarding the microbiological monitoring, the results demonstrate that it is possible to reach a high level of sterility in ORs using turbulent airflow systems, more economic and comfortable than the laminar one. This consideration of a high asepsis level can be extruded to the particulate pollution, that the verified to be conform to ISO4 classes in condition *at rest* and to ISO6 in *activity*.

The elaboration of termic stress monitoring data to define optimum microclimatic environmental conditions during an orthopaedic surgery is in progress.

The absence of SSIs case during two month of active surveillance was attributed to good functionality turbulent airflow system, good manufacturing practice of the operating staff and velocity with which the operating staff performed a surgery. Besides the operating staff followed conscientiously all guidelines that defined the prevention of NI to guarantee a high grade of environmental sterility.

The experimentation, still working, of automatic computer collecting data using RFID technology will be an important instrument for SSIs surveillance and for NI surveillance too. It will be provide in real-time any kind of sanitary information that are necessary to operating staff so reducing morbidity and mortality rates. Reducing morbidity and mortality it will be possible to pull down health-care costs   to the reduction the patient stay (LOS) time and the drugs costs.

The main step attended for the future deals with the effort to correlate the different variables (particulate and CFU concentration, ventilation systems parameters, environmental parameters and so on) with the aim to investigate the genesis of the microbiological pollution phenomena and the corresponding qualitative and quantitative trend.

References

[1]   Garner JS et al. CDC definitions for nosocomial infections, 1988. *Am J Infect Control*, 1988, 16:128–140.

[2]   Horan TC et al. CDC definitions of nosocomial surgical site infections, 1992: a modification of CDC definition of surgical wound infections. *Am J Infect Control*, 1992, 13:606–608.

[3]   Prevention of hospital-acquired infections; A practical guide 2nd edition; World Health Organization Department of Communicable Disease, Surveillance and Response; 2002

[4]   Mayon-White R et al. An international survey of the prevalence of hospital-acquired infection. *J Hosp Infect*, 1988, 11 (suppl A): 43–48.

[5]   Emmerson AM et al. The second national prevalence survey of infection in hospitals — overview of the results. *J Hosp Infect*, 1996, 32:175–190.

[6]   Gastmeier P et al. Prevalence of nosocomial infections in representative German hospitals. J Hosp Infect, 1998, 38:37–49.

[7]   Vasque J, Rossello J, Arribas JL. Prevalence of nosocomial infections in Spain: EPINE study 1990–1997. EPINE Working Group. *J Hosp Infect*, 1999, 43 Suppl: S105–S111.

[8]   Kim JM et al. Multicentre surveillance study for nosocomial infections in major hospitals in Korea. *Am J Infect Control*, 2000, 28:454–458.

[9]   Gikas A et al. Repeated multi-centre prevalence surveys of hospital acquired infection in Greek hospitals. *J Hosp Infect*, 1999, 41:11–18.

[10] Scheel O, Stormark M. National prevalence survey in hospital infections in Norway. *J Hosp Infect*, 1999, 41:331–335.

[11] Orrett FA, Brooks PJ, Richardson EG. Nosocomial infections in a rural regional hospital in a developing country: infection rates by site, service, cost, and infection control practices. *Infect Control Hosp Epidemiol*, 1998, 19:136–140.

[12] Wong E. Surgical site infections. In: Mayhall CG, editor. Hospital epidemiology and infection control. 2nd ed. Philadelphia: Lippincott Williams and Wilkins; 1999. p. 189-210.

[13] Martone WJ, Nichols RL. Recognition, prevention, surveillance, and management of SSI. *Clin Infect Dis* 2001; 33:s67-8.

[14] Martorell C., Engelman R., Corl A., Brown R.B. Surgical site infections in cardiac surgery: An 11-year perspective. Am J Infect Control 2004; 32:63-8.

[15] An YH, Friedman RJ. Prevention of sepsis in total joint arthroplasty. *J Hosp Infect* 1996; 33: 93–108.

[16] Enstone JE, Humphreys H. Monitoring infective complications following hip fracture. *J Hosp Infect* 1998; 38: 1–9.

[17] Mayon-White R et al. An international survey of the prevalence of hospital-acquired infection. *J Hosp Infect*, 1988, 11 (suppl A): 43–48.

[18] Emmerson AM et al. The second national prevalence survey of infection in hospitals — overview of the results. *J Hosp Infect*, 1996, 32:175–190.

[19] Enquête nationale de prévalence des infections nosocomiales. Mai–Juin 1996. Comité technique national des infections nosocomiales. *Bulletin Èpidémiologique Hebdomadaire*, 1997, No 36.

[20] National Nosocomial Infections Surveillance System. Nosocomial infection rates for interhospital comparison: Limitations and possible solutions. *Infect Control Hosp Epidemiol* 1991; 12:609-12.

[21] Culver DH, Horan TC, Gaynes RP, and the National Nosocomial Infection Surveillance System. Surgical wound infection rates by wound class, operative procedure, and patient risk index in U.S. hospitals, 1986-90. *Am J Med* 1991; 91(Suppl 3B): 152S-157S.

[22] Charnley J, Eftekhar M. Postoperative infection in total prosthetic arthroplasty of the hip-joint with special reference to the bacterial content of air in the operating room. *Br J Surg* 1969; **56**: 641–664.

[23] Eickhoff TC. Airborne nosocomial infection: a contemporary perspective. *Infect Control Hosp Epidemiol* 1994; **15**: 663–672.

[24] Hofstra H, van der Vossen JMBM, van der Plas, J. Microbes in food processing technology. *FEMS Microbiol Rev* 1994; **15**: 175–183.

[25] Kang YJ, Frank JF. Biological aerosols: a reveiw of airborne contamination and its measurement in dairy processing Plants. *J Food Protect* 1989; **52**: 512–524.

[26] Pierson DL, McGinnis MR, Mishra SK, Wogan CF. Microbiology on Space Station Freedom. NASA Conference Publication 3108, 1991.

[27] Whyte W, Hambraeus A, Laurell G, Hoborn J. The relative importance of the routes and sources of wound contamination during general surgery. II. Airborne. *J Hosp Infect* 1992; **22**: 41–54.

[28] Pitzurra M, Savino A, Pasquarella C. Il Monitoraggio ambientale microbiologico (MAM). *Ann Ig* 1997; **9**: 439–454.

[29] Whyte W. Sterility assurance and models for assessing bacterial contamination. *J Parenter Sc Technol* 1995; **40**: 188–197.

[30] Pitzurra M, Morlunghi P, Contaminazione microbica dell'aria atmosferica. Correlazione fra due diverse metodiche di rilevazione. *Ig Mod* 1978; **3**: 489–501.

[31] Pitzurra M. Malattie Infettive da Ricovero in Ospedale. Saronno: Ciba Geigy 1984; 295–306.

[32] Pasquarella C., Pitzurra O. and Savino A. The index of microbial air contamination. Rewiev *J of Hosp Infect* (2000) 46: 241–256.

[33] Pasquarella C., Pitzurra O. and. Savino A. The index of microbial air contamination. *J Hosp Infect* 2000; **46**: 241–256

[34] Whyte W, Lidwell OM, Lowbury EJL, Blowers R. Suggested bacteriological standards for air in ultra-clean operating rooms. *J Hosp Infect* 1983; 4: 133–139.

[35] A. Kurz, Prevention and treatment of perioperative hypothermia, *Current Anaesthesia & Critical Care*, 12, 2001, 96-102

[36] Olesen, B.W., 1982, How many sites are necessary to estimate a mean skin temperature?, *Thermal Physiology*, Raven Press, New York, 34-38.

Vibration evaluation from the effects of whole-body vibration

M. Uchikune
Department of Precision Machinery Engineering,
College of Science & Technology, Nihon University, Japan

Abstract

The purpose of this study is to make clear the physiological and psychological effects on the human body from vibration, and it aims to be a cautionary guide for the application of frequency-weighting curves with respect to health effects.

The standard is not well defined for the difference between the two effects of the human responses.

The study covers short-term exposure and assesses the risks resulting from whole-body vibrations.

For recumbent persons, tests were carried out to find the effect of whole-body vibration in a low frequency range. Physiological effects were examined by investigating the effects on the cardiovascular system, the blood flow system, the respiratory movement, and the salivation, to confirm the effects on the autonomic nervous system and on postural sways in the normal Romberg position.

Keywords: whole-body vibrations, autonomic nervous system, physiological and psychological effects.

1 Introduction

The aim of this study is to produce a guide for the physiological and psychological measurement of the human body with the vibration where the direction has vertical (z-axis) and horizontal (y-axis) uses.

The standard was shown by the psychological evaluation in relation to the frequency-weighting curves. The health effects of vibration did not show clear responses.

The guide for the application of frequency-weighting curves for principal weightings are not well defined between the mutual effects.

Concerning the exposure during the short term and the duration of exposure, risks are caused as a result of the recumbent whole-body vibrations.

The vibration dose values at which various degrees of adverse comment may be expected in buildings were based on International Standard 2631-1 [2].

The effects of vibration in buildings for workers are based on the psychological evaluation. The workers must receive the risk of exposure to whole-body vibration, and subjects are measured for the physiological effects for that purpose. In the workplace, there are several possible adverse comments, so the values of the acceleration are shown with on the Critical working areas in the acceleration of 0.2 m/s^2, Residential in 0.4-0.8 m/s^2, Office in 0.8 m/s^2, and Workshops in 1.6 m/s^2. In the traffic system, the public bus (large-sized car, small-sized car) was measured on acceleration from 0.18 to 0.60 m/s^2 and the crane and the container of dock were measured from 0.21 to 0.60 m/s^2 with operators.

The dose values in the above acceleration are applicable irrespective of age, sex, and moreover, the whole-body vibration occurs as a continuous vibration.

It was necessary that the composition of the Standard for whole-body vibration including the health effects of vibration on the autonomic nervous system were studied in this paper.

2 Method

This study was performed using multi-input vibration testing equipment in the large structure testing building at this faculty. The university students were used as the subjects of an age group (average age; 22.5 years old), all in good health, and male.

The subjects lay down in the recumbent position on the vibration table and covered their ears with earmuffs. This vibrating condition was examined from 0.04, 0.06, 0.1, 0.2, and 0.4 to 0.8 Hz with the horizontal and the vertical recumbent whole-body vibration. Such a vibration frequency can be an everyday occurrence in a workshop and may result in an occupational disease. The amplitudes of vibration table were 25, 50, 100, 125 and 150 mm in that it the accelerations of vibration ranged over 0.0067 (150mm-0.04Hz), 0.0100 (100mm-0.06Hz), 0.0279 (100mm-0.1Hz), 0.140 (125mm-0.2Hz), 0.223 (50mm-0.4Hz) and 0.447 (25mm-0.8Hz) m/s^2.

These accelerations were examined the range, including the low probability of an adverse comment in Standard.

The examination used the sinusoidal wave for z-axis (vertical) and y-axis (lateral) for a period of 15-min. Waveforms were produced by this multi-input vibration testing equipment.

Physiological effects were examined by the changes on the cardiovascular system, respiratory movement, skin temperature, blood flow, and salivation. As in our previous experiment of seated subjects, physiological changes were found, and this state acted on the sympathetic and the para-sympathetic nervous system. Table 1 shows the state of the function on the autonomic nervous system.

The physiological indicators are shown the opposite action of the physiological responses on human body for exposure to vibration.

Table 1:   Opposite action of autonomic nervous system.

Physiological indicator	state of sympathetic	para-sympathetic
Function of heart	Increase	Restraint
Function of respiration	Increase	Restraint
Function of skin temperature	Restraint	Increase

It is necessary to know the threshold level, the direction, and the exposure time in the work place. The sensors of measurement used were the thermistor, bio-amp., blood flow meter, thermometer, balance test meter, and pH meter and the outputs were replaced from the amp to be recorded onto a recorder.

The amount of the saliva secretion was measured at intervals of 3-minutes by inserting a dental cotton roll under the tongue. The heart-rate ratio and respiratory frequency were expressed as a ratio of each measured value to the reference values of the said elements with 30 seconds as a criterion value prior to vibrating (baseline value) as a criterion value. As for the measuring time in the cases of heart-rate ratio and respiratory frequency, a series of measurements were performed for 30 seconds at intervals of 3-minutes.

An introspective method used was one in which the feelings aroused in a subject's mind were described as one of the suitable items in an evaluation paper after the experiment. In accordance with a semantic differential method (SD method), the terms of adequate for the low frequencies were chosen with respect to the 7-grade evaluation.

The evaluation points were given as shown below. Psychological evaluation by the introspective method of numerical values showed that six (item of comfortable) and seven grades were converted to scale numbered 7 in which, "4" represented "normal". These grades were selected according to the twenty-one items. The words were as follows: adaptable, unpretentious, amusing, smooth, friendly, calm, sharp, active, violent, favorite, variable, fresh, strong, heavy, hard, security, speedy, aggressive, tired, unpleasant, and great.

These words were based on our previous study and it found the suitable word for this vibration among them. It used VAS (visual analog scale) method at a time.   The subjects marked the line of 100 mm with a pencil freely what the subjects felt the vibration.

3   Results and conclusions

The opposite action of the autonomic nervous system functioned to keep the human body constant, so the function of heart rate and respiratory rate increased on the state of sympathetic nervous system and was restrained on the para-sympathetic nervous system. The decreasing of the salivation is caused by sympathetic nervous system and the increasing is caused by the state of para-sympathetic nervous system.

That shows the effects of the acceleration and the frequency of the head, which are to be transmitted to the human body. The physiological indicator showed the ratio as follows and the each measured value divided by the before exposure to vibration was shown the ratio.

Table 2:   An example of the physiological responses to vibration over 15 min.

Physiological indicator	z-axis: $0.447 m/s^2$	y-axis: $0.447 m/s^2$
Heart-rate	1.01, 0.06	1.01, 0.06
Movement	2.50, 1.65	1.30, 0.62
Respiratory	1.17, 0.15 ($p<0.10$)	1.24, 0.21 ($p<.10$)
Saliva	0.46, 0.27 ($p<0.01$)	0.60, 0.38
pH	0.92, 0.06 ($p<0.05$)	0.98, 0.07
Blood flow	1.17, 0.48	1.16, 0.22
Skin temp.	0.997, 0.025	0.994, 0.015

Ratio after stimulation / before stimulation (exposure to vibration).
P: probability,   (mean, SD).

The table gives analytical results brought about from the observation referred to above.

Table 2 shows the state of the sympathetic nervous system with sinusoidal wave for z, y-axes (vertical, horizontal direction) and the acceleration of the recumbent posture was at $0.447 m/s^2$ r.m.s. These results calculated the heart rate, the movement of baseline, the respiratory rate, the saliva secretion, the pH of saliva, the blood flow of index finger and the skin temperature of middle finger during 15-min (male aged 21-26). On the sinusoidal wave for z-axis (vertical direction), the skin temperature decreased the acceleration of 0.223 and $0.447 m/s^2$ r.m.s. at 15-min. The increase was noted in the physiological indicator by the heart-rate ratio, the respiratory rate ratio and movement of baseline with heart at 0.8 Hz-25 mm ($0.447 m/s^2$), during 15-min, whereas decreased in the amount of the saliva secretion and pH in these data and the results compared these data with the baseline value. The blood flow of the index finger decreased in comparison with control and $0.0067 m/s^2$ values.

At the y-axis (lateral direction) in Table 2, it was shown that the physiological effects changed the frequent occurrence during 15-min at $0.447 m/s^2$ r.m.s.

The increase was noted in the physiological indicator by the heart-rate ratio, the movement of baseline, the respiratory rate at 0.8 Hz-25 mm ($0.447 m/s^2$), during 15-min, whereas decreases in the amount of the saliva secretion, the blood flow of index finger and the skin temperature of middle finger during 15-min at 0.8 Hz-25 mm (0.447 m/s^2), whereas decreases in the amount of the saliva secretion in these data and the results compared these data with the baseline and with control and 0.0067 m/s^2 values.

The decrease of the pH ratio was noted in the vibration frequency at 0.223 m/s^2-50 mm-0.4 Hz, 0.447 m/s^2-25 mm-0.8 during 15-min and the decrease of 2.0 % band was caused in these ranges, compared these data with the baseline value, whereas in 0.0067 m/s^2 -150 mm-0.04 Hz, and 0.0279 m/s^2 -100 mm-0.1 Hz were increased 1.0-2.4 % values.

For the recumbent persons, it considered the experimental values, and the guide for the application of frequency-weighting curves was shown for health weightings.

It was implicated that the state of value in this range was due to the transmissibility caused by the vibration frequency.

The length and the area of body sway were registered with closed eyes and opened eyes by using the balance meter, then the subjects stood on the balance meter with both feet.

It showed the ratios of the area of body sway when the subjects' eyes were closed and opened (c/o; ratio of measurements with closed eyes to measurements with opened eyes) and it tended to increase with amplitudes of 25, 50 mm, frequency of 0.4, 0.8 Hz, and acceleration at 0.223, 0.447 m/s^2.

The effects of these accelerations were shown in the movement-area of body sway when the eyes were closed and opened, then Romberg ratio as shown from 1.6 to 1.8.

Psychological evaluation by the introspective method of numerical values showed that six and seven grades were converted to scale numbered (1-6, 7) in which "4" represented "normal". It was believed that when the acceleration was "unpleasant" to exceed 0.223 m/s^2. On the subjects, 0.223 m/s^2 or 0.447 m/s^2 decreased to 4.3, 2.8 (SD method; y-axis, level: 1-7) and 4.0, 3.2 (SD method; z-axis, level: 1-7) of the evaluation value and that low frequency area which gave "normal for pleasant" in the range 0.0067, 0.010, 0.0279, and 0.140 m/s^2. Those data were shown at frequency range from 0.04 to 0.2 Hz. The uncomfortable tended to increase with increasing of acceleration to exposure vibration for lateral and vertical axes (y-and z-axes).

The assessment of the discomfort was shown a scale of vibration magnitudes (level: 1-6) and 0.223 m/s^2 or 0.447 m/s^2 decreased to 4.1 (y-axis) and 4.7 (z-axis).

In the VAS method with regard to unpleasant was noted for evaluation word and the evaluation point exhibited below 40 (scale: 100) at 0.447 m/s^2, then the tendency was shown the same data for y-and z-axes.

The same adjective of physiological tendency was "hard, great, strong, violent, active, sharp, aggressive, and speedy". The difference of the evaluation point, at which the axes were not the same values, showed contribution to the effects of acceleration for the recumbent posture.

The correlation was shown as examples in the Table 3.

There is a close relationship between the acceleration and the frequency for VAS and SD methods.

Table 3: The correlation of the psychological level.

"unpleasant"				"comfortable"			
method	axis accel. fre. amp.			method	axis accel. fre. amp.		
VAS	y 0.93 0.92 0.69			Introspective	y 0.96 0.98 0.87		
	z 0.96 0.96 0.80			(Level:1-6)	z 0.96 0.98 0.88		
S D	y 0.95 0.95 0.73						
	z 0.97 0.97 0.86						

The state of predominance of the sympathetic nervous system was shown at 0.447 m/s^2 in 15-min (z: vertical, y: lateral).

Furthermore, it showed the range of the effects of vibration on health in the directions of the z, y-axes to the human body under the environments of this vibration zone.

According to a report concerning the experiment, it was found that the health effects found in acceleration ranging from 0.223 m/s^2 in horizontal and vertical directions of the frequency ranging from 0.4 Hz, were seen when transmitted to a human body; where it was desirable to widen a frequency weighting curves.

The magnitude of whole-body vibration for health aspects may consider the weighting as the vibration frequency for recumbent posture.

The assessment must be made that the risk resulting from this experiment of whole-body vibrations are affected to the physiological and psychological level.

References

[1] Dupuis H., Zerlett G., Responses of whole-body vibration. Translation: Matsumoto T., Okada A., Ariizumi M., Nohara S., & Inaba R., Nagoya Univ.-Press, Japan, pp. 62-109, 1989.
[2] International Organization for Standardization, ISO2631 Part 1, 1997.
[3] Nakamura Y., Psychological and Social Psychology. Kosei-Press Co., Japan, 1976.
[4] Oshima M., Theory of Vibration on Human Body. Tokyo Univ.- Press, Japan, 1969.
[5] Uchikune M., Yoshida Y., Studies of the effects of low frequency vibration on the human body -Physiological and psychological effects of low frequency horizontal vibration-. Proc. of the 11th Int. Conf. On the Ergonomics Association. IEA, Paris, pp. 915-917, 1991.
[6] Uchikune M., Yoshida Y., & Shirakawa S., Studies on the effects of low frequency horizontal vibration to the human body. Low fre. noise, vibra. & active control, (13), pp. 139-142, 1994.

[7]   Uchikune M., Shirakawa S., & Yoshida Y., The effects of a low frequency range exposed to vibration on the whole-body. Proc. of the 25th Int. Conf. On occupational health. ICOH, Stockholm, p. 222, 1996.

[8]   Uchikune M., Shirakawa S., & Yoshida Y., Studies in physiological effect and psychological evaluation on a human body with the low frequency vibration. Proc. of the 13th Int. Conf. On the Ergonomics Association. IEA, Tampere, pp. 602-604, 1997.

[9]   Uchikune M., Yoshida Y., The effects on exposure of the whole-body to low frequency vibration in the range $0.01 - 0.06$ Hz. Low fre. noise, vibra. & active control, (18), pp. 77-83, 1999.

[10]   Uchikune M., Shirakawa S., Studies for the evaluation of human-body exposure to whole-body vibration at very low frequencies. Proc. of the 14th Int. Conf. On the Ergonomics Association. IEA, San Diego, p. 58, 2000.

[11]   Uchikune M., Health effects of feet vibration on autonomic nervous system. Proc. of the 26th Int. Conf. On Occupational Health. ICOH, Singapore, p.705, 2000.

[12]   Uchikune M., Development of a vibration acceleration meter for low frequency range. The Japanese society of tech. education.(42), pp.75-81, 2000.

[13]   Uchikune M., The evaluation of horizontal whole-body vibration in the low frequency range. Low fre. noise, vibra. & active control, (21), pp. 29-36, 2002.

[14]   Uchikune M., Effects on health and perception from whole-body vibration exposure. Proc. of the third Int. Conf. On Women, Work & Health, Stockholm, pp. 89-90, 2002.

[15]   Yoshida Y. (eds.), Fundamental of Human Ergonomics. Corona-Press Co., Japan, 1980.

[16]   Uchikune M., Measurement and evaluation of whole-body vibrations. Proc. of the second Int. Conf. RISK 2003, Catania, pp. 143-149, 2003.

[17]   Gurmail S Paddan, Measurement, analysis and assessment of whole-body vibration according to ISO2631-1:1997. Proc. of the 11th JGHRV2003 Meeting, Japan, pp. 174-183, 2003.

[18]   Uchikune M., Measurement of whole-body vibration strain for the standing posture. Proc. of the 11th Int. Meeting, Maastricht, pp. 359-365, 2004.

Occupational health impacts on the child waste-pickers of Dhaka City

S. Parveen[1] & I. M. Faisal[2]
[1]State University of Bangladesh, Bangladesh
[2]SouthAsia Enterprise Development Facility, Bangladesh

Abstract

This paper examines the occupational health and safety problems faced by the child waste-pickers of Dhaka City. An extensive field survey and physical examinations of the waste-pickers have been used to collect the necessary primary data. The paper tracks down the health problems to their roots with the help of an impact-pathway based analysis. The study finds that the most prevalent types of occupational risks include: bites from insects and rats, cuts and bruises, skin disease, respiratory and gastro-intestinal tract problems, eye irritation, body aches, general weakness, and frequent fever. In order to understand the type and extent of the health and safety risks faced by the waste-pickers compared to non-waste picking children with similar socio-economic and environmental profiles, a comparative epidemiological analysis was carried out using exposed and control groups. It has been found that in terms of point and period prevalence rates, waste-pickers suffer significantly more than the control-group children. Using the linear multiple regression technique, the study further finds that the link between point/period morbidity indices and the risk factor (waste-picking) is a strong one as indicated by the associated t-statistic and overall performance of the models. A number of confounding factors also seem to influence the prevalence of health problems. The regression models indicate that health problems decrease with age, increase with family size, decrease with monthly expenditure, and girls tend to suffer more compared to boys.
Keywords: solid waste, health impact, risk factor, confounding factor, prevalence rate, morbidity index.

1 Introduction

Everyday, some 4000-4500 tons of solid waste is generated in Dhaka City by its 10 million inhabitants. About half of this waste is collected by the Dhaka City Corporation (DCC) and disposed at the central landfill site at Matuail. The rest are dumped in open fields, ditches and along street sides creating a major civic health problem. The situation is made worse by fact that the there is no separate system of collection and disposal for clinical and industrial waste in the city – all the hazardous clinical and industrial wastes are dumped in the same municipal bins used for household waste disposal; eventually most of the hazardous wastes also end up in the landfill site.

In this backdrop, what is perhaps the most serious health concern is that there are a few thousand human scavengers in the city, who collect reusable and recyclable materials from garbage bins and landfill sites. A preliminary survey indicates that nearly 50% of these waste pickers are children under the age of 15, and about half of them are girls. At the landfill site, they work from dawn to dusk and sell whatever they can salvage (glass, metal, plastic, paper, animal bones) to '*Bhangaries*' (traders) at a nominal price. They earn around Taka 40 to 60 (US$ 0.6 to 0.9) a day that may constitute 20%-30% of their family income. As noted by Rouse and Ali [1], 'they enjoy little (if any) access to health services, education or legal aid of any form. In addition, they are perceived as having very low status in society and are strongly associated with criminals.'

Due to such marginal and impoverished social status, these child-workers are being compelled to work in the most unhygienic conditions without any protective measures whatsoever. Even the basic amenities such as water and sanitation are not available to them – there is only one tube well in the entire Matuail area and no sanitary toilet at the site. There is no shelter where the waste pickers could rest, or take refuge when the weather turned unbearable due to intense heat or torrential rain. This is the level of negligence and deprivation endured by the child waste pickers of Dhaka.

As a result of such exposure and negligence, the waste pickers frequently suffer from acute and chronic illnesses and injuries. This study will develop an indepth understanding of these health problems from an epidemiologfical perspective. Specifically, the study will estimate the point and period prevalence rates of the health problems through a comparative cross sectional study, and investigate the association between the health problems with the risk and confounding factors (physical, socio-economic, environmental).

2 Materials and method

2.1 Study design and data collection

During literature survey, no study could be identified (done in Bangladesh or elsewhere) that directly dealt with the health issues faced by urban waste pickers from epidemiological point of view. At the study design level, the paper by Dolk et al. [2] was found to be informative - it discusses methodological issues related to epidemiological assessment of health risks of waste management activities and offers advices on how to avoid some common pitfalls.

This study is primarily based on data and information collected through structured questionnaire survey, interview and physical examination of the respondents. Secondary information from various reports and published sources has also been used as appropriate.

2.2 Sample design

The paper is based on a comparative epidemiological study that used two study groups – exposed (waste pickers) and control (non-waste pickers from a different neighbourhood with similar socio-economic and environmental profiles). Each study group was designed as per the stratified random sampling method, where the strata constituted groups of waste pickers of different age and sex. Both groups comprised of 75 randomly selected children aged between six and fifteen; the exposed group was surveyed first and then the control group sample was designed in conformity with the exposed group.

Table 1 shows the major socioeconomic and environmental parameters for the two study groups. As seen from table 1, most of the parameter values are very similar for both groups except for the average years of schooling – fewer children from the exposed group had formal schooling (they could not afford to forego the potential income from waste picking) compared to the children from the control group.

Table 1:   Comparative parameters of the study groups.

Attribute	Exposed	Control
Sample size	75	75
Male: female	1 : 1	1 : 1.2
Average age	11	12
Avg. years of schooling	1	4
Family size	6	5
Monthly expenditure (Taka)	4,527	4,779
Access to safe water (%)	100%	100%
Sanitary latrine at home (%)	83%	88%

2.3 Descriptive statistics

Both statistical summaries and descriptive epidemiological parameters have been used in this study to identify and analyze the type and extent of various health and safety risks faced by the respondents.

This study uses point and period prevalence rates as the primary epidemiological indicators. Point prevalence gives a snapshot of the burden of disease at the time of the survey, but it misses out acutely ill individuals unless special care is taken to include them in the sample. Period prevalence rate combines the concept of incidence rate and point prevalence, and is particularly useful in testing the burden of episodic, recurrent and seasonal diseases (Bhopal et al. [3]). These rates are defined as follows:

$$\text{Point prevalence rate} = \frac{\text{(All cases of the factor at time } t)}{\text{(Population at risk at time } t)} \tag{1}$$

$$\text{Period prevalence rate} = \frac{\text{(All old and new cases of the factor over a time period)}}{\text{(Average population at risk during the same period)}} \tag{2}$$

The length of the time period used for estimating period prevalence rate was decided to be six months after some pre-testing of the questionnaire as the respondents could not reliably recollect events that took place more than six months ago.

2.4 Analysis of association

This study estimates the strength of association between point and period morbidity indices and associated risk and confounding factors using a multiple linear regression model. The morbidity indices have been calculated as the cumulative frequency of all health related problems as reported by the respondents. Dichotomous variables (dummy variables) have been used to incorporate the risk factor, and some of the independent variables, e.g., gender of the respondent, status of immunization, access to safe water and so on. The general form of the linear regression model is given by eqn. (3).

$$y_k = c + x_{1,k} + x_{2,k} + \ldots + x_{n,k} + \varepsilon_k \tag{3}$$

where, y_k = dependent variable (morbidity index)
$x_{i,k}$ = ith independent variable (risk factor, confounders)
ε_k = residual for the kth observation

Criteria for selection of variables and functional forms for regression analysis can be found in standard texts such as Kleinbaum et al. [4], Draper and Smith [5], and Palta [6].

3 Environmental health impacts

3.1 Health risks

The present mode of solid waste management by the DCC poses a number of environmental health risks. First, the city does not have separate waste disposal systems for clinical and industrial wastes. Everyday, some 500 hospitals, clinics and pathological laboratories generate 200 tons of waste, about 15% to 20% of which are extremely hazardous that include infectious waste, pathological waste, sharps, and a small amount of pharmaceutical and chemical wastes (Rahman et al. [7]). Moreover, several thousand industries located within the city (including the 'hot-spots' at Hazaribagh and Tejgaon) generate hazardous solid wastes that contain corrosives, toxic chemicals and heavy metals. Both clinical and industrial wastes are dumped in municipal landfill sites or in open fields and ditches exposing the city residents to unknown health hazards.

Second, about half of the solid waste generated in the city – some 2,250 tons a day- is not collected at all, which may include some medical and industrial wastes. Often, wastes are not collected on time and seen rolling in the streets attracting scavengers and unwanted biota.

Third, the most serious health risks are faced by the human scavengers: around 6000 to 8000 of them work in the streets and at landfill sites as waste pickers. A preliminary survey indicates that nearly 50% of them are children under the age of fifteen, and about half of them are girls. Due to their marginal and impoverished social status, these child-workers are compelled to work in the most unhygienic conditions without having access to most basic amenities such as drinking water and sanitation at workplace.

3.2 Most frequent impacts

The cumulative health impacts of all these threats on the city population are unknown – no study has so far been conducted to scientifically link these risks with health impacts. However, a number of recent studies have examined the occupation health hazards faced by the waste pickers of Dhaka, who worked in the streets or at the Matuail landfill site [8, 9, 10]. Shamsad [9], and Parveen and Faisal [10] have identified stressors (in most cases indicated by the respondents) and sources of the most common health problems faced by the waste pickers as summarized in table 2 (for prevalence rates, see table 3). The waste pickers face a whole range of health risks - from minor on-site problems such as insect bite to major health concerns such as bronchitis, hepatitis, and physical injury.

It was found that in most cases, no medication is used or doctor consulted. The waste pickers resort to over-the-counter medicine or take a day-off only if they suffer from grave and debilitating ailments.

3.3 Point and period prevalence rates

Parveen and Faisal [10] have further extended these findings by conducting a comparative epidemiological study of the health impacts using 'exposed' and 'control' groups. By comparing point and period prevalence rates for different health problems faced by these groups, they show that the child waste-pickers of Dhaka suffer significantly more compared to the 'non-waste picking' control group (table 3). It is evident from table 3 that the child waste-pickers suffered from 30% more skin problems, 40% more eye, respiratory and general health problems, 47% more aches and pains, and 20% more gastro-intestinal ailments. The difference is even greater if period prevalence rates for skin and eye related problems are compared. The most significant difference is noted for fever – 62% more waste pickers suffered from some kind of fever during a six-month period prior to this survey compared to the control group.

Table 2:   Impact pathway of common health problems.

Health problem	Stressor	Source
General health (weakness, nausea, loss of appetite etc.)	Pungent smell	Exposed organic waste
Aches and body/joint pain	Long working hours without rest	Poor work environment
Skin disease and allergy	All types of waste	All waste sources
Respiratory and eye problems	Dust, fume, smoke	Burning of plastic, tire, incineration
Gastro-intestinal problems and worms	Drinking water, dirty hand or utensils	Lack of sanitation; poor personal hygiene
Cuts and bruises, infection, physical injury	Sharp / pointed objects, heavy machineries	Hospitals and health centres, households, landfill machineries
Pain and inflammation	Insect / mosquito bites	Bare foot/hand
Fever (infection, viral, malaria, dengue etc.)	Cold, infection, mosquito bite	Poor landfill conditions
TB, bronchitis, hepatitis, AIDS etc.	Clinical waste	Hospitals and health centres
Sore, metabolic disorders, cancer	Corrosive, toxic and radioactive chemicals	Industrial or clinical waste

3.4 Influence of the risk and confounding factors

By employing the multiple regression technique, Parveen and Faisal [10] also show that there are statistically significant associations between the point and period morbidity indices and the risk factor – waste picking. This confirms the generally held view that a significant part of the health problems affecting the waste pickers are due to their hazardous occupation, and the rest of the impacts are outcomes of other socio-economic and environmental factors.

Table 4 shows the statistical associations between the point morbidity index and the confounding and risk factors: age, gender, monthly family expenditure, family size, and group of the respondent. The regression coefficients and t-statistics support a number of important conclusions: (i) the exposed group is more vulnerable to health problems than the control group; (ii) younger children tend to suffer more from health problems compared to older ones; (iii) girls suffer from more health problems compared to boys; (iv) morbidity is positively correlated to family size (crowding factor); and, (v) morbidity is negatively correlated to family expenditure (possible nutritional impact). Originally, access to water and sanitary latrine were included in the regression model but were dropped later on as they came out to be statistically insignificant. In fact, as evident from table 1 that there is little difference between the exposed and control groups in terms of these factors.

The overall goodness of fit of the linear multiple regression model for point morbidity index is satisfactory as indicated by $R^2=0.69$ and F=64.42 for a combined sample size of 150.

Table 3:   Prevalence of health problems in exposed and control groups.

Health problem	Exposed group		Control group	
	Point (%)	Period (%)	Point (%)	Period (%)
Weakness	94.67	96.00	40.00	49.33
Dizziness / nausea	88.00	90.67	6.67	9.33
Loss of appetite	85.33	88.00	30.67	36.00
Burning sensation	86.67	88.00	10.67	10.67
Swelling limbs	5.33	32.00	1.33	1.33
UTI	12.00	42.67	4.00	8.00
General health	**96.00**	**97.33**	**57.33**	**70.67**
Headache	86.67	93.33	38.67	57.33
Back pain	68.00	82.67	10.67	13.33
Pain the joint	73.33	82.67	8.00	12.00
Ache and pain	**92.00**	**94.67**	**45.33**	**69.33**
Itching	49.33	73.33	18.67	25.33
Eczema	9.33	24.00	2.67	2.67
Scabies	10.67	38.67	14.67	18.67
Abscess	2.67	56.00	0.00	0.00
Lice	80.00	81.33	30.67	32.00
Skin	**82.67**	**97.33**	**52.00**	**58.67**
Cough	66.67	82.67	32.00	42.67
Breathing problem	36.00	60.00	5.33	6.67
Blood with cough	2.67	4.00	2.67	2.67
Throat infection	24.00	46.67	4.00	6.67
Chest pain	32.00	53.33	1.33	4.00
Oral infection	29.33	49.33	1.33	1.33
Respiratory	**74.67**	**85.33**	**36.00**	**46.67**
Acidity	72.00	81.33	22.67	32.00
Loose motion & Vomiting	62.67	76.00	32.00	37.33
Blood Dysentery	13.33	64.00	2.67	4.00
Pain in stomach	62.67	76.00	18.67	29.33
Gastro-intestinal	**74.67**	**85.33**	**56.00**	**74.67**
Cuts from sharp objects	66.67	80.33	4.00	6.67
Injury caused by machines	0.00	1.00	0.00	0.00
Wound/injury	**66.67**	**80.33**	**4.00**	**6.67**
Eye irritation	34.67	53.33	6.67	10.67
Blurry vision	18.67	25.33	1.33	1.33
Eye infection	4.00	22.67	1.33	1.33
Night blindness	16.00	16.00	0.00	0.00
Eye	**45.33**	**65.33**	**6.67**	**10.67**
Fever	12.00	70.67	9.33	13.33
Fever blister	0.00	4.00	0.00	0.00
Persistent fever	6.67	9.33	6.67	8.00
Recurrent fever	21.33	32.00	1.33	1.33
Fever	**34.67**	**85.33**	**17.33**	**22.67**
Ear pain	6.67	24.00	8.00	10.67
Ear infection	6.67	29.33	5.33	6.67
Loss of hearing	1.33	1.33	2.67	2.67
Ear	**9.33**	**33.33**	**12.00**	**16.00**

Table 4: Statistical association between point morbidity index and risk/confounding factors.

Model variables	Coefficients		t	Sig.
	B	Std. Error		
(Constant)	6.274	1.665	3.768	.014
Age	-.334	.107	-3.116	.002
Gender	1.675	.564	2.970	.003
Family expenditure	.000	.000	-1.841	.068
Family size	.559	.218	2.562	.011
Group	8.681	.620	14.002	.000

Note: Dependent Variable: Point morbidity index. $R^2=0.691$, F=64.424, N=150.

A similar linear regression model has been used to test the associations between the period morbidity index and the above mentioned set of dependent variables. Results of this model are shown in table 5. The conclusions from this model are exactly the same as before (it is not entirely surprising as the point morbidity information is embedded within the period morbidity index). Particularly, the 'group' variable is strongly significant and it again indicates that waste picking as an occupation had significant influence on the overall morbidity of the children. In terms of the t-statistics, except for 'group' and 'age', other confounding factors are not significant at 95% confidence level. This may be due to the fact that period prevalence is based on mental recollection of past morbidity and therefore may not be as accurate as the point prevalence, which was verified on the spot by qualified physicians.

The overall goodness of fit of this model is quite satisfactory as indicated by $R^2=0.735$ and F=79.92 for a combined sample size of 150.

Table 5: Statistical association between period morbidity index and risk/confounding factors.

Model variables	Coefficients		t	Sig.
	B	Std. Error		
(Constant)	10.135	2.160	4.692	.000
Age	-.402	.139	-2.891	.004
Gender	.333	.732	.456	.649
Family expenditure	.000	.000	-1.407	.161
Family size	.344	.283	1.216	.226
Group	13.425	.804	16.697	.000

Note: Dependent Variable: Period morbidity index. $R^2=0.735$, F=79.922, N=150.

4 Concluding remarks

This study has identified the most frequently occurring health and safety problems faced by the child waste-pickers of Dhaka City. By comparing the statistics of waste pickers with the control group statistics, it has been found that there are significant differences between the point and period morbidity levels of these groups and these differences may be attributed to the hazardous occupation of waste picking.

This problem of health impacts on waste pickers is a much more complex one than it appears on the surface. This is really an outcome of not having an integrated and ecosystem based solid waste management plan for the city. In a recent paper, Faisal and Parveen [11] show how an ecosystem-based approach can be used to analyze the issues from a system perspective and identify a range of intervention options to address the issue in a comprehensive manner. Even then, complete alleviation of environmental health impacts is likely to take a long time; it will require preparing a detailed 'blue print' for action as well as gradual and committed implementation of the same.

Acknowledgement

This paper is based on an earlier research that was funded by the International Development Research Centre (IDRC), Canada under Ecosystem Approach to Human Health Award. The authors gratefully acknowledge this contribution of IDRC.

References

[1]   Rouse, J., and Ali, M., *Waste Pickers in Dhaka,* Water, Engineering and Development Center (WECD): Loughborough University, UK. 2001.

[2]   Dolk, H., Vrijheid, M., Armstrong, B., Abramsky, L., Bianchi, F., Grane, E., Nelen, V., Robert, E., Scott, J.E.S., Stone, D., & Tenconi, R., Risk of congenital anomalies near hazardous waste landfill sites in Europe: the EUROHAZCON study. *Lancet,* **352**, pp. 423-427, 1998.

[3]   Bhopal, R.S., Phillimore, P., & Moffat, S., Is living near a coking works harmful to health? *J. Epidemiol. Comm. Health,* **48**, pp. 237-47, 1994.

[4]   Kleinbaum, D.G., Kupper, L. L., Muller, K. E., & Nizam, A., *Applied Regression Analysis and Multivariable Methods* (3rd ed.), Brooks Cole, 1997.

[5]   Draper, N. R., & Simth, H., *Applied Regression Analysis* (3rd ed.). John Wiley & Sons: New York, 1998.

[6]   Palta, M., *Quantitative Methods in Population Health: Extension of Ordinary Regression,* John Wiley & Sons: New York, 2003.

[7]   Rahman, M. H., Ahmed, S. N., and Ullah, M. S., A study on hospital waste management in Dhaka City, *Proc. Of the 25th WECD Conference,* Integrated Development for Water Supply and Sanitation: Addis Ababa, 1999.

[8]   Khanam, K. A., Socio-Demographic Characteristics and Morbidity Pattern of Waste Pickers of Dhaka City. National Institute of Preventive and Social Medicine (NIPSOM), Dhaka, 2000.

[9]   Shamshad, R., Occupational Health Hazard of the Scavenger Children in Matuail Landfill Site, Unpublished Thesis, Department of Environmental Studies, North South University, Dhaka, Bangladesh, 2003.
[10]   Parveen, S. & Faisal, I. M., An Epidemiological Investigation of Health Impacts on the Child Waste-Pickers of Dhaka City, Unpublished working paper, State University of Bangladesh, Dhaka, 2005.
[11]   Faisal, I. M., & Parveen, S. Alleviation of Environmental Health Impacts through Ecosystem Approach – A Case Study on Solid Waste Management in Dhaka City, paper presented at Sustainable Planning 2005, Bologna, Italy, September 12-14, 2005.

Vibration exposure of workers: considerations on some technical and interpretative aspects of the EC standards recently issued

L. Baralis[1], C. Cigna[2] & M. Patrucco[2]
[1]ARES S.r.l., Torino (TO), Italy
[2]DITAG, Politecnico di Torino, Torino (TO), Italy

Abstract

The 2002/44/CE directive on occupational vibrations exposure, following the trend introduced with the recent review of the related ISO standards (ISO 2631 and ISO 5349), rises to great evidence the problem of an effective evaluation and management of the vibration related risk; but, since the aforesaid directive is not yet enforced in Italy, the new approach suggests a pause of reflection. This directive, with the necessary differences, adopts evaluation and protection criteria substantially common to those used for a number of physical risks, in particular for noise exposure assessment. However it introduces important modifications, in particular for whole-body exposure, previously commonly considered as an ergonomic problem, and now positively included in the list of occupational factors which can cause health impairment. In any case the introduction of assessment criteria adopted at European level will stimulate further investigations on this risk factor, still poorly known. It still remains in fact to fully understand the intrinsic relation between exposure parameters, related pathologies and the possibility to correlate and to quantify the interference between vibration exposure and other noxious agents (e.g. microclimatic conditions or problems related to cumulative trauma or efforts). The hope is that the compulsory respect of exposure limits now clearly defined, together with the growing conscience of the importance - even in terms of workers health protection - of the former directive 89/392/EEC will lead to a great impulse for the introduction of equipment specially engineered to reduce the vibrations emission at the source, for a revision of work organization and procedures, and for the improvement of the currently available individual protection devices. The paper discusses the results of some measurement campaigns of worker exposure recently carried out, and investigates the available updated control measures, according to the target levels provided by the new European standards; some comments are also summarized about the national situation.
Keywords: vibration exposure, occupational safety and health, machinery, EC standards, risk management.

WIT Transactions on Biomedicine and Health, Vol 9, © 2005 WIT Press
www.witpress.com, ISSN 1743-3525 (on-line)

1 Introduction

The European directive 2002/44/CE concerning occupational exposure to mechanical vibrations, closes a long administrative procedure and fills an important gap in the European normative scenario; following the recent review of ISO standards on this matter (ISO 2631 and ISO 5349), points out some problems about a correct and effective approach and risks management for workers health related to vibrations exposure.

However, though the subject is taking ever-increasing weight, there are still some problems to solve. First of all, also if vibration-related risks have been well known since a long time, control methodologies cannot yet be considered well consolidated and the approach to vibration related risk analysis and management is not yet completely shared by the whole international technical and medical community.

1.1 Relationship with other EC directives

Evaluation and protection criteria proposed by the EC directive "44" (vibrations) are substantially comparable to those defined for the assessment and control of a large number of physical risks, particularly for the noise risk assessment. This is of course not surprising, as all those documents come from the same 89/391/CEE parent directive.

In a previous draft version of the directive on physical risk assessment (draft directive 93/C77/02 CEE, that never became an official EC directive), there was the very interesting concept of "attention" threshold level (at exposure values lower than recognized action levels) to be used as a guideline and a target level in the risk management and control phase, this "attention level" could have taken great advantages in order to protect workers health, due to the statistical and epidemiological meaning of any threshold limit; unfortunately the draft directive 93/C77/02 CEE was given up and there are no signs of any attention level in final "noise" and "vibration" directives.

Anyway, according to a well established methodology, both the noise and the vibration directives adopt an evaluation approach based on the preventive estimate of the effective workers' exposure, supported by a specific measurement campaigns and a comparison with a quantitative criterion.
In comparison with the EC directive 2003/10/EC (noise), we can recognize in the vibration related document a more pronounced trend leading from an objective exposure "assessment", based on the measurement of suitable parameters, towards the "evaluation" approach, *if possible* supported by measurements. Such trend, moreover, is already supported by reference, guidelines documents and published data banks of sound pressure levels [1] and values of vibration acceleration data [2], [3] [4] from official national and international sources.

The authors are in any case deeply convinced that an exposure estimate based only on data drawn from data bases can't totally fulfill basic requirements of 89/391 European directive, where a particular situation designed risk analysis is required.

Further evaluation criteria may relate to data supplied from the machinery manufacturer in order to comply with the related European directives and national laws. From these manufacturer machinery data it should be possible to have info about typical exposure level at work place both for ordinary conditions and for different kinds of operations or machinery tools and equipment. In addition, a series of factors influencing real vibration exposure levels depend on the machinery user: these factors can be quite simple and recognizable ones, as misuse of control measures, or they can involve complex aspects, as maintenance policies (e.g. if periodic maintenance policy is considered, real exposure levels can be significantly far from the ideal estimates for most of the time).

In fact it is a well known fact that the vibratory solicitation generally cannot be defined as a particular feature arising from a specific machinery, but it is produced by the interaction of the same machinery and its working environment (roads and tracks, worked materials, accessories, etc.) and by, when pertinent, the operator actions. All these factors significantly differ from reference test condition stated for any machinery type for certification purpose. Therefore, if data supplied from the manufacturer, can avoid, in some situations, to perform expensive measurement campaigns, on the other side they introduces a wide range of uncertainty.

The following data table shows some outstanding disagree between measured and declared data, met in measurement campaigns carried out by the authors in their respective professional activities. Reference to customer, manufacturer and model of machinery are voluntarily omitted.

Table 1: Comparison between measured values following ISO 5349 standard in real working conditions and values declared by the manufacturer (*) Following national laws, "Not Declared" should be considered as "less than 2,5 m/s^2".

Equipment	Working Conditions	Measured acceleration m/s^2	Declared acceleration m/s^2
Roto-orbital grinder one-hand held air powered (case A)	Grindig wood preformed structure	4,35	Less than 2,5
Roto-orbital grinder one-hand held air powered (case B)	Grindig resins preformed objects	5,85	Less than 2,5
Electric powered drill & screwdriver	Locking iron preformed bars (screwing)	3,40	*Not Declared* (*)

In addition, we must honestly point out that, often, field measurements of vibration accelerations are not so easily repeatable, due to technical problems mainly related to the contact between vibration source and transducers and signal noise produced by cables shakings (very hard to avoid in some hand-held machinery…). So, whatever evaluation method is chosen, the uncertainty range must be evaluated and taken in account, too.

Table 2:   Comparison between measures of protection previewed from directive 2002/44/CE and other references currently used in Italy. Measured values usually are checked on more than one handle. (*) From [3] it reports a span of values; it is suggested to use the maximum values supplied to achieve a prudent evaluation. (**) From: [2] it reports average values. (***) Not found, but similar to existing data on 4x4 military vehicles.

Equipment	Measured values span m/s^2	Data bank values m/s^2
Angular grinder (working metals)	3,45 – 11,80	2,7 – **9,8**(*)
Motor chain saw (sawing timbers and branches)	3,50 – 12,30	4,0 – **13,0**(*)
Dumper (open pit mine)	0,55 – 1,00	-- (***)
Loader (tyre) open pit mine	0,70 – 1,30	1,0 ± 0,5 (**)
Electric driven carriage loader (on paved yard)	0,35 – 1,15	0,9 ± 0,7 (**) (in quarries)
Two axis bus (urban track)	0,25 – 0,80	0,5 ± 0,1 (**)

1.2 Modifications on existing rules

In any case the "44" vibration EC directive will introduce important modifications to the European legislative scenario, particularly in Italy, where vibrations related risks are at present subject to quite generic dispositions. As far as Italy is concerned, we can point out two legislative actions since years 1955 and 1956, that imposed the control of "vibrations and shakings" within suitable values, in order not to cause damages to people or things, and forced medical survey for workers employing air-powered equipment or equipped with flexible axis vibrating hand-held tools. Such actions, before the European course, were mostly used by surveillance agencies as a repressive instrument to be applied after verified health damage has happened, but they were often substantially ignored by workers and managers.

The new directive guideline points out the importance of prevention and of participated approach, and is supported by specific dispositions: information and formation of workers, study of alternative or optimized working methods aimed to reduce exposure conditions, medical surveillance if requested by suspect of real risk.

The rise of the whole-body vibrations exposure levels, previously bounded among ergonomics, to real risk factor is particularly meaningful from this point of view.

2 Applicatory technical aspects

2.1 Instrumentation

At present, we yet suffer from a generalized delay in the instrument market. First of all we feel the lack of instrumentation in full compliance with ISO or equivalent standards, suitable for an effective practical use.

Only in recent past technology has provided technically advanced PC based measurement instrumentation or multi channel analyzers with suitable features, with no need of stationary power supply, and not so delicate for daily use in potentially aggressive environments frequently met in extractive, civil, agricultural, and industrial working facilities, where they should be used for field measurement campaigns.

More handy and protected common instruments observed by the authors come from ordinary sound level meters, and lack in frequencies ranges (especially at the lower frequencies) or have a small number of effective measurement channels (normally one). This problem is sometimes solved equipping the instrumentation with a frequency scanner or, better, a multi frequency modulated signal transmission line; in this way more than one transducer at time can communicate with logical instrument in order to get all components of the acceleration vector.

Another remarkable limitation is due to relatively reduced number of weighting filters in comparison with the high number of weighting filters from ISO standards stated for the different exposure and postural conditions. Similar problems are particularly found among recording DAT equipment.

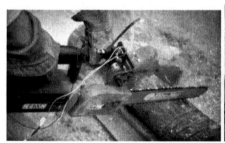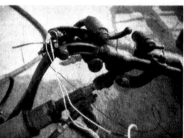

Figure 1:   Field measurement conditions.

2.2 Protection facilities

When risk analysis is performed, a series of control measures have to be carried out and, in accordance with a consolidated logical approach, they have to start form technical control measures aimed to reduce vibration generation and propagation, up to personal protective devices or organizational and procedural measures. The basic concept is, of course, vibration damping and the solutions can be applied to structures, seats or handle through which vibrations can affect users.

Currently it is quite difficult to find detailed data and info about protection gloves, damped seats and handle (for hand held tools) or about new methods and technologies designed to avoid vibration solicitation production. These difficulties may affect a properly selection of effective control measures or personal protective devices.

About damped seats, it is necessary to consider that usually these accessories can easily reduce vibration transmission at medium-high frequencies, but they are generally less effective in the lower frequency range (under 2 – 4 Hz) where the solicitation may result more damaging, according with the relevant current ISO standard.

About vibration protection gloves, we can point out that effective protection can need for relevant amount of resilient material: occasionally this can be not suitable for precise handwork and for hot environments.

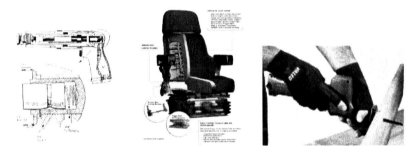

Figure 2:   Possible control measures on hand held tool, seat and protective gloves (from technical documentation of manufacturer).

2.3 Complementary factors

As it is well known that vibration exposure effects are strictly related to other factors, as at least:
- worker's age and/or his/her experience;
- his/her health condition (e.g. muscoloskeletal disorders);
- micro-climates conditions (temperature and relative humidity at work);
- contemporary working conditions with possibility of cumulative trauma or overuse;
- working time and breaks;
- further factors influencing peripheral blood circulation (e.g. alcohol drinking, some air pollutant, and may be smoke, ...);

It is clear that a deep and complete evaluation claim for a significant wide range investigation and must be accomplished with a wide competency contribute: the technical or engineering approach should be integrated with a relevant medical evaluation of environmental factors and personal health characteristics of exposed people.

3 Some examples

In the following a number of case studies is presented, in order to point out different exposure conditions, drawn form real measurement campaigns. The exposure level is given in accordance to currently available ISO standards, to be compared with EC directive requirements. Reference to manufacturer and model of machinery are voluntarily omitted.

Some picture of experimental instrumentation fitting and some result of time and frequency domain analysis are also shown (figures 3, 4, 5).

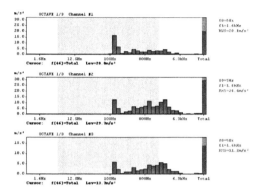

Figure 3: Back handle angular grinder: example of frequency spectra analysis in a measurement campaign.

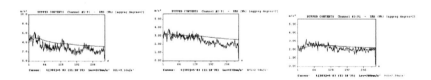

Figure 4: Back handle angular grinder: example of time history analysis in a measurement campaign.

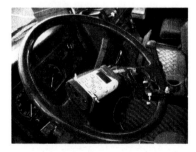

Figure 5: Steering wheel vibration measurement. Svantek mod. 948 analyzer with Triaxial accelerometer Dytran fitted in compliance with ISO 5349-2 requirements.

3.1 Case 1: Public gardens maintenance (hand-arm exposition)

Pruning season.
Activities and equipment in a standard day.

Little chain saw (usually one hand held)	time: 90 minutes	A: 3.7 m/s^2
Big chain saw	time: 15	A: 10.1 m/s^2
Motor hoe	time: 10	A: 5.0 m/s^2
Branch cutting tool	time: 5	A: 8.9 m/s^2
Remaining time: Not exposed		

A(8) calculated (ISO 5349): 2.7 m/s^2

3.2 Case 2: Public bus driver (whole body exposition)

Urban tracks, with rails crossing and partial rock slab paving roads.
Activities and equipment in a standard day.

Driving:	time: 300 minutes	A: 0.75 m/s^2
Remaining time: Not exposed		

A(8) calculated (ISO 2631): 0.59 m/s^2

3.3 Case 3: Public bus driver (hand-arm exposition)

Sub - urban tracks. Hand arm vibration on steering wheel.
Activities and equipment in a standard day.

Driving:	time: 270 minutes	A: 3.5 m/s^2
Remaining time: Not exposed		

A(8) calculated (ISO 5349): 2.6 m/s^2

3.4 Case 4: Truck driver (whole body exposition)

Activities and equipment in a standard day.

Driving (urban tracks):	time: 132 minutes	A: 0.7 m/s^2
Driving (trash container loading):	time: 240 minutes	A: 0.32 m/s^2
Driving (off road tracks – dump site):	time: 20 minutes	A: 0.49 m/s^2
Remaining time: Not exposed		

A(8) calculated (ISO 2631): $0,37 \text{ m/s}^2$

3.5 Case 5: Public bus driver (hand-arm exposition)

Hand arm vibration on steering wheel
Activities and equipment in a standard day.

Driving (urban tracks):	time: 132 minutes	A:	1.21 m/s^2
Driving (trash container loading):	time: 240 minutes	A:	0.85 m/s^2
Driving (off road tracks – dump site):	time: 20 minutes	A:	1.61 m/s^2

Remaining time: Not exposed
A(8) calculated (ISO 5349): $1,18 \text{ m/s}^2$

4 Final remarks

Finally, we have to point out that threshold limits proposed in the EC directive are quite easily reached in a normal working situation, at least for the lower threshold of action (A(8) = 2,5 m/s^2 for hand-arm exposure and A(8) = 0,5 m/s^2 for the whole body exposure). More difficult it should be in real life trespassing the upper exposure limits.

Hope is that the evaluation of exposure condition in order to respect compulsory limits now clearly defined, together with the growing conscience of the importance -even in terms of workers health protection- of the former directive 89/392/EEC will lead to a great impulse to the introduction of equipment specially engineered to reduce the vibrations emission at the source, to a revision of work organization and procedures, and to the improvement of the currently available individual protection devices.

References

[1] ISPESL; Linee guida per la valutazione del rischio rumore negli ambienti di lavoro, updated April 2003.
http://www.ispesl.it/linee_guida/fattore_di_rischio/rumore_eng.htm
[2] ISPESL; Linee guida per la valutazione delle vibrazioni negli ambienti di lavoro, updated may 2002.
http://www.ispesl.it/linee_guida/fattore_di_rischio/vibrazioni.htm
[3] AA.VV; Linee guida in materia di rischi da vibrazioni e da movimenti e sforzi ripetuti degli arti superiori. Regione Piemonte, Ass. Sanità Torino 1997.
[4] National Institute for Working Life North, Umeå, Sweden. http://umetech.niwl.se/vibration/

Measurement of hand-vibration transmissibility by non-contact measurement techniques

P. Nataletti[1], N. Paone[2] & L. Scalise[2]
[1]Centro Ricerche ISPESL, Monteporzio Catone, Roma, Italy
[2]Department of Mechanics, Università Politecnica delle Marche, Ancona, Italy

Abstract

Background: Workers who use hand-held vibrating tools may experience finger blanching attacks due to episodic vasospasm in the digital vessels. In occupational medicine, the pathological consequences to the exposure to hand-transmitted vibration are known as vibration induced white finger (VWF). In many cases, workers are recommended to use anti-vibration gloves and a standard procedure (ISO 10819) is used to test and qualify such anti-vibration gloves. Some problems and limits are known for what concerns the measurement and procedure proposed by this standard. Materials and methods: Hand-arm vibration transmissibility (ratio between rms acceleration on different points of the upper side of the hand and the handle rms acceleration) of 13 healthy subjects (main BMI: 24.3 $[kg/m^2]$) was measured using a mono-axial accelerometer on the handle and a laser Doppler vibrometer on several points on the hand. The laser vibrometer eliminates any mass loading effect on the hand tissue. Seven single frequency excitations (rms acceleration amplitude: 3 m/s^2) have been tested: 15, 20, 30, 50, 70, 90 and 110 Hz. Closed loop control of the handle acceleration is provided. Monitoring of the push force (50 ± 5.0 N) has been carried out during the test. Results: Transmissibility higher then one (1.54) has been measured at the tip of the fingers, especially for vibration frequencies lower then 70 Hz, while transmissibility lower then 1 (0.20) is reported on the hand knuckles for frequencies higher then 30 Hz. Conclusions: The measurement procedure presented a non-contact measurement of the vibration transmissibility of the human hand and in particular its spatial distribution over the hand.

Keywords: hand vibration, transmissibility, laser Doppler vibrometry.

WIT Transactions on Biomedicine and Health, Vol 9, © 2005 WIT Press
www.witpress.com, ISSN 1743-3525 (on-line)

1 Introduction

Workers operating in industrial environment and assembly lines, which operate vibrating tools, are subjected to long-term vibration exposure. This is demonstrated to be associated to vascular, neurological and muscular-skeletal symptoms and disorders (Griffin, [1]). It has been calculated (Wasserman and Wasserman, [2]) that about 10 million of workers are daily exposed to vibration during their working activities in the USA. It is estimated (Taylor [3]) that a percentage between the 30% and the 90% of the exposed population will eventually develop the disorder generally defined as hand-arm vibration syndrome (HAVS). HAVS has been especially associated to the specific vascular symptom called vibration-induced white finger (VWF). Significant positive correlation between VWF and hand-transmitted vibration levels has been demonstrated (Inaba et al. [4]) with prevalence of symptoms among woman respect to male workers (Mirbod et al. [5])).

The use of special anti-vibration gloves is considered a way to protect the worker to the exposure to the vibration. The International ISO 10819 standard was established to set a repeatable procedure to quantify the attenuation efficiency (reduction of the acceleration transmitted to the hand palm) of such gloves. According to some authors the use of such gloves is useful in the reduction of the vibration measured on the hand for specific tools such as the pneumatic chipping hammer (Goel and Rim, [6]). Nevertheless the standard itself underlines the impossibility to determine the transmissibility to the fingers. Some criticisms and "weak points" have been reported (Hewitt, [7]) especially for what concerns:

1 – Test set-up (for example: possible misalignment of the accelerometer adaptor).

2 - The impossibility to determine the transmissibility of the fingers, where the accelerometer cannot be fixed.

3 - The difficulty to carry out the tests, due to the presence of many influencing parameters.

The aim of the present paper is to propose a novel approach for the experimental setup for the assessment of the vibration transmissibility directed to the hand. Indeed such an approach could also be used to assess glove performance (contributing to improve ISO-10819). The proposed approach can provide information on the spatial distribution of the acceleration (and consequently of the vibration transmissibility) over the operators hand during the vibration exposure, without mass loading effect, that would be caused by the use of accelerometers.

2 Materials and methods

The testing procedure used in the following is based on ISO 10819. The measurement apparatus is in large part the one proposed in the same standard a part from the vibration transducer used in contact with the hand palm.

2.1 Experimental apparatus

The measurement apparatus realised for the experimental tests is schematically reported in Figure 1. The test bench is composed by: an instrumented platform with a load cell for the measurement of the push force; a electro-dynamic shaker and a closed loop controller in amplitude; a laser Doppler vibrometer; a single axis accelerometer and the signal conditioner and a control/processing unit composed by an A/D 16 bit card and a computer. The optical axis of the laser vibrometer was always aligned with the excitation direction provided by the shaker axis; a mirror was used to guarantee such condition. A detail of the experimental set-up and of the instrumented handle is reported in figure 2. The laser beam can be aimed at different points on fingers keeping the same direction of measurement.

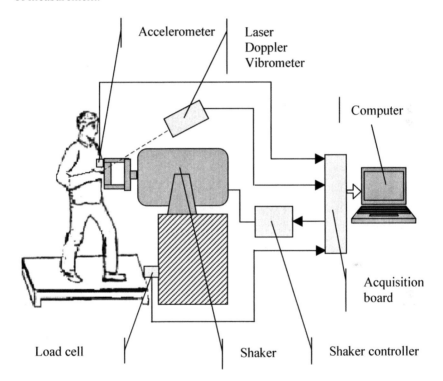

Figure 1:   Schematic of the test set-up.

2.2 Test procedure

The subjects were instructed to assume correct posture and to exercise the requested push force (50 ± 5 N); pieces of retro-reflective tape (5 x 5 mm) were attached to the subject hand in order to improve the measurement conditions for the laser vibrometer. Each test had duration of 30 s and tests were conducted during 4 days and none of the subjects performed more then 4 consecutive tests.

Each test (test duration: 30 s) has been repeated 10 times and average values have been calculated. Seven excitation frequencies were studied: 15, 20, 30, 50, 70, 90 and 110 Hz; acceleration was maintained constant at the handle (acceleration rms =3 m/s^2) during each test by means of a closed loop controller. The total number of observations for each frequency and for each subject is 120 (12 measurement points, 10 measurements).

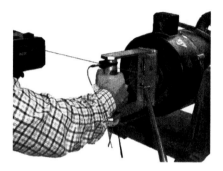 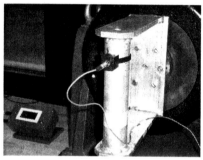

Figure 2:   Detail of the test conditions (left); The instrumented handle, the accelerometer and the display for the push force visual control (right).

2.3 Subjects and investigated variables

The study was carried out on 13 healthy, male subjects (average BMI =24.3; standard deviation= 0.9) aged 24-31 with no previous significant exposure to vibration. The study participants were recruited among the student population of the university and the technicians of the laboratory.

The transmissibility, *TR*, is calculated from the rms acceleration values as follows:

$$TR = acceleration\ measured\ at\ point\ P_{i,j}\ /\ acceleration\ at\ the\ handle; \quad (1)$$

Where $P_{i,j}$ ($i=1 \ldots 3$, number of points along each finger; $j=1 \ldots 4$, number of measured fingers) are the 12 measurement points on the hand reported in figure 3.

Each subject, during the tests, maintained the push force at 50 N ± 5 N looking to voltmeter display connected to the reference load cell (Figure 2, right). The grip force was not controlled and the subjects were asked to maintain a strong grip and full contact between the hand palm and the handle during tests. In order to improve test repeatability each subject is asked to release the handle and relax for 60 s between each test; this reduces the variability intra-subjects Hewitt, [7]. Even if it is considered not necessary to use a controlled loop feed back system to maintain constant acceleration level on the handle, Hewitt [7], we have used such closed loop control and used a 3 m/s^2 rms acceleration at the handle for all the tests, so to perform all tests at the same vibration input to the hand.

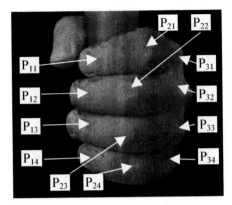

Figure 3:   Measurement point $P_{i,j}$ on the hand during grasping.

No temperature and humidity control was performed during the tests. By this procedure, all measurement of the hand vibration will be performed in the direction of the laser beam which is aligned with the shaker vibration axis. Misalignment of accelerometers used to measure transmissibility is a known problem, which can leads up to 20% of underestimation of the transmissibility with a misalignment of 40° (Hewitt, [7]).

3   Results

The average transmissibility (over 10 measurements) as function of the single frequency excitations, are shown in figure 4 for some of the measured point (all knuckles and distal joints). It is possible to verify how the transmissibility varies as function of the vibration frequency and as function of the measurement point. In our experiment, we measured a maximum average *TR* of 1.54 (point $P_{1,3,}$ at 90 Hz) and a minimum average *TR* of 0.29 (points $P_{3,3}$ at 70 Hz and $P_{3,4}$ at 90 Hz). The average *TR* over all the measured point is 0.98 and the standard deviation is 0.30 (table 1 and 2).

In figure 5 it is reported the map of average transmissibility (over the 13 subject measured) for the third finger as function of the frequency and of the position along the finger. The higher values of *TR* are measured on the distal joint at 70 and 90 Hz (1.14 and 1.54, respectively); the lower values are at the knuckles at 70 and 90 Hz (0.29 and 0.32, respectively).

Figure 6 reports the same analysis of the average transmissibility (over 13 subject) for the fourth finger. Even for this finger the higher values of the *TR* are in correspondence of the distal joints at 70 and 90 Hz (1.41 and 1.31, respectively); while the lower *TR* are in correspondence of the knuckle at the frequencies of 70 and 90 Hz (0.66 and 0.29, respectively).

The influence of the grip force exerted by the operators during the tests has been investigated asking two subjects to repeat the tests operating both an high grip (about 90 % of the subject maximum grip) and a low grip (about the 50% 0f the subject maximum grip). In figure 7, we report the *TR* (point $P_{3,1}$) as function of the frequency for the 2 subjects and the grip force exerted. It is possible to note how, for the two subjects, the high grip cause an higher *TR* respect to the low grip for the frequencies 15 and 30 Hz while there is an inversion (lower TR at high grip) at 70 and 90 Hz.

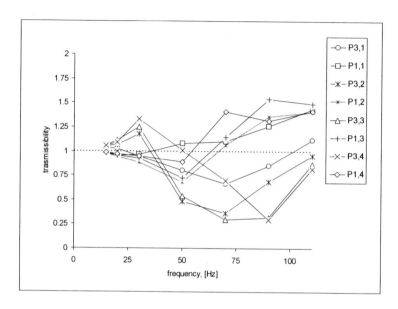

Figure 4:   Average transmissibility as function of the excitation frequency for some of the measured points (see figure 3); data from all the 13 subjects.

Table 1:   Mean transmissibility values for third and forth finger as function of the frequency.

Finger position	15 Hz	20 Hz	30 Hz	50 Hz	70 Hz	90 Hz
P1,3	0.98	0.95	0.93	0.72	1.14	1.54
P2,3	0.99	1.01	1.02	1.04	1.06	1.02
P3,3	1.06	1.11	1.25	0.54	0.29	0.32
P1,4	0.99	0.97	0.95	0.89	1.41	1.31
P2,4	1.00	1.01	1.06	0.92	0.84	0.79
P3,4	1.06	1.09	1.33	1.01	0.66	0.29

Finally we report in figure 8 the standard deviation of the calculated TR for all the measured point of the 13 subjects as function of the frequency. It appears clear how the dispersion of the data increases for high frequencies.

Table 2. Standard deviation of the transmissibility values for third and fourth finger as function of the frequency.

Finger position	15 Hz	20 Hz	30 Hz	50 Hz	70 Hz	90 Hz
P1,3	0.00	0.02	0.06	0.28	0.10	0.19
P2,3	0.01	0.01	0.00	0.29	0.14	0.19
P3,3	0.05	0.03	0.05	0.17	0.08	0.09
P1,4	0.01	0.01	0.03	0.24	0.13	0.15
P2,4	0.02	0.01	0.02	0.39	0.18	0.09
P3,4	0.06	0.06	0.07	0.45	0.33	0.24

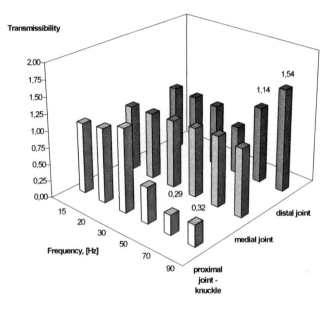

Figure 5: Transmissibility along the third finger as function of the frequency.

4 Discussion

The novel method for the measurement of vibrational transmissibility has been proposed, the experimental campaign carried out over 13 subjects has been described and the results are reported.

The method proposed allows to investigate the transmissibility over the fingers, the hand and over other anatomy district (not shown in this paper). Another important feature of the proposed method is the absence of the contact and mass loading effect obtainable by the use of the laser Doppler vibrometer.

The results show a distribution of the measurable acceleration over the fingers joints and the knuckles which demonstrate the difficulty to assign a single transmissibility value for one tests if the measurement point is not defined (for example, at 90 Hz the average TR over the third finger is 0.96 while the max TR is 1.54 on the distal joint).

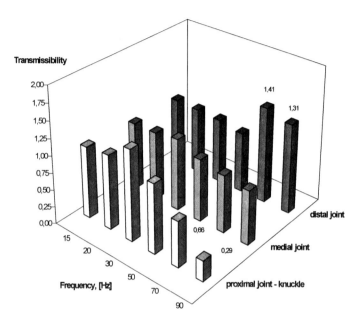

Figure 6: Transmissibility along the fourth finger as function of the frequency.

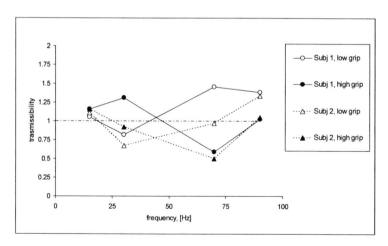

Figure 7: Transmissibility for two subjects as function of the frequency for two level of grip force (low and high).

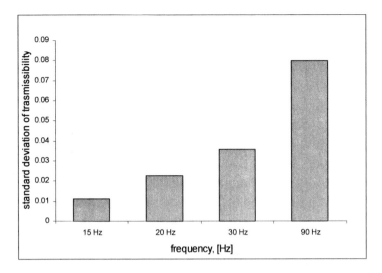

Figure 8:   Standard deviation over all transmissibility values as function of the frequency.

The results show a reduction of the transmissibility in correspondence of the knuckles at 70 and 90 Hz (up to -71%) and an increase of the transmissibility (up to +54%) for the third and fourth distal joints.

As shown by other authors (Hewitt, [7]; Smutz et al. [9]; Dong et al. [11]), there is a clear dependence on frequency of the transmissibility. In particular it has been reported a TR>1 for frequencies higher then 50 Hz for all the distal joints. The third and fourth distal joints showed the highest TR.

TR < 1 for frequencies higher then 5o Hz have been reported for measurements on all the knuckles with the lowest TR measured on the third and fourth knuckles.

Taking into account the limited number of frequencies tested a resonance on the TR seems to be present at 30 Hz and a minimum is reported at 70 and 90 Hz for the knuckles.

Despite the opinion of some other authors (Hewitt, [7]), the effect of the grip force looks to be important (data only from 2 subjects). It is the opinion of the authors, that the influence of such parameter should be considered when transmissibility is measured.

Acknowledgment

This work as been carried out with the financial support of the Istituto Superiore per la Prevenzione e la Sicurezza del Lavoro - ISPESL (Contract: C17/DIL/02).

References

[1]   M. J. Griffin (1990), Handbook of human vibration. Academic Press, London.

[2]   D. E. Wasserman and J. F. Wasserman, The nuts and bolts of human exposure to vibration, Sound and Vibration, 35th ann issue, Jan 2002.

[3]   W. Taylor (1989), The hand-arm syndrome-objective tests. *Proc. Inst Phys*, **2(9)**, 425–33.

[4]   R. Inaba, S. Mirbod, H. Iwata., Pathophysiology of Vibration-induced White Finger and safety Levels for Hand-Transmitted Vibration, J. Occup Health, 1996, 38, 1-5.

[5]   S. Mirbod, R. Inaba and H. Iwata (1997), Operating vibrating tools an prevalence of subjective complaints in vibration syndrome. *Cent. Eur. J. Publ. Health*, **3**, 97–102.

[6]   V. Goel and K. Rim (1987), Role of gloves in reducing vibration: An analysis for pneumatic chipping hammer. *Am. Ind. Hyg. Assoc. J.*, **48**(1), 9–14.

[7]   S. Hewitt (1998), Assessing the performance of anti-vibration gloves—a possible alternative to ISO 10819, 1996. *Ann. Occup. Hyg.*, **42**(4), 245–52.

[8]   T. Shenk and F. Gillmeister, Measurement of hand-arm vibration: errors and uncertainties, Proc. of 9th Int Conf on Hand-Arm Vibration, 5-8 June 2001, Nancy.

[9]   W. P. Smutz, R. Dong, B. Han, A. W. Schopper, D. E. Welcome and M. L. Kashon, A Method for Reducing Adaptor Misalignment when Testing Gloves Using ISO 10819, *Ann. Occup. Hyg.*, **46**(3), 3009–3015, 2002.

[10]   ISO 10819:1996—Mechanical vibration and shock—Hand-arm vibration —Method for the measurement and evaluation of the vibration transmissibility of gloves at the palm of the hand. International Organization for Standardization.

[11]   R. G. Dong, T. W. McDowell, D. E. Welcome and W. P. Smutz (2005), Correlations between biodynamic characteristics of human hand-arm system and the isolation effectiveness of anti-vibration gloves. *Int. J. of Industrial Ergonomics*, **35**(3), 205–216.

Air pollution control for occupational health improvement

L. Santarpia, F. Gugliermetti & G. Zori
Department of "Fisica Tecnica", Rome University "La Sapienza", Italy

Abstract

Indoor air pollution can make workplaces worse. Mechanical or natural ventilation systems, impelled by thermal gradients or wind pressure, can reduce indoor pollution levels by introducing adequate indoor air changes; moreover airflows can drag pollutant gases both from the external environment and among internal spaces. An air curtain system can reduce the airflow through openings of adjoining spaces and, as a consequence, can realize a system to control pollution. Flux reduction, gaseous and particulate pollutant control and human exposure time produced by air curtain ventilation systems are investigated by theoretical and advanced CFD analysis in order to improve their design by general guidelines.
Keywords: air curtain, pollution control, free air jet, pollutant flux.

1 Introduction

Human exposure to particulates has recently received considerable attention as a result of epidemiological studies showing associations between environmental particle concentration and mortality. These associations have been initially demonstrated for total suspended particles (TSP) and PM_{10}; however, results from later studies suggest that fine particles ($PM_{2.5}$) and particle components, such as sulphate (SO_4^{2-}) and aerosol strong acidity (H^+), may also be associated with increased mortality and other adverse health impacts.

From studies of indoor environments, it is clear that significant fraction (50–90%) of outdoor PM_{10}, $PM_{2.5}$, SO_4^{2-} and H^+ penetrate indoors. Once indoors, these particulate species may be depleted through deposition onto surfaces, or, in the case of H^+, through reactions with other indoor pollutants.

The vehicle emissions are one of most important outdoor PM sources. The pattern of particles concentration is function of the distance from the roads and change around the building envelope; besides street canyon effects, local air-flow patterns, reciprocal building locations can largely influence concentration and size particles distributions. Particles emitted from vehicles can penetrate indoors, and the degree to which this occurs depends on the characteristics of the buildings.

The multiplicity of factors involved in the process of penetration of particles produces large variations in the expected outcomes, i.e. in terms of vehicle-affected indoor particle concentration levels. Therefore, various studies, in which particle concentration levels were measured indoor and compared with the outdoor concentrations, have led to different conclusions regarding the extent of vehicle impact. This great spread in results indicates the complexity of the processes involved and thus the need for a good understanding of the specific urban setting in the assessment either of the human exposure or of the risk related to vehicle emission contributions to indoor particle concentration levels.

2 Background

A study of indoor and outdoor PM_{10} and $PM_{2.5}$ concentrations was carried out in the indoor and outdoor environmental of 28 houses in the area of Huddersfield, England [1], with the objective to identify the effect of road emissions on particle concentrations. The houses were selected both to provide a range of different locations in terms of distance from main roads and to be consistent in their ventilation, internal emission sources, and overall design. The houses within 50 m from the main road were classified as 'proximity' group, while the others as 'background' group. The mean indoor and outdoor PM_{10} and $PM_{2.5}$ concentrations measured for 'proximity' and 'background' houses, with their median ratios for each couple of 'proximity' and 'background' houses are presented in Tab. 1.

Table 1:   Measured concentration at 'proximity' and 'background' houses.

Pollutant	Location	'Proximity' homes ($\mu g/m^3$)	'Background' homes ($\mu g/m^3$)
PM_{10}	Indoor	35.36	34.91
$PM_{2.5}$	Indoor	17.81	19.52
PM_{10}	Outdoor	36.25	33.70
$PM_{2.5}$	Outdoor	18.91	23.31

The decrease in these mass concentrations between the values at the minimum distance from the road and the background levels ranged up to about 25-30% and was noticeable in the first 20-30 m from the road. Considering this relatively small gradient, and that many of the 'proximity' houses were already at the roadside, little impact of vehicle emissions on indoor PM_{10} and $PM_{2.5}$ concentration levels indoor is to be expected.

Time distribution of PM_{10} concentrations were performed in Hong Kong [2] for two indoor sites located next to main roads; measurements, only for one site, showed two peaks, one at around 7 am and the second at around 5 pm, corresponding to the peak-hour traffic on the street. The lowest concentration was measured at about midnight.

A different example is provided by a study conducted by Jamriska et al. 2000 [3] on the fifth floor of an office building located about 100 m from a busy road. Particles in the range 0.016 to 0.626 μm were measured by an SMPS; in this study, the presence of significant indoor pollutant sources was not identified and it was shown that the indoor airborne particles distribution followed outdoor air pattern, in which the vehicle combustion aerosols represented the main pollution source. Fig. 1 compares outdoor particles size distribution with filtered air though a battery of Pyracube deep-bed filters (with an efficiency of approximately 30% according to classification by the AS1132 No. 1 dust methylene blue test), and with filtered and air conditioned air.

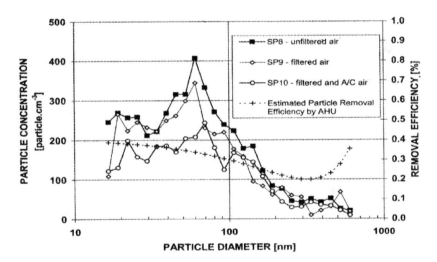

Figure 1:   Particles size distribution measured for different ventilation system and particle removal efficiency.

Figure 1 shows similar distributions of particulate sizes for all the considered cases, also if concentrations are lower in filtered and air-conditioned; also the peak of distributions, due to the vehicle emission, is clearly visible in all the indoor distributions.

Studies on air curtain dynamic efficiency, respect both to the improvement of indoor air quality and to reduction of human exposure to hazardous fumes, has been conducted by Santarpia et al. [4, 5, 6, 7] for different geometry and thermo fluid dynamic boundary conditions.

3 Experimental methodology

A 2D meshed (5000 nodes) model has been built (Fig. 2) and an isothermal fluid-dynamic analysis has been carried out for different boundary conditions:

- the outdoor atmosphere (3 x 4m) and the indoor atmosphere (2.1÷10.5 x 4 m) constitutes the calculation domain;
- the wall are set adiabatic;
- the doorway allows indoor-outdoor airflows;
- the air curtain is installed on the communicating door;
- the air curtain operates with external filtered air (0.4 m³/h x m);
- a variable height (0÷1.2 m) window is installed on bottom wall.

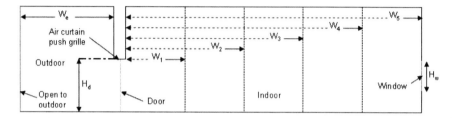

Figure 2: Simulation layout.

A k-ε model, implemented in a commercial software (FLUENT), is used to solve the fluid-dynamic field in the calculation domain.

The standard k-ε model is a semi-empirical model based on model transport equations for the turbulence kinetic energy (k) and its dissipation rate (ε). In the derivation of the k-ε model, it was assumed that the flow is fully turbulent, and the effects of molecular viscosity are negligible. The standard k-ε model is therefore valid only for fully turbulent flows. The k and ε are obtained from the following equations (Einstein notation):

$$\frac{\partial}{\partial t}(\rho k) + \frac{\partial}{\partial x_i}(\rho k u_i) = \frac{\partial}{\partial x_j}\left[\left(\mu + \frac{\mu_t}{\sigma_k}\right)\frac{\partial k}{\partial x_j}\right] + S_k + S_b - \rho\varepsilon - Y_M + S'$$

and

$$\frac{\partial}{\partial t}(\rho\varepsilon) + \frac{\partial}{\partial x_i}(\rho\varepsilon u_i) = \frac{\partial}{\partial x_j}\left[\left(\mu + \frac{\mu_t}{\sigma_\varepsilon}\right)\frac{\partial\varepsilon}{\partial x_j}\right] + C_1\frac{\varepsilon}{k}(S_k + C_2 S_b) - C_3\rho\frac{\varepsilon^2}{k} + S''$$

In these equations, S_k represents the generation of turbulence kinetic energy due to the mean velocity gradients. S_b is the generation of turbulence kinetic energy due to buoyancy. YM represents the contribution of the fluctuating dilatation in compressible turbulence to the overall dissipation rate. C_1, C_2 and C_3 are constants. σ_k and σ_ε are the turbulent Prandtl numbers for k and ε, respectively. S' and S'' are user-defined source terms. The turbulent (or eddy) viscosity , μ_t , is computed by combining k and ε as follows:

$$\mu_t = \rho C_4 \frac{k^2}{\varepsilon}$$

where C_4 is a constant.

The CFD simulation has been used to esteem the air curtain airflows distribution. In figure 3 the entrained airflows notation is presented.

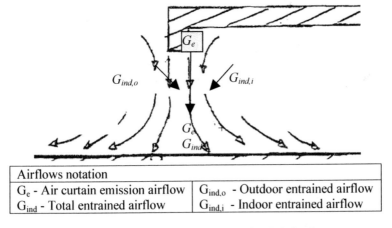

Airflows notation	
G_e - Air curtain emission airflow	$G_{ind,o}$ - Outdoor entrained airflow
G_{ind} - Total entrained airflow	$G_{ind,i}$ - Indoor entrained airflow

Figure 3:   Confined air jet entrained airflows.

The theoretical indoor concentration, C_{in}, can be carried out by the mass balance equation (Fig. 4):

$$\frac{d(V \cdot C_{in})}{dt} = G_3 \cdot C_M - (G_4 + G_5) \cdot C_{in}$$

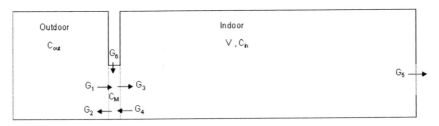

Figure 4:   Indoor mass balance notation.

The C_M value is carried out assuming a perfect mixing of entrained air:

$$C_M = \frac{G_1 C_{out} + G_4 C_{in} + G_6 C_e}{G_2 + G_3}$$

Integrating and setting $C = C_0$ at $t = 0$:

$$C_{in} = \left(C_0 - \frac{K_2}{K_1} \right) e^{-\frac{K_1}{V} t} + \frac{K_2}{K_1}$$

$$K_1 = G_4 + G_5 - \frac{G_3 \cdot G_4}{G_2 + G_3} \quad ; \quad K_2 = G_3 \frac{G_1 \cdot C_{out} + G_e \cdot C_e}{G_2 + G_3}$$

4 Results

Based on CFD numerical data the entrained airflows (Fig. 3) are presented in table 2. In last column is presented the external entrained airflow to total air curtain entrained airflow ratio, ψ, as:

$$\psi = \frac{G_{ind,o}}{G_{ind}} \quad ; \text{ with } G_{ind} = G_{ind,i} + G_{ind,o}.$$

Table 2:   Entrained airflows.

H_w/H_d	W/H_d	$G_{ind,o}$	$G_{ind,i}$	G_{ind}	ψ	H_w/H_d	W/H_d	$G_{ind,o}$	$G_{ind,i}$	G_{ind}	ψ
0.00	1	0.092	0.279	0.371	0.25	0.43	1	0.101	0.114	0.215	0.47
0.00	2	0.092	0.274	0.366	0.25	0.43	2	0.101	0.117	0.218	0.46
0.00	3	0.095	0.286	0.381	0.25	0.43	3	0.101	0.117	0.218	0.46
0.00	4	0.098	0.292	0.390	0.25	0.43	4	0.102	0.119	0.220	0.46
0.00	5	0.100	0.294	0.393	0.25	0.43	5	0.103	0.118	0.221	0.47
0.14	1	0.094	0.215	0.309	0.30	0.57	1	0.105	0.109	0.214	0.49
0.14	2	0.092	0.270	0.362	0.25	0.57	2	0.108	0.108	0.216	0.50
0.14	3	0.095	0.286	0.381	0.25	0.57	3	0.110	0.111	0.220	0.50
0.14	4	0.098	0.293	0.392	0.25	0.57	4	0.113	0.114	0.226	0.50
0.14	5	0.091	0.216	0.307	0.30	0.57	5	0.122	0.115	0.237	0.52
0.29	1	0.098	0.118	0.215	0.39						
0.29	2	0.097	0.121	0.218	0.36	H_d, H_w - Door and window height (m)					
0.29	3	0.096	0.122	0.218	0.37	W - Indoor space length (m)					
0.29	4	0.096	0.124	0.220	0.39	G_{ind}, $G_{ind,o}$, $G_{ind,i}$ - Total, outdoor and indoor					
0.29	5	0.097	0.125	0.221	0.43	entrained airflow (m^3/h x m)					

The indoor volume extension not affect the ψ ratio, instead the indoor natural ventilation through the window have an influence on the entrained airflows (fig. 5). The airflows distribution reach the free jet conditions ($\psi = 0.5$) for larger window surface.

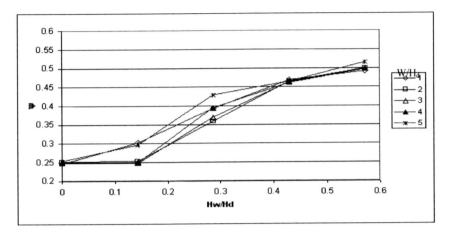

Figure 5: Ψ ratio vs. window height and indoor space length.

The indoor particle concentration as been theoretically carried out using the same model of Fig. 4. The outdoor concentration and the efficiency of the air curtain filter has been derived from Jamriska et al. [3] and are reported in table 3 for each particle diameter.

Table 3:   Outdoor particle concentration and filter removal efficiency.

D (nm)	20	30	40	50	60	70	80	90	100	200	300	400	500	600
C_{out} (particle/cm^3)	270	210	270	320	400	340	270	250	230	90	50	45	30	20
η (%)	39	38	36	35	34	33	32	31	30	24	20	21	28	36

The particle indoor concentrations vs. particle diameters are presented in Fig. 6. The outlet window airflow not affect the air curtain efficiency for H_w/H_d ratio lower than 0.15. The air curtain operates with external filtered air can reduce the indoor particle concentration up to 50%.

5 Remarks

During the last two decades, there has been increasing concern over the effects of indoor contamination on health. Changes in building design intended to improve energy efficiency have meant that modern homes are frequently more airtight than older structures. This has led to more comfortable buildings with lower running cost, but has also caused indoor environments in which contaminants may build up to much higher concentrations than before. Indoor air and dust, besides food and workplace, are significant sources of exposure for the general population, especially children. Indoor pollution has been ranked by the United

States Environmental Protection Agency Advisory Board (EPA) and the Centres for Disease Control (CDC) as a high environmental risk [8].

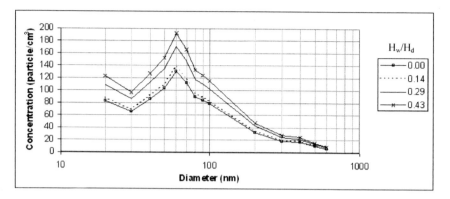

Figure 6:   Particle indoor concentration.

Besides outdoor air (vehicle-related emission), smoking has been found to be the most important source of $PM_{2.5}$ in indoor air, and cooking has been identified as the second strongest source of fine PM in indoor air [9]. As a result of these sources, indoor particle concentrations are often higher than the corresponding outdoor levels. These findings, in conjunction with the fact that people spend the majority of their time indoors, suggest indoor sources to be important contributors to personal exposure to PM_{10} and $PM_{2.5}$.

The air curtain system can effectively hinder the outdoor-to-indoor contaminant diffusion and the indoor-to-indoor air exchange between two confined adjoining spaces. The filter pack installed inside the air curtain device have a 31% average removal efficiency in consequence the indoor diameter distribution of particles is different from outdoor, with variation between -7% and 15% (fig. 7).

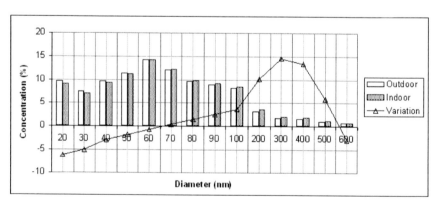

Figure 7:   Particle diameter distribution and indoor-outdoor variation.

Acknowledgement

This work has been supported with the economical contribute of the "Fondazione Cassa di Risparmio di Roma" in the frame of a national program devoted to the human health protection.

References

[1]   Kingham S., Briggs D., Elliot P., Fischer P., Lebret E., 2000. Spatial variations in the concentrations of traffic-related pollutants in indoor and outdoor air in Huddersfield, England. Atmospheric Environment 34, 905-916.

[2]   Chao M.L., Mao I.F., 1998. Spatial variations of airborne particles in metropolitan Taipei. Science of the Total Environment 209, 225-231.

[3]   Jamriska M., Morawska L., Clark B., 2000.The effect of ventilation and filtration on submicrometer particles in an indoor environment. Indoor Air 10, 19-26.

[4]   Santarpia L., Gugliermetti F., 2002. Smoke movement and management in larges spaces. Heat and Technology (Vol.1). - International Journal of heat and technology.

[5]   Santarpia L, Gugliermetti F., 2000. Air curtains to reduce outdoor pollutants infiltration through buildings aperture. Proc of Intren Conf. HB2000, Helsinki, August 5-10.

[6]   Santarpia L. Gugliermetti F., 1999. A phenomenological approach to the performance of shutter type air curtains Proc. Of Air pollution 99, 27-29 July, San Francisco.

[7]   Santarpia L., Gugliermetti F., Zori G., 2005. Dynamic efficiency of air curtain systems. HEFAT2005, 4th International Conference on Heat Transfer, Fluid Mechanics and Thermodynamics. 19-23 September 2005, Cairo, Egypt.

[8]   USEPA (United States Environmental Protection Agency), 2001. Exposure factors handbook Vol III, Chapter 17. Natural Center for Environmental Assessment. Whashington, D.C.

[9]   Monn C., Fuchs A., Hogger D., Junker M. Et al. 1997. Particulate matter less than 10 µm (PM_{10}) and fine particles less than 2.5 µm ($PM_{2.5}$): relationship between indoor, outdoor and personal concentrations. Science of the Total Environment 208, 15-21.

Health and safety in the workplace: prevention of hazards to reproductive health

C. Ferradans-Caramés[1] & F. González-Bugatto[2]
[1]Department of Labour Law, Cádiz University, Spain
[2]Department of Obstetrics and Gynaecology,
"Puerta del Mar" Teaching Hospital, Cádiz, Spain

Abstract

Occupational exposure figures are inexact, and environmental levels are even more difficult to document. Exposure usually involves chemical mixtures, and individuals may not be aware of all the chemicals with which they come into contact. Thus, the effect of individual chemicals is difficult to assess, and cause-and-effect relationships are nearly impossible to establish. The action plan, which should be drawn up by every employer, should specifically take into account when assessing the hazards involved in carrying out a particular job in a specific working environment, the factors which can have a bearing on the ability of the individual to have children, making a distinction between hazards which can affect women, and those which can affect men. Objective risk assessment should be made more specific, taking into consideration both the characteristics of the job and the individual by whom the said job is done.
Keywords: reproductive health, workplace, chemical hazards, labour risks prevention.

1 The right to reproduction and occupational health

The objective of our study is to analyse, from both a physiological and a legal perspective, the problems which arise at work which may be harmful to reproduction due to the characteristics of a working environment, the facilities, the chemical, physical or biological substances present, etc. The treatment of this question has to be distinct depending upon whether the potentially affected subject is female or male, given that the effects of these possibly detrimental factors could be different according to the gender variant [1].

Once the objective of this paper has been set out, we are going to endeavour to demarcate, from a constitutional perspective, the extent of the right to have children, and on what precepts that right to be protected is based.

To this end, it is essential to mention several Articles of the Spanish Constitution of 1978 (hereinafter SC). Thus in Article 15, the right to life and physical and moral well-being is declared as one of the most important and fundamental of constitutional rights. In Article 39 it is established that the authorities ought to guarantee social, economic and legal protection for the family, and in 39.3, specifically mothers. It is clear that in this Magna Carta, in a similar manner to those of our fellow European nations, the right to have children is not expressly recognised. Nevertheless, it is necessary to clarify that in all events the right to have children is one of the primordial manifestations of the right to physical well-being, for both men and women, just like their right to freedom, as the decision whether to have children or not is an exercise of the free will of the individual [2].

The right to have children is a right of autonomous choice for the individual, which brings about the birth of a series of rights and obligations and a necessity to avoid the obstacles which might arise in a working environment. In particular we refer to the protection which should be implemented as decreed by Article 40.2 of the SC, which establishes that the authorities will take care of safety and hygiene at work and Article 43, which recognises the right to health and safety.

This affirmation arises from the hypothesis that the right to have children forms part of health of an individual. Article 43 decrees the right to well being in a generic manner without defining what that consists of, thus permitting a flexible interpretation conditioned by the evolution of social and cultural factors in a given moment. To this end, the reason behind the prescription of the World Health Organisation (WHO) is obvious, as it considers that health is not only the absence of illness, but also "physical, psychological and social well-being" which, representing an ambitious goal, could be the outcome of an appropriate adaptation between the environment and the person.

Occupational health is defined more precisely in the in-session document of the first joint ILO (International Labour Organization)/WHO committee as "the requirements for establishing and maintaining a safe and healthy working environment which will facilitate optimal physical and mental health in relation to work and the adaptation of work to the capabilities of workers in the light of their state of physical and mental health." As such, occupational health is not only sustaining the absence of immediate risks for the worker, but also to progressively improve the wellbeing of said worker [3].

From the above, the framework of occupational health should be understood to encompass the protection of the reproductive facet of all workers, be they male or female, leading to the development of preventative measures, both individual and collective, in the face of multiple hazards which may confront the worker in a work environment [4]. However, this objective must also take into account the diversity in the prevention and protection required, depending upon the gender of the potentially affected subject, as the incidence of the different risks present can vary due to biological differences (hormonal, genetic, anatomical…).

2   Chemical exposure and reproductive toxicity

2.1 Introduction

The endocrine function of the gonads is primarily concerned with perpetuation of the species. The survival of any species depends on the integrity of its reproductive system. Genes located in the chromosomes of the germ cells ensure the maintenance of structure and function in the organism in its own lifetime and from generation to generation.

The twentieth century has undergone an industrial renaissance; through scientific and technical advances, there has been a significant extension in life expectancy and generally an enhanced quality of life. Concomitant to this industrial renaissance, an estimated 50,000 to 60,000 chemicals have come into common use. Approximately 600 or more new chemicals enter commerce each year [5].

The impact of new chemicals on the reproductive system was tragically accentuated by the thalidomide disaster in the 1960s [6]. This episode led to increased awareness on a worldwide basis and brought forth laws and guidelines pertaining to reproductive system safety and testing protocols.

The potential hazards posed to human reproduction by chemicals, and human risks from chemical exposure are difficult to assess because of the complexity of the reproductive process, the unreliability of laboratory tests, and the quality of human data.

The effects of environmental agents on sexual differentiation and the development of reproductive capacity are largely unknown. Of the chemicals that have been studied, it is worth noting that they possess a wide diversity in molecular structure and that they may affect specific cell populations within the reproductive system.

2.2 Chemicals

- Workers in waste incinerators are exposed to *1,2-dibromo-3-chloropropane (DBCP)* and suffer oligo-spermia, azoospermia, and germinal cell aplasia [7].
- Factory workers in *battery plants* in Bulgaria, *lead mine* workers in the U.S. state of Missouri, and workers in Sweden who handle *organic solvents (toluene, benzene, and xylene)* suffer from low sperm counts, abnormal sperm, and varying degrees of infertility.
- *Diethylstilbestrol (DES), lead, chlordecone, methyl mercury,* and many *cancer chemotherapeutic agents* have been shown to be toxic to the male and female reproductive systems and possibly capable of inflicting genetic damage to germ cells.
- Environmental estrogen mimics (e.g., *DDT*).
- Not only are there compounds in the environment that possess estrogenic properties, but there are also environmental antiandrogens (e.g., *vinclozolin*).

2.3 Biotransformation of exogenous chemicals

When chemicals reach blood circulation they can be distributed by any tissue or organ of human economy. Often these chemicals suffer biotransformation reactions in metabolic organs, such as the liver or kidneys, becoming in some cases more potent toxics than the original substances. Some cases which affect the functioning of the testes are:

- *N-hexane,* yields *2,5-hexanedione (2,5-HD)*, an environmental toxicant, and this metabolite, that can be detected in urine from workers in the shoe industry, causes peripheral polyneuropathy and testicular atrophy [8].
- In workers of semiconductor manufacturing plants who are exposed to *Ethylene glycol ethers*, along with its metabolites, such as *2-methoxy-ethanol (2-ME)* and *2-ethoxy-ethanol (2-EE)* was found a increased risk of spontaneous abortion [9].
- *Several heavy metals* are known to adversely affect testicular function; *Cadmium* causes testicular toxicity.
- *Esters of o-phthalic acid (phthalate esters* or *PAEs)* are used extensively in medical devices and other consumer products as plasticizers. Because the PAEs are not convalently bound to the plastic, they can leach into the environment.
- *Ethanol* also causes delayed testicular development and may affect the Sertoli cell and/or the Leydig cell. *Trifluoroethanol and trifluoroacetaldehyde* produce specific damage to pachytene and dividing spermatocytes and round spermatids in rats.
- Antibiotics: Metabolites of *cephalosporin* reportedly cause testicular toxicity in rats. Testicular degeneration from analogs of cephalosporin is most likely to occur with *cefbuperazone, cefamandole, and cefoperazone. Cyclosporine* can also inhibit testosterone biosynthesis in the rat testes.

Less is known about how chemicals or drugs interfere with ovarian metabolism because of its more difficult and complex hormonal relationships.

Nevertheless, several chemotherapeutic agents can inhibit ovarian function: *prednisone, vincristine, vinblastine, 6-mercaptopurine, nitrogen mustard, cyclophosphamide, chlorambucil, busulfan, methotrexate, cytosine arabinoside, L-asparginase, 5-fluorouracil* and *adriamycin* [10].

2.4 Targets for chemical toxicity: gonads

The gonads are also targets for a host of drugs and chemicals [Table 1]. The majority of these agents are representatives of major chemical classes of cancer chemotherapeutic agents, particularly the alkylating agents. A number of endocrine agents are of value in the treatment of certain cancers. *Antiestrogens* (e.g., *tamoxifen*), aromatase inhibitors (e.g., *aminoglutethimide*), GnRH agonists and *antagonists*, and *antiandrogens* (e.g., *flutamide*) can interfere with the endocrine system.

Table 1:   Drugs that are gonadotoxic in humans.

MALES	FEMALES
Busulfan	Busulfan
Chlorambucil	Chlorambucil
Cyclophosphamide	Cyclophosphamide
Nitrogen mustard	Nitrogen mustard
Doxorubicin	
Corticosteroids	
Cytosine-arabinoside	
Methotrexate	
Procarbazine	
Vincristine	
Vinblastine	Vinblastine

Procarbazine, an antineoplastic drug, causes severe damage to the acrosomal plasma membrane and the nucleus of the sperm head in hamsters. Alkylating agents (*ultraviolet and x-rays)* can damage DNA molecules and are effective against rapidly dividing cells. Not surprisingly, the division of germ cells is also affected, leading to arrest of spermatogenesis.

2.5 Human risk factors affecting fertility

Most humans are exposed to a vast number of chemicals that may be hazardous to their reproductive capacity. Many chemicals have been identified as reproductive hazards in laboratory studies [11]. Although the extrapolation of data from laboratory animals to humans is inexact, a number of these chemicals have also been shown to exert detrimental effects on human reproductive performance. The list includes drugs, especially *steroid hormone*s and *chemotherapeutic agents*; *metals* and *trace elements*; *pesticides*; *food additives* and *contaminants*; *industrial chemicals*; and *consumer products*.

2.5.1 Male fertility
It has also been suggested that the human male is more vulnerable to environmental and occupational toxins than other mammals. It is noteworthy that chronic illness may have a profound affect on gonadal function [12]. Several systemic illnesses can reduce spermatogenesis, including *thyrotoxicosis, hypothyroidism, renal failure, mumps, and Crohn's disease*. A large number of nonhormonal diseases can likewise decrease serum testosterone as well as gonadotrophins. *Aging, nutritional deficiencies*, and *obesity* can affect fertility. Thus, a host of both endocrine and nonendocrine diseases can affect male fertility.

2.5.2 Female fertility
Many factors can affect the normal function of the female reproductive system, as evidenced by variations in the menstrual process. Hence, *physiologic,*

sociologic, and psychological factors have been linked with menstrual disorders. Factors that are already known to affect menstruation are for the most part completely unrelated to occupational settings include *age, body weight extremes, liver disease, thyroid dysfunction, intrauterine contraceptive devices, stress,* and *exercise.* It is, therefore, obvious that a number of factors can affect menstruation and that these factors do not even include such things as therapeutic drugs, so-called recreational drugs, or potentially toxic substances present in occupational environments.

2.6 Extrapolation of animal data to humans and epidemiologic studies

It is considerably easier to extrapolate controlled drug studies in animals to exact therapeutic regimens in humans than it is to simulate a chemical's exposure in an animal to a presumed environmental exposure in humans.

Epidemiology is increasingly important in establishing cause-and-effect relationships. Epidemiology and risk assessment are inextricably related. There is a need for more well designed studies in order to implicate any individual chemical because in most occupations, workers are exposed to raw, intermediate and finished products and there are also confounding factors associated with lifestyles responsible for reproductive dysfunction. Occupational exposure are always higher than environmental exposures, so that epidemiological studies should be conducted on chemicals which are reported to have adverse effects on reproduction in the experimental system [13]. By closely monitoring worker exposures to industrial/environmental toxicants, safer conditions will be established.

3 Preventative and protective measures

Health and safety are essential elements of the quality of work and represent one of the more important fields of the regulatory activity of the ILO and the social policy of the European Union [3]. This, evidently, should be reflected in the legal system of each of the Member States, among them Spain. In this respect it is necessary to bring up Spanish Act 31/1995, of 8 November, ruling occupational risks, the content of which has been complimented and/or modified by Act 54/2003, of 12 December. This Act reforms the regulatory framework dealing with the prevention of hazards in the workplace claiming, in accord with the statement of its motives, that the planning of preventative measures should not be a merely formal act. This action plan should, therefore, be produced at the same time as the design of a managerial project assessing the inherent hazards in a job and being updated periodically, as the circumstances and conditions of the job change, all this being presented in a coherent and integrated ensemble of preventative measures, appropriate to the nature of the hazards and effectively controlling the same, in order to reduce the accident rate in the workplace.

With the objective of obtaining the desired result, the preventative policy is reinforced by the specification in Article 16 of the APOR of a new measure. The action plan for the prevention of occupational risks is a document which ought to be drawn up by all employers. This will then be integrated into the general managerial system of the business, in both the complete range of activities and in all hierarchical levels. This plan should detail the organisational structure, the processes, and the resources necessary to carry out the precautionary measures required to prevent occupational risks within the business.

Risk assessment plays a fundamental role in the action plan, in accordance with that made mandatory in Article 16.2 of the APOR. This plan should programme an initial evaluation which takes into consideration, in a general manner, the nature of the duties involved, the characteristics of the existing jobs, and of the workers who perform them. The plan should be updated when the working conditions change and due to these changes injuries to workers' health have occurred. Additionally, at the end of Article 16.2.a, it specifies that "when the result of the assessment makes it necessary the employer will make periodical inspections of the working conditions and the duties of the workers in services rendered, in order to detect potentially dangerous situations."

It will therefore be obligatory to carry out an objective survey of the hazards which could combine in a determined place of work, but this is not sufficient as the result obtained should have to be made specific, in other words its efficiency should be confirmed in the moment of being applied to a specific worker [14], with the objective of complying with the general principle which claims that it is the place of work which ought to be adapted to the worker (Article 15.1 of the APOR) and not vice versa.

Working on this principle, in regard to the occupational risks which can harm the right to have children, we should mention what is established in Article 25.2 of the APOR [15,16] which emphasises that when it comes to risk assessment the exceptional way in which hazards can harm this aspect of the worker should be taken into consideration. The precept, using scientific terminology, establishes that "the employer ought to take into consideration in risk assessment the factors which may influence the procreative capacity of the workers, in particular from exposure to physical, chemical and biological agents which may cause children to be born with deformities or have a toxic effect on procreation, both in the area of fertility and in the development of offspring, with the objective of introducing the necessary preventative measures".

In accordance with the aforementioned, in the first place we should emphasise that this specific protection should be applied to all workers who can have children, unless the impossibility of their so doing is reliably corroborated [15]. We make this precise distinction because the reference in Article 25 of the APOR to the "protection of workers who are particularly sensitive to certain risks," could lead to an error, as Article 25.2 demands an disinterested protection against certain risks, and not the selective protection of some groups of workers.

Secondly, we should underline that the assessment of risks which can affect procreation may encounter certain difficulties as, to-date, there have not been enough medical studies which confirm the existence of a cause-effect relationship between the execution of a job within certain working conditions and fertility problems or deformation in offspring [1]. Due to this, as established by the European Council [3], in order to implement a culture of prevention it is necessary to improve awareness of the risks posed by the agents involved, systematically gathering information and scientific reports, and coordinating the respective programmes with research centres, in order to direct them to the solutions of problems and to transfer the results to business. It should be highlighted that in the year 2000, a Communication from the Commission was adopted. This Communication provided guidelines for the assessment of chemical, physical and biological agents, as well as the industrial procedures considered to be dangerous to the health of a pregnant worker, one who has recently given birth or who is breast-feeding [17] which could be useful material for assessment, even if the toxic agents which affect pregnant or breast-feeding women at work are not the same as those which affect fertility.

When dealing with risk assessment it is essential to bear another important question in mind. We have clarified that protection against the harmful effects on procreation is too generic and consequently needs to be differentiated from the general potential harm which could be caused to men and women. In other words, the gender variant should be taken into account as a criterion of diversity [4], to show clearly that some risks can affect both males and females alike, while others will have a more virulent effect on only one of the sexes. Consequently, an action plan ought to take into account this relevant circumstance, as is highlighted in Article 16.1.a of the APOR which specifies that the initial risk assessment will take into consideration "the nature of work, the characteristics of the existing jobs and the workers who do them." In order to achieve this the employer could be given professional advice by the prevention services (Article 31.3.a of the APOR), and by the Health and Safety Committee (the specialist body for the representation of workers regulated by Article 39.1.a of the APOR), bodies which have the possibility of a more direct contact with the affected wage-earners allowing the workers themselves to contribute, from their own experience, anything which may have a bearing on the matter.

Thirdly, according to Article 16.2.b of the APOR, if the results of the assessment make certain hazardous situations clear, for example if after readings are taken it is concluded that the exposure to certain chemical or physical elements exceeds the exposure limit values, the employer must take such measures as are necessary to eliminate or reduce and control this exposure. In other words, if after the appropriate assessment the existence of risks which may affect the right of the workers to have children are detected, such risks must be eliminated. However, if that is not a possibility, they should reduced and monitored by means of, for example, the use of the appropriate individual equipment or the preparation of a catalogue of products and techniques which involve a risk for the worker, with an attachment detailing the necessary protective measures for the evasion or reduction of risk. To this effect, it will be necessary to analyse the alternatives to prevention which exist, in accordance with the context in which the potentially affected worker is found. Article 16.2.b of the APOR states that preventative activities will be a planning objective for the employer, including for each action "the deadline for appointing a person to be in charge and the human resources and equipment necessary for their fulfilment" which will require a prior study, such as that which we have discussed. The employer will then be obliged to detect inadequate measures as a consequence of planned periodical inspections, which will then be modified to meet the level of protection required.

In the worst case scenario where, even if an action plan exists and the appropriate assessment has been carried out, discovering certain risks for procreation but, despite this, the hazardous elements have not been eliminated or replaced, or the necessary preventative measures have not been introduced, the employer could be charged as liable for a serious or very serious administrative sanction, depending upon the magnitude of the risk to the worker.

4 Conclusions

- Industrial processes imply that an estimated 50,000 to 60,000 chemicals have come into common use. Approximately 600 or more new chemicals enter commerce each year.
- Occupational exposure figures are inexact, and environmental levels are even more difficult to document. Exposure usually involves chemical mixtures, and individuals may not be aware of all the chemicals with which they come into contact. Thus, the effect of individual chemicals is difficult to assess, and cause-and-effect relationships are nearly impossible to establish.
- The action plan, which should be drawn up by every employer, should specifically take into account when assessing the hazards involved in carrying out a particular job in a specific working environment, the factors which can have a bearing on the ability of the individual to have children, making a distinction between hazards which can affect women, and those which can affect men.
- Objective risk assessment should be made more specific, taking into consideration both the characteristics of the job and the individual by whom said job is done.
- If, after due assessment, the employer detects situations which pose a risk to the fertility of workers, measures must be introduced which eliminate, reduce or control said hazards, otherwise said employer will be incumbent to a serious, or very serious, administrative liability, according to the magnitude of damage caused.

References

[1]   Pérez del Río, T. & Ballester Pastor, M.A., *Woman and Health at Work*, La Ley, Madrid, p. 46, 2000.
[2]   Gómez Sánchez, Y., *The Right to Human Reproduction*, Marcial Pons, Madrid, p. 40, 1994.
[3]   Decision of 3 June 2002, On a new strategy for health and safety in the workplace (2002-2006), Official Journal of European Community, 161, 5 June 2002.

[4]   Arial Calama, I., Occupational health for women: beyond reproductive health. *New situations for Labour Law: family, immigration and the concept of the worker,* ed. J. López López, Marcial Pons, Madrid, p. 183, 2001.

[5]   Thomas, M.J. & Thomas, J.A., Toxic responses of the reproductive system. *Casarett & Doull's Toxicology: The Basic Science of Poisons,* ed. C.D. Klaassen, McGraw-Hill, 6th ed., 2001.

[6]   Lenz, W., Thalidomide and congenital abnormalities. *Lancet,* 1, p. 1219, 1962.

[7]   Bakoglu, M., Karademir, A. & Ayberk, S., An evaluation of the occupational health risks to workers in a hazardous waste incinerator. *J Occup Health,* 46(2), pp. 156-64, 2004.

[8]   Prieto, M.J., Marhuenda, D., Roel, J. & Cardona, A., Free and total 2,5-hexenedione in biological monitoring of workers exposed to n-hexane in the shoe industry. *Toxicol Lett.,* 145(3), pp. 249-60, 2003.

[9]   Correa, A., Gray, R.H., Cohen, R., Rothman, N., Shah, F., Seacat, H. & Corn, M., Ethylene glycol ethers and risk of spontaneous abortion and subfertility. *Am J Epidemiol.,* 143(7), pp. 707-14, 1996.

[10]   Gorospe, W.C. & Reinhard M., Toxic effects on the ovary of the nonpregnant female. *Reproductive Toxicology,* ed. R.J. Witorsch, 2nd ed., New York, Raven Press, pp. 141–157, 1995.

[11]   Clegg, E.D., Perreault, S.D. & Klinefelter, G.R., Assessment of male reproductive toxicity. *Principles and Methods of Toxicology,* ed. A.W. Hayes, 4th ed., Philadelphia, Taylor & Francis, pp. 1263-1300, 2001.

[12]   Turner, H.E. & Wass, J.A.H., Gonadal function in men with chronic illness, *Clin Endocrinol,* 47, pp. 379–403, 1997.

[13]   Kumar, S., Occupational exposure associated with reproductive dysfunction. *J Occup Health,* 46(1), pp. 1-19, 2004.

[14]   Fernández Marcos, L., *Comments on the Act for the prevention of occupational risks and regulatory guidelines,* 2nd ed., Dikynson, Madrid, 2001.

[15]   Rodriguez Ramos, M.J. & Pérez Borrego, G., Groups at Particular risk in the Act on the prevention of occupational risks. *Occupational Risk Prevention,* eds. A. Ojeda, M.R. Alarcón & M.J. Rodríguez Ramos, Aranzadi, Pamplona, p. 409, 1996.

[16]   García-Perrote Escartín, I., Protection of workers who are particularly sensitive to certain hazards. *Health and Safety at Work,* eds. M.E. Casas, M.C. Palomeque & F.Valdés Dal Ré, La Ley, Madrid, p. 41, 1997.

[17]   European Community Communication COM (2000), 466, 5 October 2000.

Section 5
Water quality issues

Validity of coliphages as indicators of viral pollution of water in the Aral Sea area, Uzbekistan

D. K. Fayzieva, I. A. Usmanov, E. E. Bekzhanova,
F. B. Kadirkhodjaeva & F. B. Shadijanova
Institute for Water Problems, Academy of Sciences, Uzbekistan

Abstract

Hygienic standards of microbial contamination of water in water-bodies for different types of water consumption have been developed to prevent intestinal infections amongst the population. The current methods of microbiologic examination of water in water-bodies used for different types of water sources in Uzbekistan do not always meet the ISO requirements. This sets the goals of studying the validity of the bacteriological and viral indicators as well as implementing appropriate methods of laboratory analysis.

Timely identification of microbial contamination of water is of special importance for correct and quick arrangement of anti-epidemic and sanitation activities. Among all other activities aimed at the reduction and prevention of viral infections, early and prompt identification of viral pollution of water is of top priority. According to the Uzbek State Standard 950:2000 "Drinking Water" a number of plague forming units (PFU) of coliphages in water was recommended as an indirect indicator of water pollution by enteroviruses.

The study conducted in Khorazm and Karakalpakstan (in the Aral Sea area) could find no correlation between the rate of viral hepatitis A (VHA), percentage of tap-water samples that do not meet the standard and the quality of water from surface water-bodies tested for coliphages. This makes questionable the sanitary-indicative value of coliphages and their usefulness for evaluation of epidemiological safety of water regarding viral infection.

It is necessary to set modern and more representative direct methods revealing the indicators of viral pollution of water in water-bodies and tap-water in Uzbekistan.

Keywords: water pollution, indirect indicators of viral contamination, coliphages, the Aral Sea area.

1 Introduction

Given the fact that even one viral unit of few viruses is able to cause of serious case of disease, the evidence of their presence in water should be provided [1]. The results of last investigations show, coliphages can not represent itself as indicators of virus pollution of water, as their presence not always correlates with presence of the virus agents [2, 3, 4, 5]. It was demonstrated that if to test water-samples for the presence of enteroviruses, antigens of viral hepatitis A and rotaviruses, the number of even of tap-water samples defined as unsafe water by the microbiological indicators can rise by 30-40% [2, 3]. The enteroviruses can be isolated from water on a background when coliphages are not detected (~ in 2-3% of assays) [2]. All above stated puts under doubt sanitary - indicative importance of coliphages and opportunity of their use while estimation of epidemic safety of water concerning virus infections [3, 4, 5].

Now identification of viral pollution of water in water-bodies is being regulated in Uzbekistan by the State Standard Uz 950:2000 "Drinking water" that recommends to use number of plague forming units (PFU) of coliphages in water as an indirect indicator of its viral pollution [6]. However, no special research was conducted in the country to study the indicator value of PFU of coliphages.

The objectives of the present research was to study the dynamics of viral hepatitis A rate among the population of Khorezm province and the Republic of Karakalpakstan (the Aral Sea area) and to find its correlation with the quality indicator of water, namely the coliphages level in water-bodies of different types of water-consumption.

2 Data and methods

Hepatitis A morbidity has been analyzed on its rate (per 100,000 of population) among the population of areas under study. Every case of the disease or a suspected case registered in official reporting documents was taken as a unit of evaluation. The percentage of water-samples with coli-phages was calculated in every area under study. The statistic materials of the province centers for sanitary and epidemiological surveillance for 2000-2004 were used.

3 Results

As Table 1 shows, viral hepatitis A (VHA) rates are still high in the areas under study. The intensive indicator of VHA morbidity in Khorezm province was 375.9 in 2000 having reduced by 2004 to 287.6 per 100,000 of population. In Karakalpakstan, in 2000 it was 464.9 having reduced in 2004 to 356.6 per 100,000 of population.

During the whole period of the research the percentage of tap-water samples that did not meet the standard by the presence of coliphages had ranged from 3.8 to 5.7 per cent. The fact of coliphages identification in tap-water indicated both insufficient sanitary and technical efficiency of the facilities and insufficient sanitary surveillance of their functioning (Table 2). The share of non-standard by coli-phages samples in water of surface water-bodies was large and ranged from 14 to 34 per cent (Table 3).

Table 1: Dynamics of VHA morbidity rates among the population of the Aral Sea area (per 100,000 of population).

Provinces	Years				
	2000	2001	2002	2003	2004
Khorazm	375.9	394.6	415.0	384.4	287.6
Karakalpakstan	464.9	398.4	657.1	397.8	356.6

Table 2: Findings of the sanitary and virological analysis of tap-water in the Aral Sea area

Province	Years	plaque-forming units of coliphages		
		Number of samples	Among them positive samples	% of positive samples
Khorazm	2000	250	11	4.4
	2002	215	12	5.6
	2004	196	8	4.1
Karakalpakstan	2000	310	12	3.8
	2002	280	16	5.7
	2004	295	14	4.7

Table 3: Share of non-standard by coliphages water-samples from surface water-bodies (river, irrigation ditch) in the Aral Sea area.

Province	Years				
	2000	2001	2002	2003	2004
Khorazm	30.0	14.0	18.0	17.2	16,5
Karakalpakstan	34.0	17.0	20.2	23.0	19.4

In the epidemiology of viral hepatitis A, the leading etiologic role is played by a "water factor" that is why we have studied the correlation between the VHA rates among the population and the share of non-standard by coliphages water-samples in tap-water and in water of open sources i.e. from surface water-bodies (river, irrigation ditch).

The findings shown in Table 4 demonstrate a significant scattering of the correlation coefficient depending on the type of water-consumption in the areas under study. Poor correlation was found between the VHA rates in Khorezm province and the percentage of non-standard samples: for tap-water it was 0.37; for surface water-bodies – 0.39. The similar data were obtained when treating the findings obtained in Karakalpakstan. In this area, the correlation coefficients were 0.40 and 0.35, respectively.

Table 4: Correlation coefficients between the VHA rates in population and the share of non-standard by coliphages water samples (%).

Province	Tap water	Open sources
Khorazm	0.37	0.39
Karakalpakstan	0.40	0.35

Thus, the research of coliphages failed to evaluate objectively viral pollution of water in different types of water-consumption. This makes questionable the sanitary-indicative value of coliphages and their usefulness for evaluation of epidemiological safety of water regarding viral infection.

A certain part in this is, probably, played by imperfection of the existing methods identifying coliphages because they are made using agar-layers. This method implies identification of the number of plaque-forming units in 1.5 ml of water-sample in which enterobacteria are able to give negative colonies on the bacterial "lawn". It is evident that in order to raise representativeness of the method it is necessary to work out a specific technique that would imply concentration of certain volumes of water, the minimum volumes being 100 and 1000 litres.

It should be also taken into account that the existing method is indirect while the only reliable method to have virologically safe water is to eliminate human pathogenic viruses that can be identified by direct virological tests.

4 Conclusions

Ensuring epidemiological safety of water regarding human viral infection requires up-dating the indicators and order of sanitary and epidemiological surveillance of water quality for different types of water-consumption.

Modern and representative indicators of viral pollution of water used for drinking and household needs have to be studied in local conditions and implemented into practice.

Amendments to the existing regulating documents and instructions used in the practice of virological laboratories within the system of the state sanitary and epidemiological surveillance of environment need to be made.

Acknowledgements

This investigation was carried out in the frame of the research project No 13.40 on "Ecological and epidemiological assessment of anthropogenic impact on drinking water sources", in 2003-2005, funded by the State Scientific and Technology Program of the Republic of Uzbekistan. Authors express their gratitude to the Center of Science and Technologies at the Cabinet of Ministers of the Republic of Uzbekistan for given opportunity in organization of the investigation on validity of coliphages as indicators of water pollution by viruses. We feel sincere gratitude to the Embassy of France in Uzbekistan for great support in organization of expert evaluation travel to the Aral Sea area and study of local laboratory conditions and data on microbial water quality and water-borne diseases rates in collaboration with Head of Environment and Water Department of Pasteur Institute in Lille, Dr. Tristan Simonart in August-September of 2003.

References

[1] Vinogradova L.A., Luzin, P.M., Korovka, V.G. *Urgent problems of medical virology*, pp. 69-72, Moscow, 1985.
[2] Amvrosieva, T.V., Diakonova, O.V., Poklonskaya, N.V. To a problem of an adequate estimation of epidemic safety of water concerning viral infections. *Proceedings of the 4th International Congress: "Water, Ecology, Technology - ECWATECH"*, p.740-741, Moscow, 2000.
[3] Amvrosieva, T.V., Diakonova, O.V., Boguch, Z.F., Kazinetc, O.N. Main directions to improve sanitary virological control of drinking water quality. *Proceedings of the 5th International Congress: "Water, Ecology, Technology - ECWATECH"*, p.487, Moscow, 2002.
[4] Kaskarova, G.N., Blagova O.E. Significance of coliphages in assessment of viral pollution of water. *Proceedings of the 5th International Congress: "Water, Ecology, Technology - ECWATECH"*, p.681, Moscow, 2002.
[5] Nedachin, A.E., Sanamyan, A.G., Dmitrieva, R.A. Comparative estimation of efficiency allocation of viruses from water with use of a membrane filtration method. *Proceedings of the 5th International Congress: "Water, Ecology, Technology - ECWATECH"*, p.479, Moscow, 2002.
[6] *Drinking water. The hygienic demands and the quality surveillance*, Uz DSt (Uzbek State Standard), 950:2000.

Solving simultaneous risk equations: waste water recycling and fresh water sustainability in an arid continent

G. K. Smith[1] & A. Smith[2]
[1]School of International Studies, University of South Australia
[2]Clean Ocean Foundation, Australia

Abstract

Two separate sets of entrenched environmental mal-practices in Australia have created serious health risk issues. The risk equations are becoming clearer and are interlinked. Solving one of these equations can assist in solving the other. Equation 1: Major Australian cities have dealt with the growing human and industrial waste water flows produced over the last century of growth by utilising coastal proximity and piping partially treated effluent into the oceans. As the volume and toxicity of the outfalls has multiplied, so have adverse health effects. Equation 2: The mainly European settlers of an arid continent increased their fresh water consumption at a prodigious rate. All major Australian cities are in water supply crisis and irrigations schemes and depleted rivers threaten agricultural sustainability. Tradeable water rights are to be granted to farmers but it has become potentially unaffordable for governments to buy back sufficient water rights to restore major river flows. Solutions: The Clean Ocean Foundation established the campaign to "close ocean outfalls" and invest in advanced technology recycling of all waste water to standards suitable for an array of agricultural and industrial uses, without health risks. Such an investment, which would be well supported by urban populations, takes the pressure from river systems and assists the affordability of water for farmers, industry, and for environmental buy-backs schemes alike.
Keywords: water recycling, water policy, environmental risk, environmental campaigns, Australia.

1 Introduction

Two apparently separate sets of entrenched water practices in Australia have created severe environmental, economic and social problems, and sets of risk equations whose interactive dimensions have only recently begun to be identified. Both sets of risk issues have struggled to impact on the public policy process, but new political and policy dynamics are developing from local community and elite scientific activism. This paper looks at the linkages between two initially separate sets of issues, and how awareness of health risks of waste water disposal at the local community level are interacting with the science-led debate about the environmental risks of unsustainable water usage in the agricultural and urban economy. The idea of a single water cycle has real policy implications which have begun to be explored: solutions in waste water recycling will contribute to solutions to the highly stressed state of rivers and groundwater.

The more familiar Australian story is about the diversion of water from fragile river systems to support the demands of urban and rural economies: how the European occupants of the arid continent of Australia increased fresh water consumption at a prodigious rate, especially since the second half of the last century.

A less familiar story, or one certainly less discussed in polite society and influenced by cultural taboos, is about how major Australian cities have dealt with the growing human and industrial waste water flows from the last 60 years of growth – by utilising coastal proximity and piping untreated or partially treated effluent into the oceans. With all of Australia's major cities and most of its minor cities located on or near the coast, this was the "lucky country" version of urbanisation and industrialisation. Where many other countries used their rivers for this purpose, Australians could put most of the waste water further out of sight and mind into the oceans, and this continued through into the 21st century. But as the volume and toxicity of the ocean outfalls have increased remorselessly, so have the documented cases of adverse environmental and health effects, and concern for unmeasured hazards. The visible plumes of pollutants have increased, shocking not only the citizens of Sydney at Bondi beach, but also those of Melbourne, at the equally iconic surf beach Gunnamatta (a Koori word for beach and sand hills).

Each of these narratives of risk is explored and the potential links between them are examined in the Australian context, together with an analysis of the different forms of political activism for policy change. Advanced waste water treatment which produces water with potential for recycling has become urgent for its own set of growing health risk reasons: there is no safe ocean dump for such a dangerous cocktail of pollutants. The economic costs of effective and sustainable solutions for the rivers may be partly offset by the potential for water recycling from the ocean waste outfalls to meet specified industrial, agricultural and domestic water needs. The risk investigation needs to be comprehensive, open, and with an appropriate sense of urgency – so that the economic investments, from public sector infrastructure and private sector policy settings, can be focused and implemented without the procrastination that accompanies partial approaches.

2 Risk equation A: the emerging health crisis of ocean waste outfalls

The planning mindset in Australia that has led to the creation of an estimated 143 ocean waste water outfalls was no different to that which generally accompanied the growth of cities in the industrial revolution, and which accompanies the rapid growth of cities in parts of the developing world today. The water task for the narrowly focused city planner was/is to bring in potable or safe water in for human and industrial uses, get rain water drained off the streets to mitigate flooding, and send sewage waste somewhere beyond the city limits. A comprehensive sewerage system was a matter of pride in engineering accomplishment and urban modernity, solving the great public health crises that the open sewer represented, both in reality, and also in folk memory of plague and pestilence. It was as though the very act of moving the waste somewhere else was such an achievement that the matter of where it went and what was happening there was for smaller minds.

In the Australian states, large public utilities, Boards of Works, operated through the 20th century. They built the system and the state enforced the laws of sewerage on property owners, with pipes inscribed on land titles and checked on sale of property. The initial perception of risk was very simple: the waste removal system had transformed a high health risk system into a no-risk one, and the community's champions were the engineers who build the pipes to take it all away. Sydney and Melbourne took slightly different paths to the same endpoint over the twentieth century as urban and industrial growth continued. Sydney, being more proximate to the ocean, chose largely to pour it straight in. Melbourne, on an extensive bay, and with a more socially progressive self-image, developed a major sewage farm for 'treated' effluent around a significant part of the bay near the town of Werribee, to grow pastures to raise cattle. But, overwhelmed by growing volume, and disturbed that much still flowed or overflowed into the bay near the city, the Melbourne and Metropolitan Board of Works in the 1960s set about building the great pipe to the ocean to get to the no-risk final solution that the vastness of the oceans seemed to offer. Community opposition at the time saw the planned pipe moved from Westernport Bay (on the south-eastern side of the city) to Gunnamatta, much further south on the ocean. To allay concerns of landholders and ocean users in the area of the outfall, it was claimed that new treatment technologies installed on the way to the ocean would deal with all pollution issues [2]. At the opening of the major treatment plant for the pipe in 1975, the Board's Chairman is reputed to have declared that the water from the plant was "good enough to drink".

This completion of the pipe marked the transition by a public body from engineering works utility to political spin agent (to the point of outright denial), in the face of concerns over emerging health risks. It foreshadowed an inertia, and a defensive politicisation, which 33 years later, in 2005, saw the same pipe with little improved treatment plant producing nothing more than what is defined in Australia as Class C level of treatment [3], while the evidence of risks, identified, probable and possible has steadily mounted [4].

Over this period there have been dramatic changes in the volume and composition of the outfall. Focussing on Melbourne as illustrative case study, the volume of outfall has expanded rapidly with population and industrial growth, leading to a typical discharge at Gunnamatta of 450 ML per day. This was a greater daily flow that that typical of the Murray River in its course. Furthermore, and of crucial importance to environmental health risk, the composition of the outfall continued to change as industrial, domestic and human pharmaceutical practices changed: new chemical and bio-chemical components waste entered the waste system. Some of the practices were shaped by government policies; industries including hospitals & abattoirs wanting to dispose of their waste through the sewerage system were able to do so through entering trade waste agreements with the Environment Protection Agency, and paying a fee. These "licenses to pollute" represent the demise of agencies set up after the first wave of environmentalism in the late 1960s, coopted into the normalised politics of pollution.

The general scientific literature on the array of health risks associated or potentially associated with various components of waste water and the potential for technologies to address these risks is growing rapidly. In Australia, the work of the Oz-AQUAREC team at University of Wollongong (a partner of the EC initiative for Integrated Concepts for Reuse of Upgraded Wastewater) provides an important clearing house [5]. Its 2005 conference on *Integrated Concepts in Water Recycling* focussed directly on issues of water quality and water usage options, and a previous one on *A Triple Bottom Line Approach to Water Recycling* explored not only the complex technical issues of water risk, but also the institutional and social settings that can inhibit or facilitate change.

Growing scientific awareness of the potential health risks has been met in some States with a degree of resistance by the institutions that evolved from the Boards of Works, now with contemporary names such as *Melbourne Water* and *Sydney Water*. These organisations, who once saw their duty as being to provided unlimited fresh water to the city at minimal cost, were in the most recent 5 years, demonstrating their new profile as water conservers, charging urban consumers ever more for their water and using the revenue to fund campaigns to create social pressure on individuals who wasted water, who were to be defined as "Water Wallies", thoughtless wasters. Most of these newly rebranded water authorities have been unable to focus sharply on the health risks of waste water disposal into the oceans, and on the issues of public and financial responsibility which these risks raise. Comprehensive studies on Australian ocean outfalls have generally been slow to develop, and there is little public confidence in the benchmarks being set by EPAs often reporting to the same Ministers as the water authorities, and sharing a budgetary allocation between them. There is a significant lag between identifying potential risk elements, developing a notion of acceptable levels and then monitoring for those levels and reporting in a meaningful way.

The driver for change has come instead from community organisations [6]. These organisations have in turn been boosted by the expansion of human settlement and recreational activity to geographical areas near ocean outfalls. For Melbourne, the pipe was taken to Gunnamatta at the end of the once remote Mornington Peninsula in the 1970s. The Mornington Peninsula today is a leading region of wine-making, recreational activity and life-style settlement. The outfall is are no longer out of sight; and so no longer out of mind. The Clean Ocean Foundation [1] was originally by local surfers concerned about their health, and partly inspired by the UK group *Surfers Against Sewerage.* It has become intensely engaged in campaigning activities at the local, state and national levels, but deeply connected to a political base in the Mornington Peninsula

In the absence of sufficient testing by the water authorities, the Foundation began to conduct its own tests, with sampling identifying problematic bacteria and viruses e.g. enterococci, faecal coliforms, streptococci, hepatitis C, and chemical contaminants e.g. N, P, phthalates, dioxins. Surveys of beach users identified numerous reported health problems e.g. throat, ear, gastric infections, viral meningitis and hepatitis, and a database of health reports was accumulated. The evidence was sporadic, ad hoc, indicative not conclusive – but sufficient to demonstrate the reality and potential of significant health risks.

The Clean Ocean Foundation developed a campaign over the last four years to contest the technology and politics of outfall inertia, creating a political dynamic for policy change. In response to the myriad of identified, probable, and possible health risks, it adopted the most challenging of all alternatives to the old pipe-it-to-the-ocean paradigm: a demand to commit to closing the pipe altogether in 10 years. This would allow time the time to identify, test and invest in recycling usable water for a range of purposes.

3   Risk equation B: the crisis of fresh water supply in an arid country

The exponential growth in water consumption over the last century, and in particular the last 40 years, was driven not only the rapid growth of cities based on the English suburban garden and American swimming pool, but ever expanding irrigation schemes which permitted and encouraged farmers to tap the rivers for irrigation projects oblivious to the consequences. As a result, all of Australia's major cities face fresh water crises of varying but growing proportions, as dams fail to provide the quantity of water required and with quality in sharp decline. On the agricultural side, irrigators' overuse of water has been at the expense of other rural interests, with damaged groundwater and rising salinity a persistent theme of scientific documentation [7]. The fate of the great Murray-Darling system is the most analysed, and it no longer carries enough water to keep its ocean entrance open without regular dredging.

Analysing and forecasting the state of rivers, groundwater, salinity and the total effect on sustainability requires the knowledge and skills of complex science. The pressure for change in water use policies has come principally from the environmental scientific community, and increasingly from it leaders, felt driven by the urgency of the situation to act in common to deliver a message on necessary changes. The unsustainability of the practices of damming and draining rivers was spelt out most recently in *Blueprint for a National Water Plan*, [8] the report of the "Wentworth Group" of eminent scientists to a meeting of all Australian state and federal governments. The Blueprint focused on three reforms:

1. Protecting river health and the rights of all Australians to clean usable water, prioritising environmental needs;
2. Establishing a national water entitlements and trading system, and funding the return of at least 100GL to the Murray river each year;
3. Engaging local communities to ensure a fair transition, including Environmental Water Trusts to manage stressed river systems

Initial public policy responses to the water supply crisis reflect the power and perceptions of different sectors. In the cities, the price increases and water saving campaigns of the water authorities achieved a degree of inevitable response from the public, who in their process of re-education were not at all engaged over the industrial, agricultural and wastewater issues and were led to believe that the full solution lay in their own profligate hands. In agricultural industry, where 70% of water consumption occurs, water was instead turned into a gift not a tax – farmers who had helped themselves to the rivers over the previous decades were to be given commercial water rights, and if governments now wished to "restore environmental flows", they would have to buy these rights from those farmers who had been given them. But it has become expensive for governments to buy back sufficient water rights to restore major river flows, with Quiggin estimating up to $3 billion to restore the Murray River [9,10]. Rewarding those who have pursued the most unsustainable farming practices also appears to create a situation of moral hazard, which some fear might lead to further demands for governments to pay to cease other unsustainable practices such as excessive land clearing [11].

4   Achieving change: contrasting campaign styles

Damage to the rivers, with all its long term consequences, has become the focus of a scientific politics, characterised by increased activism of larger and larger groups of the most eminent scientists, based on rational principles of evidence and argument. Some of these scientists at times seem angry and baffled at the obduracy of the political and economic system, in the face of their compelling arguments. Ocean outfalls, with all their consequences, have by contrast, become the focus of community politics, characterised by a direct demands for policy change at the local/state level based on the precautionary principle. This is expressed most notably the demand by the Clean Ocean Foundation for a commitment to "close ocean outfalls" within 10 years.

The idea that there is a single water cycle in the real world of the biosphere is a compelling intellectual reason for bringing the two water campaigns and water constituencies together and provides an impulse to coordinate with each other in shaping policy change. In particular, the community campaign may have some lessons for the elite science campaign on how to affect public policy.

When faced by seemingly transfixed water authorities, the Clean Ocean Foundation responded by instead lobbying the political authorities that could direct the water agencies. The Foundation used a mixture of traditional and highly innovative strategies to put the issue on the agenda. It worked on a marginal seat strategy in state and federal elections to mobilise support in both major political parties, while making sure the Greens and environmental parties were on message, as some of these groups had been slow to prioritise the issue. It linked local community events to the campaign and enlisted support of wine growers, vegetable growers, singers, and advertisers. It secured *pro bono* support from major advertising and billboard companies and featured a dramatic giant billboard with 'floating Nemo' above Melbourne's major southbound highway, in which a clown fish of uncanny likeness to a Disney creation was depicted floating in polluted water. It ran an information rich website and regular enews. It conducted public education campaigns through the purchase of a police "booze bus" converted into an "ooze bus", full of interactive displays on the reality and risks of outfalls. When running low on funds it asked twelve significant Australian artists to contribute to a fundraiser by painting on surfboards, and ran a highly successful auction at Christies, with commission waived.

As a result of its campaigning the Clean Ocean Foundation has achieved major successes with impacts at both the Victorian state and federal level of politics and policy making. The State opposition party (Liberal) accepted the Foundation's policies in full and the State government (Labor) has committed to a multimillion dollar water recycling feasibility study in response to the campaign [12]. The federal opposition (Labor) and the federal Greens have adopted key policy recommendations, and the Howard Governments $2 billion Water Trust announced during the 2004 election campaign, included a particular focus on water infrastructure and recycling which the Foundation had influenced, in part through the local federal MP who had become an active member of the Foundation [13].

By contrast, the Wentworth Group of scientists, named inauspiciously after the hotel they met in rather than the vision they pursued, has sought to capture the heights of scientific consensus and operate on policy through the strength of rational argument. Their *Blueprint for a National Water Plan* was received by the Premiers and the Prime Minister at an inter-governmental meeting. But the policy proposals it has put forward require wider constituencies to secure the government funding commitments that are identified as necessary, and it is not clear how they will build these constituencies. It appears that the reform process they have sought to initiate has yet to gather momentum. Perhaps the report which gives community forces a role in the implementation of the plans and in ensuring 'fairness' will need to involve those groups in ensuring, first, the acceptance of the plan. This would require that such groups 'own' the plan, and to be assured that the water rights system is the means to achieve the objective.

The Wentworth Group of Concerned Scientists included a single paragraph on recycling waste water in its otherwise extensive report, merely to note some of the targets that have been set by some urban centres. That they touched base with the issue can be seen as conceptually inclusive, but for a group who see themselves advocating "radical and fundamental reform", it is a very light touch in an area where the Group could be setting targets and estimating potential impacts.

The Clean Ocean Foundation established the community-based campaign to close ocean outfalls <u>and</u> invest in hi-tech recycling of all waste water to a standard, suitable for a large variety of agricultural and industrial uses, without health risks to workers, consumers or the public at large. It has sought commitments from political parties to achieve this over a 10 year period, confident that water which is clearly safe for many specific uses can be secured by detailed investigation of water hazards and strong investments in best practice technologies to deal with particular risks. Here the scientific community will need to be fully engaged. At the same time, management of inputs into the system would be directly addressed and alternative waste processes developed for industry, rather than ongoing licenses to use the system never build for such purposes.

Such an investment in recycling is an investment in the essential infrastructure of the society, as essential today as the sewerage system was to the city 100 years ago – and is no more than the unfinished business of the construction of that system. Such investments need to be undertaken by governments as part of their responsibility to the community and cannot be expected to be profit making in the strict commercial sense. But they will create a saleable water output given the water market that is increasingly coming into effect, and this will produce some financial return (and of course user-pays taxes for water treatment is already part of the property tax mix). Public infrastructure investments, which would be well supported by urban populations, can ease the pressure on river systems and assist the affordability of water to farmers, and to environmental buy-backs schemes alike. It is a major contribution towards solving two environmental health risk problems simultaneously.

References

[1]   www.cleanocean.org.
[2]   Treatment Plants: Case Study, www.cleanocean.org/index_general. asp?menuid=040.060.040.
[3]   Guidelines for environmental management: Uses of reclaimed water, EPA Victoria,
       http://epanote2.epa.vic.gov.au/EPA/Publications.nsf/d85500a0d7f5f07b4a 2565d1002268f3/64c2a15969d75e184a2569a00025de63/$FILE/464.2.pdf
[4]   Kevekordes, K. & Clayton, M.N., Development of Hormosira Banksii (Phaeophyceae) embryos in selected components of secondarily-treated sewage effluent. Journal of Phycology, 36(1), pp. 25 -33.
[5]   www.uoe.edu.au/eng/cem/research/ozaquarec.html.

[6]   Jordan, A. & Greenaway, J., Shifting agendas, changing regulatory structures and the 'new' politics of environmental pollution: British coastal water policy 1955-1995. Public Administration, 76(4), pp. 669-685, 1998.

[7]   Australian Dryland Salinity Assessment 2000, National Land and Water Resources Audit,
http://audit.ea.gov.au/ANRA/land/docs/national/Salinity_Contents.html.

[8]   The Wentworth Group of Concerned Scientists, Blueprint for a National Water Plan, WWF, Sydney, 2003.

[9]   Quiggin, J., Let's clear muddy waters, Australian Financial Review, 22 October 2003.

[10]   Quiggin, J., Risk and water management in the Murray-Darling Basin, Murray Darling Program Working Paper: M05#$4, Risk and Sustainable Management Group, University of Queensland.

[11]   Gleeson, T., Have the environmental scientists got it right this time? On line opinion, www.onlineopinion.com.au/view.asp?article=1182.

[12]   Our Water Our Future: Securing Our Water Future Together, Department of Sustainability and Environment, Victoria, Australia,
http://www.dse.vic.gov.au/dse/nrenlwm.nsf/LinkView/BF55F9AC10B38 71FCA256EA200255F883018EEC1F535E3A84A2567D7000B1794.

[13]   Koutsoukis, J., Gunnamatta priority in push to end ocean outfalls, The Age, August 13, 2004,
www.theage.com.au/articles/2004/08/12/1092102596047.html.

The role of urban lake sediments as historical archives of industrial pollution and health linkages: an example from Daresbury pond, north Cheshire, UK

A. L. Power[1], A. T. Worsley[1], C. A. Booth[2], N. Richardson[1] & A. Bedford[1]
[1]Natural, Geographical & Applied Sciences,
Edge Hill University College, UK
[2]Environmental and Analytical Science Division,
Research Institute in Advanced Technologies (RIATec),
University of Wolverhampton, UK

Abstract

Research in Halton, northwest England, recognises the health effects of environmental pollution due to the extensive amount of industrialisation the area has experienced since the industrial revolution. The chemical industry still dominates this region, and concerns have arisen over potential links between industrial pollution and high morbidity and mortality in Halton. Recent commissioned work suggests that unhealthy life style and material deprivation are factors affecting health. However due to insufficient data a direct comparison has not been made between temporal pollution patterns and health records to assess impacts of pollution on health. A methodology using characteristics of lake sediments has provided proxy records of atmospheric pollution variations dating from pre-industrial times to present day. Preliminary mineral magnetic results are presented demonstrating the pollution profile of the area, giving a detailed record of changing atmospheric pollution since the lake was formed. In the future this can be compared to health records to identify possible relationships between pollution trends and disease patterns.
Keywords: atmospheric pollution, public health, palaeolimnology, Halton Borough Council.

1   Introduction

Effects of environmental pollution on human health are an increasing concern to local, regional, national and international communities [1]. The sources of pollution are many. However, it is those areas where large-scale industrial activity occurs, especially chemical industries, which are commonly attributed to air, land and water contamination and, as a consequence, are frequently associated with public health issues [1].

The Halton area of north Cheshire (UK), which encompasses the towns of both Runcorn and Widnes, has been an industrial heartland for the national chemical industry for many years (mid 1700s) [2], (Figure 1). As a consequence, contemporary and temporal pollution of the Halton environment, and its associated health implications for local communities, are concerns that have prompted Halton Primary Care Trust (part of the National Health Service) to commission a cross-disciplinary (medical and environmental scientists) research investigation into linkages between the environment and notably high rates of mortality and morbidity in the local area.

This work presents the first analytical results collated from the interrogation of lake sediment stratigraphies retrieved from Daresbury Pond (an urban lake), north Cheshire, UK, establishing them as archives of temporal pollution. The project aims to ascertain if mineral magnetic methodologies can be employed to distinguish local/regional environmental pollution episodes and therefore, ultimately assist examination of linkages between human health histories and those of local/regional pollution.

2   The Halton area

2.1 Industry in Halton

Extensive industries were initiated in Runcorn during the mid 1700s, which included stone, shipping, brewery, skin-yards and quarries [3]. Due to its location, docking facilities on the Mersey Estuary and general improvements in transport facilities (particularly the construction of the Transporter Bridge and Manchester Ship Canal), the area quickly became a haven for chemical industries. By 1855 Runcorn had the reputation of a one-industry town due to a boom in chemical trade [2]. This meant, chemical industries continued to dominate the local area (both Runcorn and Widnes). Unfortunately, the various manufacturing processes emitted malodorous chemicals, gases and black smoke from chimneys of inadequate heights, which began to heavily pollute the area [4]. As a consequence, in 1888, Runcorn was described as the "dirtiest, ugliest and most depressing town in England" [3].

The environmental implications of extensive air pollution, land contamination, chemical waste, drainage problems and the death of vegetation; led to health concerns about premature mortality and ill health of chemical workers, plus health complaints from communities residing to near chemical works [5]. As a consequence, to reduce pollution levels in Runcorn, Alkali Acts were established in 1863. These introduced stringent standards for working conditions in chemical plants and control of by-products produced from chemical processes [2].

Types of industry widened within the area in 1964, when Runcorn was designated as a 'New Town' [3]. However, despite development and reconstruction, Runcorn remains a predominately chemical-based industrialised town. Nowadays, pollution levels are considerably less than in the historical past [7]. In the main, this is due to the introduction of air quality standards [6]. However, that said, a wide range of chemical processes still occur around Runcorn and heavy pollution loads are experienced [8]. For instance, in 2003, over 50 industrial businesses were operating at circa 15 sites in Widnes and Runcorn [7].

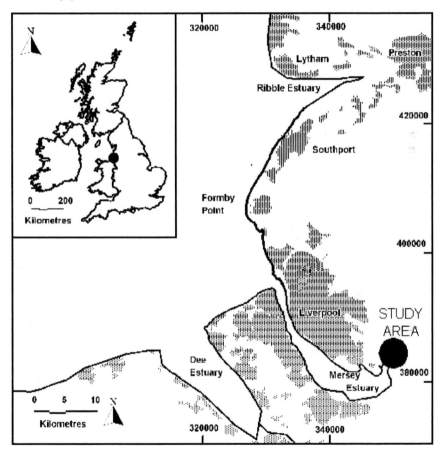

Figure 1:   Location map of the Halton study area, northwest U.K.

2.2 Media attention

In 1999, the national media brought attention to the discovery that a quarry at Weston Point, Halton, formerly used for chemical waste disposal until 1972, contained the toxic gas HCBD (hexachlorobutadiene), and was now contaminating nearby homes [9]. Local public concerns arose over the potentially serious health implications of this incident. Given the substantive industrial history of Runcorn and consequential contamination, this has affected public health perceptions, with many neighbouring communities questioning the effects of environmental pollution on their own health [8]. To address these matters, the Halton Prime Care Trust has recognised the importance of understanding local and regional linkages between environmental pollution and human health, and instigated this research.

3   Health in Halton

Halton experiences higher cases of mortality and morbidity than similar areas [8]. Compared to Standard Mortality Ratios (SMRs) for the rest of England, Halton demonstrates higher SMRs from all causes, all cancers, lung cancer and coronary heart disease (Table 1). This illustrates the importance and urgency for investigating attributable health factors in Halton.

Table 1:   Health in Halton indicator table using SMRs for all age ranges (1998 to 2000). Data adapted [8].

Health problem	England	North West	Halton
All causes	100	115.20	**120.02**
Asthma	100	100.04	91.60
All cancers	100	109.42	**127.90**
Lung cancer	100	124.17	**159.60**
Bronchitis & Emphysema	99	94.78	**95.14**
Coronary Heart Disease	99	115.65	**133.26**
All circulatory diseases	100	113.69	113.35

4   Urban lake sediments as proxy historical pollution indicators

Amongst other sources, lakes receive atmospheric particulate pollution from industrial and vehicular emissions. Over time the process of lacustrine sedimentation, may allow the development of a pollution record within the sediments [10]. Consequently, urban lakes are unique pollution sinks for measuring, monitoring and modelling industrial environmental contamination [11, 12]. In that sense, urban lake sediment magneto-chemical stratigraphies have been successfully used as proxy indicators of high-resolution atmospheric pollution records in the north Cheshire area (unpublished), for circa 250 year profiles [12].

5   Case study of Daresbury Delph Pond

5.1 Field methodology

Daresbury Delph pond (SJ 574 819), immediately east of Runcorn, is situated near to an urbanised area, adjacent to a busy dual carriage way (4 lane traffic) and a motorway (6 lane traffic). As such, with consideration of prevailing winds (westward) and its urbanised setting, the lake was selected as a site appropriate for holding a long-term pollution record, due to its appropriate location, small size and minimal management history (minimal sediment disturbance). With aid of a small boat, a sediment core (52 cm length, 6 cm diameter) sample was retrieved from the deepest and central part of the lake using a Gilsen corer (plate 1).

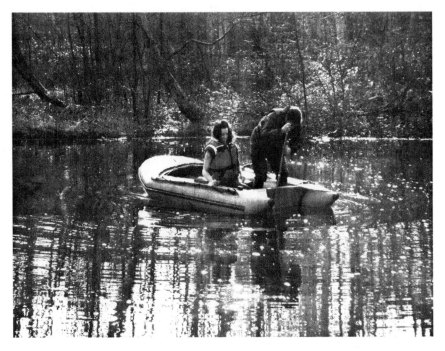

Plate 1: Sediment corer being forcefully inserted into soft muddy sediment, deposited on the lake bottom, before its removal under vacuum conditions from Daresbury Delph Pond.

5.2 Laboratory methodology

Sediment was extruded from the core at 5 mm intervals to provide a high-resolution stratigraphic sequence. After drying at 35°C, samples were prepared for mineral magnetic analyses [13]. Initial, low-field, mass-specific, magnetic susceptibility (χ_{LF}) was measured using a Bartington (Oxford, England) MS2 susceptibility meter. Anhysteretic Remanence Magnetisation (ARM) was induced with a peak alternating field of 100 mT and small steady biasing field of 0.04 mT using a Molspin (Newcastle-upon-Tyne, England) A.F. demagnetizer. The resultant remanence created within the samples was measured using a Molspin 1A magnetometer. The samples were then exposed to a series of 'forward' and 'reverse' field sizes up to a maximum 'saturation' field of 800 mT

(SIRM), and the isothermal remanent magnetisation (IRM) measured on the magnetometer. Table 2 summarises the parameters presented in this work.

Table 2:   Mineral magnetic parameters and their interpretations [13–16].

Magnetic Parameters	Interpretations
χ_{LF}	Mass specific low frequency magnetic susceptibility: this is measured within a small magnetic field and is reversible (no remanence is induced). Its value is roughly proportional to the concentration of ferrimagnetic minerals within the sample, although in materials with little or no ferrimagnetic component and a relatively large antiferromagnetic component, the latter may dominate the signal.
ARM	Mass specific anhysteretic remanent magnetisation: for this work ARM was induced in the samples by combining a peak AF field of 100 mT with a DC biasing field of 0.04 mT. It is particularly sensitive to the concentration of magnetic grains of stable single domain size, e.g. ~0.03-0.06 µm.
SIRM	Mass specific saturated isothermal remanent magnetisation: this is the highest amount of magnetic remanence that can be produced in a sample by applying a large magnetic field. It is measured on a mass specific basis. In this study a saturating field of 0.8 T has been used and will produce saturation in most mineral types. However, some antiferromagnetic minerals may not be saturated in this field (e.g. goethite) and therefore this parameter is often called IRM_{800mT}. The value of SIRM is related to concentrations of all remanence-carrying minerals in the sample, but is also dependent upon the assemblage of mineral types and their magnetic grain size.

5.3 Results and discussion

Magnetic profiles, for the Daresbury Delph Pond core, display notable downcore changes in the magneto-sediment characteristics (Figure 2). For instance, the lowest section of each profile (23 - 52 cm) shows notably lower values than the upper section. That said, there are both differences and similarities between the upper sections of the profiles. The χ_{LF} and SIRM profiles are similar, with peaks at (2 cm and 8.5 cm), whereas ARM is different to both of the other profiles, with a single peak (2 cm). It is proposed that these observations indicate a pre-industrial background period of minimal or natural pollution in the lower corer. In contrast, the upper core observations indicate an industrial period, where pollution increases above background levels to a peak industrial time of maximum pollution. However, if this is the case, the upper core contains two pollution episodes because the χ_{LF} and SIRM profiles show two peaks. Whereas, the ARM profile shows only the upper of the two peaks. Since ARM measurements reveal the presence of ultrafine ferrimagnetic grains, this indicates that the proposed upper pollution episode contains a magnetic fingerprint, which is different to the lower pollution episode. Therefore, these preliminary measurements already suggest that, historically, there have been two different pollution sources, which have been dominant at different times.

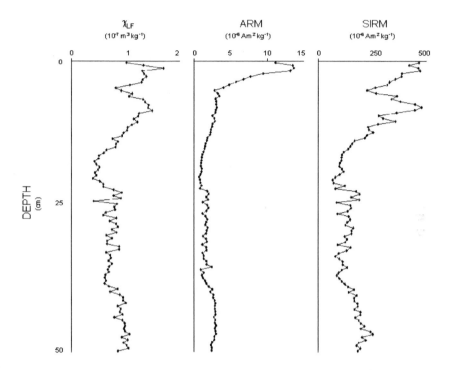

Figure 2:   Magnetic profile data for Daresbury Delph Pond.

It is noteworthy to mention that similar pollution profiles have been identified in south Merseyside [12], suggesting that both urban lakes retain a regional pollution signal. If the stratigraphy dates for the south Merseyside work (unpublished ^{210}Pb) are similar to this case study, then the lower pollution episode occurred at circa. 1850, a time of boom industrial activity in the Halton area. The decline in values, recorded above this point in the core, is probably attributable to the reduction in pollution concentrations after the introduction of the Alkaline Acts (1863), which encouraged safer and less wasteful techniques to be introduced by the chemical industry. With this timeframe in mind, it is probable that the upper peak is attributable to the introduction and increased use of modern road vehicles, especially as the site is adjacent to two major regional transport networks. However, these interpretations require further analytical testing [17].

6 Ongoing and proposed future work

By combining these preliminary magnetic results with further analyses (i.e. laser-diffraction, x-ray fluorescence and spheroidal carbonaceous particle counts, together with radiometric dating), a more detailed record of atmospheric pollution change over the past *ca.* 250 years will be achievable. Subsequently, pollution profiles will be compared with archive health records. This will be accomplished in tandem with consultants from the Halton Public Health team and hopefully will reveal some interesting correlations between pollution episodes and disease patterns.

7 Conclusions

In an area dominated by the chemical industry for more than 150 years the Halton Health Project [8] has highlighted the need for a consideration of the historical impact of atmospheric pollution on local populations. While there is much work currently being done on the contemporary monitoring of atmospheric pollution (in particular with regards to disease patterns) and significant research into the health and social histories, there is no research focussing upon its temporal nature. If we are to gain a clearer understanding of the relationship between human health and atmospheric pollution the temporal dimension must be considered. This research, coupled with the work in South Merseyside [12], establishes an important initial, sedimentary record of atmospheric pollution that can be used as the basis for further work and demonstrates clearly, the importance of small, anthropogenic, urban lakes to the local community as well as to research in environmental science. The work therefore has begun to fulfil the need highlighted by public health organisations [8] by producing the first coherent archive of historical atmospheric pollution for Halton itself.

Acknowledgements

All authors gratefully thank Dr Julia Miller (formerly of Halton Primary Care Trust) for her foresight to fund this research and Dr Charlie Orton for her ongoing assistance. Thanks are also extended to Mr Paul Oldfield of Halton Borough Council for his assistance in obtaining permission to use Daresbury Pond for this investigation and Mr Bill Hardman who granted authorisation. Finally, ALP acknowledges the receipt of a research bursary paid by Halton Primary Care Trust and also the receipt of PhD studentship fees paid by Edge Hill University College.

References

[1]   McCally, M., Life support: the Environment and Human Health. MIT press, Cambridge, 2002.

[2]   Warren, K., Chemical Foundations: The Alkali Industry in Britain to 1926. Clarendon Press, Oxford, 1980.

[3]   Jones, A.D., Industry & Runcorn 1750 to 1960. Publicity & Information services Department, Halton Borough Council, January 1969.

[4]   Allen, J.F., Journal of the Society of Chemical Industry. 29th June 1881.

[5]   Royal Commission on Noxious Vapours, Report of the Royal Commission on Noxious Vapours, 1878.

[6]   Chester City Council, A Review of Pollution 1986 to 1990. The Cheshire District Councils, pp. 68-82, 1991.

[7]   Environment Agency, Pollution Inventory <http://www.environment-agency.gov.uk> accessed on 17/05/2005.

[8]   Department of Geography and Institute for Health Research Lancaster University, Understanding the factors affecting health in Halton: Final Report. 2003.

[9]   Vidal, J., Toxic Shock, The Guardian - Newspaper, 11th February 2000.

[10]   Foster, I.D.L, & Charlesworth, S.M., Heavy metals in the hydrological cycle: trends and explanations. Hydrological Processes, 10, pp. 227-261, 1995.

[11]   Charlesworth, S.M., & Lees, J.A., The use of mineral magnetic measurements in polluted urban lakes and deposited dusts, Coventry, UK. Phys. Chem. Earth., 22, pp. 203-206, 1997.

[12]   Worsley, A.T., Booth, C.A., Power, A.L., Appleby, P.G. & Wright, E.J., Atmospheric pollution and health: the significance of datable archives from a small, urban lake in Merseyside, UK. (Published in this volume), 2005.

[13]   Walden, J., Oldfield, F., & Smith, J.P., Environmental Magnetism: A Practical Guide, Technical Guide No. 6, Quaternary Research Association, Cambridge, England, pp 243, 1999.

[14]   King, J., Banerjee, S.K., Marvin, J. & Ozdemir, O., A comparison of different magnetic methods for determining the relative grain size of magnetite in natural materials: some results from lake sediments. Earth & Planetary Science Letters, 59, pp. 404-419, 1982.

[15]   Maher, B.A., Magnetic properties of some synthetic sub-micron magnetites. Geophysical Journal, 94, pp. 83-96, 1988.

[16]   Yu, L. & Oldfield, F., A multivariate mixing model for identifying sediment sources from magnetic measurements. Quaternary Research, 32, pp. 168-181, 1989.

[17]   Shilton, V.F., Booth, C.A., Smith, J.P., Giess, P., Mitchell, D.J. & Williams, C.D., Magnetic properties of urban street dusts and their relationship with organic matter content in the West Midlands, UK. Atmospheric Environment, (in press), 2005.

Residual radioactivity from the treatment of water for urban domestic applications

R. Kleinschmidt
Queensland Health Scientific Services, Queensland Department of Health, Brisbane. Australia

Abstract

An assessment of radiologically enhanced residual materials generated during treatment of domestic water supplies in southeast Queensland, Australia was conducted. Radioactivity concentrations of ^{3}H, ^{210}Po, ^{222}Rn, $^{226/228}$Ra, uranium and thorium in water sourced from both surface water catchments and ground water resources were examined both pre- and post-treatment under typical water treatment plant operations. Surface water treatment processes included sedimentation, coagulation, flocculation and filtration, while the groundwater was treated using cation exchange resins. Waste products generated during treatment included sediments, filtration media, used ion exchange resin, backwash and wastewaters. Elevated residual concentrations of radionuclides were identified in these waste products. The waste product activity concentrations were used to model the radiological impact of the materials when either utilised for beneficial purposes, or upon disposal. The results indicate that, under current water resource exploitation programs, reuse or disposal of the treatment wastes do not pose a significant radiological risk, however, regulatory disposal limits may be exceeded for disposable carbon filters from household point-of-use treatment systems. The impact of population growth and changes in water supply sources are also considered.
Keywords: water treatment, radioactivity, TENORM, waste.

1   Introduction

As the population of southeast Queensland, Australia, continues to increase, the need for adequate water resources will continue to expand. Alternative supplies will be required to meet the demands for water as traditional sources become stressed, and technology based intervention and treatment will become more common as poorer quality alternative water supplies are exploited.

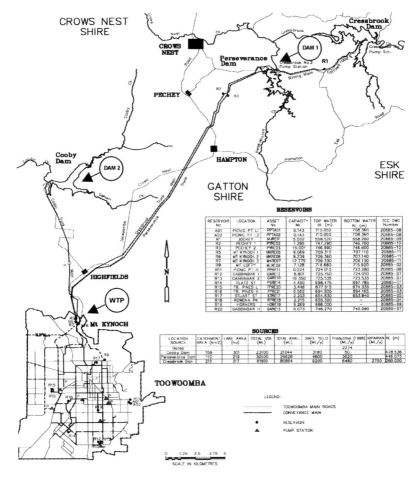

Figure 1: Toowoomba surface water supply and water treatment plant locations.

While radiological water quality is addressed at considerable length by local guideline documents (drinking water – NHMRC/ARMCANZ [1]; Irrigation, recreational and stock watering – ANZECC/ARMCANZ [2]) and globally (WHO [3], USEPA [4], EU [5] and Kocher [6]), the impact of contaminants, either naturally occurring or artificially introduced, removed from water upon treatment, and discharge of waste waters that may have become radiologically contaminated, is limited. The subject of generation of Technologically Enhanced Naturally Occurring Radioactive Materials (TENORM) during water resource exploitation is a current topic both locally (Cooper [7], RHSAC [8]) and internationally (IAEA [9]). Cooper [7] concedes that local information is extremely limited and recommends an investment in defining the magnitude of TENORM generation.

This study was based on the small city of Toowoomba, with a population of approximately 117000 people. Toowoomba is situated about 130 km west of Brisbane, the capital of Queensland, and is situated on the eastern rim of the Australian Great Dividing Range. Toowoomba was chosen for the study as it is typical of small cities in the region, undergoing continued growth (1.4% per annum, QDLGPSR [10]) and drawing its water supply from a combination of both surface and groundwater, specifically three surface water catchment and storage dams, and thirteen groundwater bores (Figure 1). Table 1 provides data relevant to the study. Current water consumption is approximately 14500 ML per annum, with 89% provided from the storage dams and the remaining 11% from bores (QHSS [11]).

The surface water treatment plant (WTP) consists of a series of stages including flocculation (aluminium sulphate and polydadmac), settling, filtration and post filtration chemical dosing. Supernatant from the settling tanks is recycled to the head of the plant for reprocessing. The filtration system consists of a bed of anthracite filter coal over graded sand and fine gravel. Backwash from the filter beds is recycled to the head of the plant for reprocessing. Dried sludge generated from the plant is stockpiled on site and removed for beneficial land-use applications, including use as a soil conditioner.

The groundwater bores are located throughout the city and tap into a number of disjointed aquifers. Only 2 bores were in use at the time of this study. In both cases the groundwater is passed through a cation exchange resin prior to injection into the city water distribution system. Wastes generated by the system include old exchange resin and regeneration backwash. Disposal of the expired resin is achieved by controlled landfill while the regeneration backwash fluids are discharged to the sewer.

There are no local nuclear industries other than limited unsealed medical and sealed industrial sources and it is assumed that naturally occurring radionuclides are the predominant species.

Table 1: Water statistics and treatment data for this assessment.

Description		REF
Total water supplied – 2004	14587 ML/year	QDNRM [12]
Total connections	44878	QDNRM [12]
Total litres/connection/day	936 L/day	QDNRM [12]
Total litres/drinking-cooking-washing up/day	100 L/day	Lawson [13]
Number of Dams	3	QDNRM [12]
Number Bores (in use)	13 (2)	QDNRM [12]
Solid waste – WTP	290 tonne/year	QHSS [11]
Solid waste – bores	12.8 tonne/year	QHSS [11]
Liquid waste - bores (1300 L/regen x 300/year)	390000 L/year	QHSS [11]
Number of POUs in use (15% of connections)	6700	Lawson [13]

2 Experimental/materials and methods

2.1 Sampling

Water samples were collected in 10 L acid washed polyethylene bottles for ^{3}H, ^{210}Po, ^{226}Ra, uranium and thorium radionuclide assay methods. Samples were acid preserved in the laboratory after filtration and sub-sampling.

Samples for dissolved ^{222}Rn analysis were collected in either 20 mL glass scintillation vials (groundwater) or 1 litre acid washed glass Erlenmeyer flasks (surface water). Environmental samples were collected by gently submerging the 1 L flask beneath the water surface to the desired sampling depth. The cap was removed and the flask filled to capacity, the cap being replaced while still submerged to eliminate any headspace. Sampling of water from distribution systems was conducted using a plastic hose immersed in the flask and adjusting the flow rate until a constant, turbulence-free flow of water was established. This flow of water was maintained until the sample bottle overflowed and at least 3 volumes of water had washed through the system. The hose was gently removed and the vial capped ensuring elimination of headspace. Samples were then chilled on ice and returned to the laboratory for analysis as soon as possible.

Sediment, sludge, ion exchange resin and filter bed samples were collected in either 1 L detergent washed glass bottles or clean plastic bags.

2.2 Methods

2.2.1 Water

2.2.1.1 Tritium (^{3}H) Tritium in water measurement was conducted using a method described in ISO 9698 [14]). Samples were counted on a Packard 3170 TR/SL liquid scintillation analyser (LSA). A minimum detection level of 1.5 Bq.L^{-1} was obtained for the method using a 400 min count time.

2.2.1.2 Radon (^{222}Rn) Two methods were used for ^{222}Rn analysis depending on the required minimum detection level. Direct counting was conducted on 15 mL aliquots of water after addition of 5 mL of a mineral oil based scintillation cocktail.

The ^{222}Rn samples collected in 1 L Erlenmeyer flasks were opened and 20 mL of water removed and discarded. The void was replaced with 15 mL of mineral oil scintillator and the flask recapped. The flask was then vigorously shaken for 15 minutes to allow for the preferential transfer of dissolved radon into the scintillation cocktail. After separation of the aqueous phase (24 hours), the scintillator was extracted for counting. All samples were sealed and allowed to sit for a minimum of 3 hours to allow in-growth of decay progeny.

Counting of samples from either method was conducted using the LSA. Respective minimum detection levels of 80 mBq.L^{-1} and 12 mBq.L^{-1} were obtained using these methods for a count time of 250 minutes.

2.2.1.3 Radium (^{226}Ra) The ^{222}Rn emanation method was used for ^{226}Ra determinations. Samples were prepared by pre-concentrating 1000 mL of water sample to 15 mL by evaporation. The concentrated samples were transferred to Teflon coated poly vials and 5 mL of mineral oil scintillator added to trap the radon gas. The vials were capped and stored for a minimum of 15 days to allow ingrowth of ^{222}Ra. Analysis was conducted as for the ^{222}Rn method. A minimum detection level of 1.4 mBq.L^{-1} was obtained using this method for a 180 minute counting period.

2.2.1.4 Polonium (^{210}Po) ^{210}Po was determined using a method published by EML [15]. Water samples of 1000 mL were pre-concentrated by evaporation to a volume of 200 mL before ^{210}Po deposition on 20 mm diameter nickel foil discs. The foils were transferred to a 20 mL polyethylene scintillation vial, cocktail added and then counted with the LSA. Extraction and alpha counting efficiency were observed to be greater than 60% for the method with a minimum detection level of 8 mBq.L^{-1} for a counting time of 180 minutes.

2.2.1.5 Uranium Uranium analysis was conducted using direct measurement of ^{238}U by ICPMS (Agilent 7500 ICPMS Chem Station) using in-house methods (QHSS [16]).

2.2.1.6 Thorium Thorium was determined as ^{232}Th by ICPMS simultaneously with ^{238}U analysis.

2.2.2 Waste solids

Radioactivity concentrations in solid wastes were determined using high resolution gamma-ray spectrometry (EG&G Gamma-X, ~40% rel. eff. + EG&G Dspec Plus spectrometer). The spectrometer was calibrated using IAEA RGU-1 reference material in a standard geometry. Samples were dried to constant mass and sealed in 100 mL polyethylene jars for a minimum of 20 days (to allow ^{238}U series decay progeny to reach secular equilibrium) before counting. Typical counting times were 100000 seconds.

2.3 Models

Two models were used to determine the impact of residual radioactivity associated with water treatment. The models used were RESRAD (ANL [17]) and CARBDOSE (USEPA [18]). RESRAD was used to model the potential radiological dose associated with the beneficial land application of solid wastes derived from the water treatment plant (WTP), and with landfill of spent ion exchange resins from the groundwater treatment plants (GWTP).

The CARBDOSE model was used to estimate the residual activity present on granulated activated carbon point-of-use (POU) filters.

3 Results and discussion

Table 2 provides a summary of results for water sampled at the WTP and GWTPs, while Table 3 provides solid waste radioactivity concentrations.

Table 2:   Radioactivity concentrations in water samples.

Sample	Bq.L^{-1}		mBq.L^{-1} (2σ uncertainty)			
	^{3}H	^{222}Rn	^{226}Ra	^{210}Po	^{238}U	^{232}Th
Dam 1 (Persev)	1.1 (1.3)	0.02 (0.01)	1.6 (1.1)	11.5 (5.7)	0.78 (0.06)	< 0.04
Dam 2 (Cooby)	1.5 (1.3)	0.15 (0.07)	10 (2)	6.5 (5.2)	2.93 (0.23)	< 0.04
WTP – Raw	0.1 (1.3)	0.08 (0.02)	2.0 (1.2)	6.7 (5.3)	1.23 (0.10)	< 0.04
WTP – Supernatant	-	-	1.1 (1.0)	4.7 (5.0)	1.87 (0.15)	< 0.04
WTP – Treated	0.2 (1.3)	0.03 (0.02)	0.5 (1.0)	9.3 (4.9)	1.77 (0.14)	< 0.04
Bore 1 – Raw	0.6 (1.3)	13.0 (0.7)	1.5 (1.1)	253 (13)	0.15 (0.01)	< 0.04
Bore 1 – Treated	0.3 (1.3)	10.6 (0.6)	1.0 (1.0)	24 (7)	0.15 (0.01)	< 0.04
Bore 2 – Raw	0.2 (1.3)	17.2 (0.9)	0.1 (0.9)	52 (9)	0.77 (0.06)	< 0.04
Bore 2 – Treated	1.0 (1.3)	14.6 (0.8)	2.7 (1.3)	2.1 (4.9)	0.78 (0.06)	< 0.04
Bore 2 – Regen	1.3 (1.3)	4.2 (0.5)	21 (10)	3.8 (4.9)	3.18 (0.25)	< 0.04
Consumer Pt 1	-0.7 (1.2)	0.03 (0.02)	3.0 (1.3)	9.0 (5.5)	1.07 (0.08)	< 0.04
Consumer Pt 2	-	8.9 (1.0)	-	-	1.25 (0.10)	< 0.04
Consumer Pt 3	-	0.21 (0.08)	-	-	0.70 (0.06)	< 0.04

Table 3:   Radioactivity concentrations in solid waste material.

Sample	Bq.kg^{-1} - dry weight (2σ uncertainty)					
	^{238}U	^{226}Ra	^{210}Pb	^{228}Ra	^{40}K	^{7}Be
WTP sludge < 30 d	140 (50)	37 (6)	89 (32)	46 (5)	110 (30)	170 (35)
WTP sludge > 60 d	134 (33)	39 (3)	77 (15)	50 (5)	85 (14)	20 (6)
WTP f/coal – New	63 (15)	13 (3)	12 (10)	16 (4)	60 (20)	< 11
WTP f/coal – Used	31 (12)	16 (2)	15 (8)	12 (2)	< 18	< 7
Bore 1 resin – New	< 11	< 2	< 12	< 4	< 21	< 8
Bore 1 resin – Used	< 16	6 (4)	113 (16)	< 8	57 (27)	< 14

3.1   Surface water treatment plant

It was observed that the ^{238}U concentration in treated water was higher than the raw water entering the treatment plant. Subsequent investigation established that a proportion of the excess ^{238}U present within the system is associated with leaching of uranium from the anthracite filter coal utilised in the plant and recycling of supernatant from the sludge settling tanks.   Activity-balance calculations for ^{210}Po, ^{226}Ra and ^{238}U accounted for ^{210}Po to within 5% and ^{238}U to within 20%, however, it was observed that there is retention of ^{226}Ra in the system with 85% being held back in the WTP.

3.1.1   Sludge
The RESRAD model was used to calculate the additional radiation dose to a critical group (small crop farmer) associated with the beneficial use of the sludge

produced from the WTP. Radionuclide concentrations used in the model are based on the residual activities derived from the *>60 day old sludge* (Table 3). Results are calculated assuming that the total annual inventory of 290000 kg of sludge is applied in a 50 mm layer to the surface of a 4000 m^2 field. Table 4 shows the calculated results. A maximum dose of 78 µSv.y^{-1} was calculated for a time period of less than 1 year, decreasing to ~30 µSv.y^{-1} after 10 years and 0 µSv.y^{-1} at 100 years.

Table 4:   RESRAD dose results for beneficial reuse of sludge.

Contribution from:	Effective Dose (µSv.y^{-1})	% of total dose
Ground	40.3	52
Inhalation (excluding radon)	0.7	1
Radon	20.7	26
Ingestion (soil)	1.7	2
Remainder (plant/meat/milk)	14.5	19
TOTAL	*77.9*	*100*

3.2   Groundwater treatment plants

3.2.1   Ion exchange resin

The cation exchange resin used in the two operational bores is not changed regularly, and may be used for up to 10 years. The waste resin (~6500kg/bore) is buried in a controlled landfill with a minimum cover of 1000 mm of clean fill. The RESRAD model was used to calculate radiation dose to a landfill operator critical group. It is assumed that the controlled landfill site has been designed to minimise contamination of local surface and groundwater. Table 5 shows the calculated results. A maximum dose of 4.4 µSv.y^{-1} was calculated for a time period of less than 1 year, decreasing to 2.8 µSv.y^{-1} at 100 years. The total contribution arises from ^{222}Rn emanation.

Table 5:   RESRAD dose results for controlled landfill of spent resin.

Contribution from:	Effective Dose (µSv.y^{-1})	% of total dose
Radon	4.4	100
Remainder (ground/inhalation/plant etc.)	0	0
TOTAL	*4.4*	*100*

3.2.2   Resin regeneration

Regeneration is conducted on the bore 2 GWTP on a daily basis determined by water flow & volume. The regeneration waste (390000 L/year) is directly discharged to the domestic wastewater system. For the radionuclides examined, the most restrictive sewer disposal criterion is for ^{210}Po at 2.04 kBq.m^{-3} (OQPC [19]). Results in Table 2 indicate that in all cases the activity concentrations for ^{210}Po are significantly less than the specified release criteria.

3.3 Point-of-use granulated activated carbon filters

Granulated activated carbon filters (GAC) in POU units are known to effectively remove ^{222}Rn and are installed in up to 15% of households (Lawson [13]). The units are fitted as under-sink units and treat water used for drinking, cooking and washing up, typically treating 100 L of water per day. Toowoomba groundwater contains ^{222}Rn concentrations up to 15 Bq.L^{-1} at the pump stations and 9 Bq.L^{-1} at consumer points throughout the city (Table 2). CARBDOSE was used to model ^{222}Rn activities present on GAC filters for radon activity concentrations of a maximum of 10 Bq.L^{-1} and a mean of 3 Bq.L^{-1} at 95% removal efficiency and 100 L per day (Table 1).

Table 6:   CARBDOSE results for activity retained on GAC filters.

Supply ^{222}Rn Concentration (Bq.L^{-1})	222Rn activity on filter @ 100 days (kBq)	Progeny activity concentration on filter @ 100 years (kBq.kg^{-1})
3	15.7	1.8
10	52.4	49.9

Landfill disposal criteria for ^{210}Pb + decay progeny is 5 kBq.kg^{-1} (OQPC [19]). The data in Table 6 indicates that the disposal criterion is exceeded for situations where expired GAC filter cartridges are placed in municipal landfills after use in filtering water with ^{222}Rn concentrations of 10 Bq.L^{-1}.

4   Conclusions

An assessment of radiologically enhanced residual materials generated when treating water for a small city was conducted. The water supply was drawn from both surface and groundwater resources. All radioactive constituent concentrations monitored fell within current Australian drinking water guideline values (NHMRC/ARMCANZ [1] & ANZECC/ARMCANZ [2]).

Activity balance calculations were performed for radionuclides within the WTP and inventories of ^{210}Po and ^{238}U could be accounted for within measurement uncertainty constraints. An as yet unidentified ^{226}Ra retention mechanism is holding back greater than 80% of the radionuclide. It was identified that filter media and recycled process waters may act as temporary sinks for radionuclides within the surface water treatment plant. Further work is required to fully characterise the ^{226}Ra activity balance of the system.

Sludge generated during surface water treatment contained enhanced concentrations of ^{238}U, ^{226}Ra and ^{210}Pb. Modelling the additional dose to a small crops farmer (as the critical group) using the sludge as a soil conditioner provides a maximum dose of 78 µSv per year.

Additional dose associated with the disposal of exhausted ion exchange resin from the groundwater treatment plants to a controlled landfill was calculated for landfill plant operators. Results indicate that an additional dose of less than 5 µSv per year can be attributed to the practice.

Regeneration wastes derived from the groundwater treatment plants are discharged to the sewer. Current radionuclide concentrations in the regeneration waste do not exceed regulatory limits for discharge to the sewer (OQPC [19]).

Granulated activated carbon filter cartridges used in household point-of-use water treatment filters may contain ^{222}Rn decay progeny at levels that exceed regulatory disposal criteria for landfill disposal. Individual GAC filter compliance with regulatory waste disposal criteria will be determined by the location of the user within the city supply area, the status of groundwater supplementation and mixing of surface and groundwater within the distribution system.

Additional work is underway to further characterise ^{222}Rn concentration in the water distribution system by sampling a larger number of consumer outlets. This data will be used to further assess regulatory compliance issues.

This study forms a preliminary stage of a broader study assessing the impact of waterborne radioactivity in urban and rural environments. This data will be used in validating a computer model developed to assess the radiological impact of water supply, treatment, distribution, wastewater collection and treatment processes, and ultimate discharge to the environment as either waste or a beneficial material, particularly with a view to future increases in resource exploitation and population growth.

Acknowledgements

The author is indebted to the management and staff of Toowoomba Water, Toowoomba City Council for providing access to sampling locations, infrastructure and information relevant to their water treatment plants and distribution systems. Acknowledgement is also extended to Mr Allan Burton, of Queensland Health Scientific Services for his assistance in sample preparation.

References

[1]   NHMRC/ARMCANZ. Australian Drinking water Guidelines 1996 – Update 2001. National Water Quality Management Strategy Paper No. 6, National Health and Medical Research Council & Agricultural and Resource Management Council of Australia and New Zealand, Australian Government Publishing Service, Canberra. 2001

[2]   ANZECC/ARMCANZ. Australian and New Zealand Guidelines for Fresh and Marine Water Quality. National Water Quality Management Strategy Paper No. 4. Australian and New Zealand Environmental and Conservation Council & Agricultural and Resource Management Council of Australia and New Zealand. Australian Government Publishing Service. Canberra. 2000

[3]   WHO. Guidelines for drinking-water quality, 3rd Edition. World Health Organisation. Geneva. 2004

[4]   USEPA. National Primary Drinking Water Regulations; Radionuclides; Final Rule. Environmental Protection Agency 40 CFR Parts 9, 141 and 142: Washington, USA. 2000

[5]   EU. Drinking Water Directive. Council Directive 98/83/EC on the quality of water intended for human consumption. European Commission. 1998

[6]   Kocher, DC. Drinking water standards for radionuclides: the dilemma and a possible resolution. *Health Physics* 80: 486-490. 2001

[7]   Cooper, MB. Naturally Occurring Radioactive Materials (NORM) in Australian Industries – Review of Current Inventories and Future Generation. Report prepared for the Radiation Health & Safety Advisory Council, ERS-006 EnviroRad Services Pty Ltd. Australia. 2003

[8]   RHSAC. Naturally Occurring Radioactive Material (NORM) in Australia: Issues for Discussion. Radiation Health & Safety Advisory Council Report to the CEO, ARPANSA. Australia. 2004

[9]   IAEA. Extent of Environmental Contamination by Naturally Occurring Radioactive Material (NORM) and Technological Options for Mitigation. Technical Report Series No. 419. Vienna: International Atomic Energy Agency. 2003

[10]   QDLGPSR. Population and Housing fact Sheet – Toowoomba City. Queensland Government, Department of Local Government, Planning, Sport and Recreation, Brisbane. Australia. 2004

[11]   QHSS. Water Treatment Survey - Toowoomba City Council. Conducted by Queensland Health Scientific Services, unpublished data. Brisbane. Australia. 2004

[12]   QDNRM. Annual water statistics report 2003 - 2004, Queensland Department of Natural Resources and Mines. Brisbane. Australia. 2004

[13]   Lawson, B. Personal communication, 20 April 2005, Aqua Fresh Water Purifying Systems, Brisbane. Australia

[14]   ISO9698. Water quality – Determination of tritium activity concentration – Liquid scintillation counting method. International Standard 9698. International Organisation for Standardisation, Geneva. Switzerland. 1989.

[15]   EML. Environmental Measurement Laboratory Procedures Manual, HASL-300, 28th Edition. US Department of Energy. New York. 1997

[16]   QHSS. Trace Elements in Clinical Samples, Waters and Digests by ICPMS, Method. QIS Document No. 18229R2. Brisbane. Australia. 2000

[17]   ANL. RESRAD Version 6.22 Computer Model. ANL, Argonne. USA

[18]   USEPA. CARBDOSE Version 5.0 Computer model. USEPA, Boston. USA

[19]   OQPC. Radiation Safety Regulation 1999, Reprint No. 2H, April 2005. Office of the Queensland Parliamentary Counsel, Brisbane. Australia.

Section 6
Electromagnetic fields

UMTS network planning using genetic algorithms

F. Garzia, C. Perna & R. Cusani
INFOCOM Department, University of Rome "La Sapienza", Italy

Abstract

The continuously growing of cellular net complexity, that followed the introduction of UMTS technology, has reduced the usefulness of traditional design tools, making them quite unworthy.

The purpose of this paper is to illustrate a design tool for UMTS optimized net planning based on genetic algorithms. In particular, some utilities for 3G net designers, useful to respect important aspects (such as the environmental one) of the cellular net, are shown.

Keywords: UMTS network planning, genetic algorithms.

1 Introduction

The extraordinary growth of mobile telecommunication sector of the last years has implied strong economical investments of enterprises that operate in this vital sector, in particular way from the net infrastructure point of view.

The development of third generation mobile communication (3G) such as UMTS, with the related advanced allowed services, has increased the need of an efficient network planning that could keep into account all the aspects of complexity which are typical of this new technology, changing the traditional approach to this kind of problem [1-3].

In fact, even if the WCDMA techniques used by UMTS reduces the problems related to the frequency management, the capacity of the net represents a vital problem since the capacity of each radio cell is strongly related to the signal – interference ratio (SIR), that is a function of the number and of the kind of active users inside each communication cell [2-3].

The need of reduction of radiated power, due to environmental restrictions, and the need of guaranteeing a good quality of services, requires a capillary distribution of Radio Base Stations (BSs) on the territory to be covered. Nowadays, due to the reduced availability of BSs placement zones, it is necessary to seek new and efficient methods to optimize the cellular coverage services.

Different and interesting solutions have already been proposed [3-9]. One of the most interesting is based on a technique inspired to the natural evolution, represented by the Genetic Algorithms (GAs) [8-10], which are good candidates, thanks to their versatility, to solve a complex and multi-parametric problem such as the considered one.

The purpose of this work is to illustrate a new GAs based method to solve the optimization coverage and capacity problem of UMTS system, keeping into account its specific features and the typical restrictions found in real situations, such as the environmental one.

2 The genetic algorithms

Genetic algorithms are considered wide range numerical optimisation methods, which use the natural processes of evolution and genetic recombination. Thanks to their versatility, they can be used in different application fields.

The algorithms encode each parameters of the problem to be optimised into a proper sequence (where the alphabet used is generally binary) called a gene, and combine the different genes to constitute a chromosome. A proper set of chromosomes, called population, undergoes the Darwinian processes of natural selection, mating and mutation, creating new generations, until it reaches the final optimal solution under the selective pressure of the desired fitness function.

GA optimisers, therefore, operate according to the following nine points:
1) encoding the solution parameters as genes;
2) creation of chromosomes as strings of genes;
3) initialisation of a starting population;
4) evaluation and assignment of fitness values to the individuals of the population;
5) reproduction by means of fitness-weighted selection of individuals belonging to the population;
6) recombination to produce recombined members;
7) mutation on the recombined members to produce the members of the next generation.
8) evaluation and assignment of fitness values to the individuals of the next generation;
9) convergence check.

The coding is a mapping from the parameter space to the chromosome space and it transforms the set of parameters, which is generally composed by real numbers, in a string characterized by a finite length. The parameters are coded into genes of the chromosome that allow the GA to evolve independently of the parameters themselves and therefore of the solution space.

Once created the chromosomes it is necessary choose the number of them which composes the initial population. This number strongly influences the efficiency of the algorithm in finding the optimal solution: a high number provides a better sampling of the solution space but slows the convergence.

Fitness function, or cost function, or object function provides a measure of the goodness of a given chromosome and therefore the goodness of an individual within a population. Since the fitness function acts on the parameters themselves, it is necessary to decode the genes composing a given chromosome to calculate the fitness function of a certain individual of the population.

The reproduction takes place utilising a proper selection strategy which uses the fitness function to choose a certain number of good candidates. The individuals are assigned a space of a roulette wheel that is proportional to they fitness: the higher the fitness, the larger is the space assigned on the wheel and the higher is the probability to be selected at every wheel tournament. The tournament process is repeated until a reproduced population of N individuals is formed.

The recombination process selects at random two individuals of the reproduced population, called parents, crossing them to generate two new individuals called children. The simplest technique is represented by the single-point crossover, where, if the crossover probability overcome a fixed threshold, a random location in the parent's chromosome is selected and the portion of the chromosome preceding the selected point is copied from parent A to child A, and from parent B to child B, while the portion of chromosome of parent A following the random selected point is placed in the corresponding positions in child B, and vice versa for the remaining portion of parent B chromosome.

If the crossover probability is below a fixed threshold, the whole chromosome of parent A is copied into child A, and the same happens for parent B and child B. The crossover is useful to rearrange genes to produce better combinations of them and therefore more fit individuals. The recombination process has shown to be very important and it has been found that it should be applied with a probability varying between 0.6 and 0.8 to obtain the best results.

The mutation is used to survey parts of the solution space that are not represented by the current population. If the mutation probability overcomes a fixed threshold, an element in the string composing the chromosome is chosen at random and it is changed from 1 to 0 or vice versa, depending of its initial value. To obtain good results, it has been shown that mutations must occur with a low probability varying between 0.01 and 0.1.

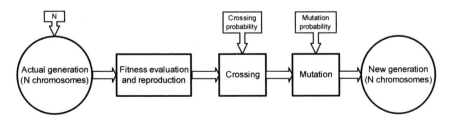

Figure 1:   Operative scheme of a GA iteration.

The converge check can use different criteria such as the absence of further improvements, the reaching of the desired goal or the reaching of a fixed maximum number of generations.

3 Definition of the problem

It is evident that, thanks to their versatility, GAs represent good candidates to solve the typical optimization problem of UMTS cellular net planning.

GAs have already been used for this kind of problem [5-9], even if their application is limited only to territory coverage. On the contrary, in this paper, other parameters (such as SIR), that strongly influence the results in real situations, are considered, generating a powerful tool for optimal net planning.

Some general criteria have been adopted, without reducing the generality of the problem that are:

1) it has been considered a suburban area whose dimensions are 3 km x 3 km with an inhomogeneous traffic distribution;
2) high gain BSs, placed at the same height, are considered;
3) circular irradiation diagrams of BSs, instead of three-lobe diagrams, are considered. This assumption, made to simplify the implementation of the algorithm, does not influence the final result;
4) a consolidated electromagnetic propagation model [11] has been adopted;
5) the SIR has been calculated using the following formula [3]:

$$SIR = SF \times \frac{P_r}{I_{in} + I_{out} + \eta} \tag{1}$$

where SF is the Spreading Factor, P_r is the received power, I_{in} is the intra-cells interference, I_{out} is the inter-cells interference, η is the thermal noise.

4 Proposed algorithms for optimization problem

Since a plenty of goals and restrictions must be respected in a UMTS net, the design can be made following different criteria.

The designer can therefore have different optimization tools that allows him to consider, in each real situation, the predominant aspects.

For this reason, in this paper, the different mentioned real situations have been considered, showing the great flexibility of the proposed method.

4.1 Case 1

A situation without information about traffic level, without restrictions about the maximum number of BSs that can be used and without restrictions about their territorial placement is considered.

The goal of this case is the optimization of territorial coverage, neglecting the performance of the service aspects.

To reach this target it is necessary to find a proper fitness function of GA and a proper chromosome.

The BSs are coded, inside the chromosome, by means of 2 double vectors, that represents the coordinates of each BS on the territory. To determine the length of the chromosome, related to the number of considered BSs, the minimum number of BSs necessary to ensure the coverage of a given percentage p_T of the territory, is calculated as:

$$n\_bs_{min} = \lceil p_T \times A_{Tot}/C_{BS} \rceil \tag{2}$$

where A_{Tot} represents the area of the considered territory; p_T is the percentage of territory that must be covered; C_{BS} is the maximum coverage area of each BSs.

Due to the usual not regular shape of the territory to be covered and to the impossibility of perfectly matching the coverage diagram of near BSs, the value calculated by means of eq.(2) may be not sufficient and it is necessary to consider a proper multiple n, generally equal to two. In the considered situation, we have $n\_srb_{min}=23$.

Each gene of the chromosome, representing a BSs, is composed by a number k of variables equal to 3: 2 are used for the position of the BSs on the territory and 1 is used to represent the state of activation /deactivation of the BSs.

The length λ of the chromosome (in term of number of variables) in the considered situation is expressed by the following formula:

$$\lambda = n \times n\_bs_{min} \times k. \tag{3}$$

Substituting the numerical values, we have: $\lambda= 138$.

The fitness function (F_{fit}) to minimize is, in this situation:

$$F_{fit} = \alpha \times \frac{A_{Tot} - A_{Cov}}{A_{Tot}} + \beta \times \frac{O_L}{A_{Tot}} + \gamma \times \frac{n\_bs}{n \times n\_bs_{min}}, \tag{4}$$

where A_{Cov} is the sum of the coverage areas of the BSs placed on the territory, O_L is the sum of the superposition areas of radiation diagram of BSs, n_bs is the number of BSs placed on the territory, α, β e γ are weight coefficients that are varied as a function of the project goals.

4.2 Case 2

In real situations, the traffic inside a territory is not distributed in a homogeneous way. The concentration users' zone are named hot spots. It is evident that, to guarantee a certain QoS level, it is necessary to reduce, as more as possible, the intra-cells and inter-cells interference. As a consequence, placing a BS in a hot spot represents a first significant step in net optimization.

Given a non homogeneous traffic distribution and an initial numbers of BSs, calculated according to eq.(2), the algorithm is capable of maximizing coverage and capacity and of minimizing cost.

The fitness function to minimize in this case is:

$$F_f = \alpha \times \frac{A_{Tot} - A_{Cov}}{A_{Tot}} + \beta \times \frac{O_L}{A_{Tot}} + \gamma \times \frac{n\_bs}{n \times n\_bs_{min}} + \delta \times \frac{U_{Tot} - U_{Cov}}{U_{Tot}} \tag{5}$$

where U_{Tot} is the number of estimated users inside the territory and U_{Cov} is the number of users covered by the active BSs.

4.3 Case 3

In real situation, for environmental reasons, it is not possible to place BSs anywhere. In this case, only a limited number of zones is available and it is necessary to find a function that accepts, as inputs, not only information concerning traffic but also information concerning the available installation zones (in particular their coordinates). The function must optimize the net considering these limitations that is a cost vinculum. Its structure is therefore equal to the one of eq.(5) less the cost factor.

4.4 Case 4

Another crucial factor in UMTS system is represented by the radiated power (environmental restrictions), with particular respect to the QoS. Therefore the net needs, sometimes, to place the BSs on the territory to reduce, as more as possible, the emitted power, guaranteeing an acceptable level of QoS.

In this case the power of each BS is considered as input parameter (which can be properly changed), that influences not only the coverage area but also the transmission capacity.

The fitness function is therefore:

$$F_f = \alpha \times \frac{A_{Tot} - A_{Cov}}{A_{Tot}} + \beta \times \frac{O_L}{A_{Tot}} + \gamma \times \frac{P_{Tot}}{n\_srb \times P_{Max}} + \delta \times \frac{U_{Tot} - U_{Cov}}{U_{Tot}} \qquad (6)$$

where P_{Tot} is the total power of BSs and P_{Max} in the maximum power radiated by each BS.

5 Performance of the algorithms and results

In the following the results of each situation considered above are shown.

5.1 Case 1

Purpose of case 1 is the optimization of the net considering only the coverage of the territory, keeping into account the cost factor. The results obtained are shown in the following.

A first situation has been obtained considering the following values for the weights of fitness function: $\alpha = 0.6$, $\beta=0.1$, $\gamma=0.3$. The results are shown in figs.2. It is possible to see that the presence of a strong cost component has heavily penalized the coverage maximization.

A second situation has been obtained considering the following values for the weights of fitness function $\alpha = 1$, $\beta=0$, $\gamma=0$, that is to maximize coverage considering the cost as a quasi-neglectable factor.

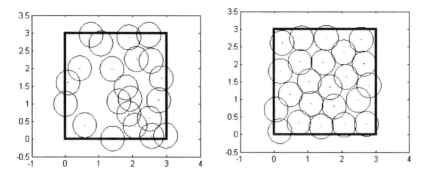

Figure 2:   Initial situation (left) and final results after 300 generations (right).

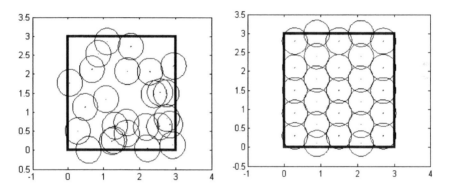

Figure 3:   Initial situation (left) and final results after 300 generations (right).

Due to the structure of fitness function, it always tends to limit the number of BSs on the territory, evaluating each time if the coverage gain justify the increase of the number of BSs.

5.2 Case 2

In this case, given a non homogenous traffic distribution, the fitness function tends to maximize capacity and coverage, trying anyway to reduce costs.

A first situation has been obtained considering the following values for the weights of fitness function: $\alpha=0.3$, $\beta=0.1$, $\gamma=0.2$ e $\delta=0.5$, that is to consider mainly the capacity component. The results are shown in figs.4.

A second situation has been obtained considering the following values for the weights of fitness function: $\alpha=0.5$, $\beta=0.1$, $\gamma=0.2$ e $\delta=0.3$, that is to consider complementary situation with respect to the previous one. The results are shown in figs.5.

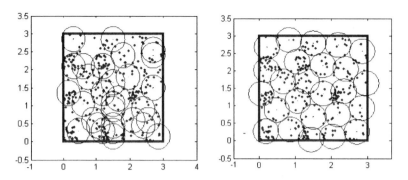

Figure 4:   Initial situation (left) and final results after 1000 generations (right).

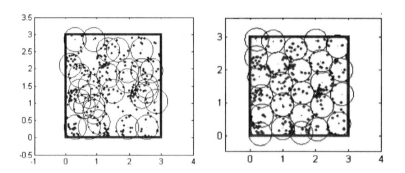

Figure 5:   Initial situation (left) and final results after 1000 generations (right).

5.3 Case 3

In this case, given a limited numbers of zones to place BSs (environmental restrictions) and a limited number of BSs (26 for example), the maximum coverage is desired. The obtained results are shown in figs.6

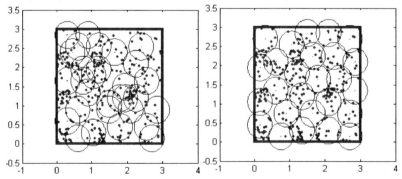

Figure 6:   Initial situation (left) and final results after 600 generations (right).

5.4 Case 4

In this situation, the maximization of coverage and capacity is desired, with a reduction of the emitted power (environmental restrictions).

The results are shown of figs.7. It is possible to see that the GA places the BSs in the zones where the traffic density is higher, to reduce, as more as possible, the radiated power, reducing, obviously, also the coverage area of the BSs, as it is possible to see from figs.7).

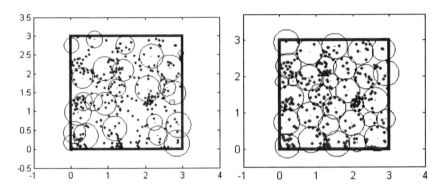

Figure 7:   Initial situation (left) and final results after 1000 generations (right).

5.5 Results

The results are shown in table 1.

Table 1:   Table of performances of each considered situation.

Fitness function (Case)	Number of BSs	Coverage	Capacity
1 A	23	89,3%	-
1 B	27	98.1%	-
2 A	25	92.3%	99.06%
2 B	25	96.8%	98.12%
3	26	96.9%	98.75%
4	31	94.9%	98.75%

From tab.1 it is possible to see that in the most of considered situations, the obtained solutions are satisfying from both coverage and capacity point of view. The results demonstrate that the GA ensures always high quality results, whose performances increase with the precision of input data.

In particular, a significant reduction of number of BSs is always present (cost reduction) even if their initial number is not a given data. This number is always a bit greater than the minimum number of BSs of the considered territory, calculated with eq.(2), due to the impossibility of perfectly matching the circular radiation diagrams of near BSs.

It is also possible to see a certain variability from the coverage point of view while a quasi constant behaviour from the capacity point of view.

The computation time is also quite short, since the most of good solutions are obtained after 150-200 generations of GA: the other subsequent generations give only little improvement of quality of solutions.

6 Conclusions

A genetic algorithm based technique to optimize the design of UMTS cellular nets has been presented.

The proposed method keeps into proper consideration the most of limits imposed by the installation of the BSs necessary to guarantee an optimal service, also including environmental restrictions.

Even if some simplifications were made, the considered technique is capable of ensuring good results from any point of view, representing a useful tools for UMTS initial optimization.

References

[1]   J. C. S. Cheung, M. A. Beach, J. McGeehan, "Network Planning for Third- generation Mobile Radio Systems", IEEE Commun. Mag., vol. 32, pp. 54-59, Nov. 1994.

[2]   E. Berruto, M. Gudmundson, R. Menolascino, W. Mohr, M. Pizarroso, "Research Activities on UMTS Radio Interface, Network Architectures, and Planning", IEEE Commun. Mag., vol. 36, pp. 82-95, Feb. 1998.

[3]   E. Amaldi, A. Capone, F. Malucelli, "*Planning UMTS Base Station Location: Optimization Models With Power Control and Algorithms* - IEEE transactions on wireless communications, vol. 2, pp. 939-952, no. 5, September 2003

[4]   B. Chamaret, S. Josselin, P. Kuonen, M. Pizarroso, B. Salas-Manzanedo, S. Ubeda, D. Wagner, "*Radio Network Optimization With Maximum Independent Set Search*", Proc. IEEE VTC '97, pp.770-774, May 1997.

[5]   P. Calegari, F. Guidec, P. Kuonen, D. Wagner, "*Genetic Approach to Radio Network Optimization for Mobile Systems*", IEEE, pp.755-759. (1997)

[6]   I. Laki, L. Farkas, L. Nagy, "*Cell Planning in Mobile Communication Systems Using SGA Optimization*". IEEE, pp. 124-127. (2001)

[7]   K. Lieska, E. Laitinen, J. Lahteenmaki, "*Radio Coverage Optimization With Genetic Algorithms*", IEEE, pp. 318-322. (1998).

[8]   F. Garzia, R. Cusani, "*Optimisation of Cellular Base Stations Placement in Territory With Urban and Environmental Restrictions By Means of Genetic Algorithms*", Proc. of EETI 2004 Energy, Environment and Technological Innovation, Rio de Janeiro, Brasil, (2004).

[9]   F. Garzia, R. Cusani, *"Wireless LAN optimal design in the underground Gran Sasso mountain laboratories of Italian National Institute of Nuclear Physics"*, Proc. of EETI 2004 Energy, Environment and Technological Innovation, Rio de Janeiro, Brasil, (2004).

[10]   D.E. Goldberg, *"Genetic Algorithms in Search, Optimisation and Machine Learning"*, Addison Wesley, 1989.

[11]   M. Hata, *"Empirical Formula for Propagation Loss in Land Mobile Radio Services"*, IEEE Transactions on Vehicular Technology, Vol. VT-29, No. 3, pp. 317-325, August 1980.

Long-term and low-thermal biological effects of microwaves

D. Adang[1,2], C. Remacle[3] & A. Vander Vorst[1]
[1]*EMIC Microwave Laboratory, Université Catholique de Louvain, Louvain-la-Neuve, Belgium*
[2]*ACOS Well-Being, Defence, Brussels, Belgium*
[3]*BANI Biologie Animale, Université Catholique de Louvain, Louvain-la-Neuve, Belgium*

Abstract

There is evidence that radio frequencies (RF) and microwaves directly affect living systems, as indicated by in vivo absorption experiments. Evidence is also provided by in vitro studies, revealing effects at various frequencies and intensities, on a number of cellular endpoints, including calcium binding, proliferation and alteration in membrane channels. There is ambiguity, however, about the relative contribution of direct and indirect non-thermal, i.e. low-thermal effects, as well as the possibility of direct low-thermal interactions. In this study, a possible causal link between microwave radiation (radar, cellular phone) and physiological and cellular changes is being evaluated by an epidemiological animal study on 128 rats, for 1.5 year. In order to assess the possible biological long-term effects of microwaves, we selected among others the following blood and hormonal parameters: lymphocytes, monocytes, granulocytes, erythrocytes, platelets, cytokines, corticosterone and ACTH (adrenocorticotrophic hormone). There is lack of knowledge about the biological mechanisms of the exposure to such low-level electromagnetic fields.
Keywords: electromagnetic fields, long-term biological effects, low-thermal, radar, cellular phone, microwaves, environmental risk.

1 Introduction

Radio frequencies (RF) and microwaves are non-ionizing, unlike much higher frequency waves above the visible range. The interaction of RF/microwaves with cell tissue can be considered as the result of three processes: penetration by electromagnetic waves and their propagation into the living system, primary interaction of the waves with cell tissue, and possible secondary effects of the primary interaction.

The word 'interaction' is important. It signals that end results depend not only on the action of the field but are influenced by the reaction of the living system. Living systems have a great capacity for compensating the effects induced by external influences, including electromagnetic sources. While it is often overlooked, it is one main reason why conclusions derived from computer models must be approached with caution. Guidelines for limiting the exposure provide protection against known adverse health effects; low-thermal long-term effects are not considered until today.

The thermal effects of microwaves are well known. There exists, however, a lot of uncertainties about the low-thermal long-term effects. This lack of scientific consensus led the World Health Organization to state that more scientific research is needed on this issue [1]. Very few people are exposed to thermally significant levels of microwaves. The big majority of exposures occur at levels at which weak-fields interactions would be the only possible source of any adverse health response. On the other hand, there is a major deficiency in the understanding of the effects of pulsed fields. Only a few isolated reports on pulsed fields are available while it is not possible to identify either the frequency or the peak power domains of importance [2]. Today, the general use of radar systems for navigation, together with the extension of radio communication links, satellite communications and cellular phone technology into the microwave frequency range, has implied a wider need for engineers and physicians to investigate the possible harmful effects of microwaves on the human environmental health. An increased or decreased presence of a biological marker does not necessarily indicate any pathological process, but may be a useful index for biological dosimetry of microwave exposure. The question of the microwave syndrome at low exposure level was raised several decades ago in Eastern Europe. It involves a number of signs like headache, perspiration, emotional instability, tiredness, somnolence, sexual problems, loss of memory, concentration and decision difficulties, insomnia, depressive hypochondriac tendencies, etc. Evaluation is difficult because of the absence of a control group and lack of reliable dosimetric data. A paper dated a few years ago supports RF sickness syndrome as a medical disorder [3].

2 Objectives

The objective of the present study consists in verifying the possible physiological modifications and anatomopathological changes due to low-level microwave exposure (1 GHz and 10 GHz), using both continuous and pulsed waves. In a first phase, this study focuses on selected blood and hormonal parameters as biological indicators of changes in the immune system of the animal. In a second phase, the possible carcinogenic effects will be investigated and microscopic study will be performed on all vital tissue.

3 Methods

3.1 An animal study

There is an increasing concern about the possibility that radiofrequency exposure may play a role in the causation or promotion of cancer, especially related to the blood-forming organs [4].

A possible causal association between microwave exposure and biological effects of this kind of non-ionizing radiation is evaluated by an experimental study on a population of 128 *Wistar albino* rats, subdivided into 4 groups, depending on frequency and mode exposure, sham as well. To reduce as much as possible the stress factor, we have chosen for a collective exposure in an exposure unit, suitable for 32 rats, instead of an individual exposure where the rat is caged in a small waveguide. The different groups of rats are exposed two hours a day, seven days a week during eighteen months, to microwaves at 1 GHz and 10 GHz, continuous and pulsed mode, at an average power density of 200 µW/cm² and 500 µW/cm² respectively. This is explained in section 6 of this paper. In order to determine the possible biological long-term effects of microwaves, we selected the following parameters: blood cells, stress-induced hormones (adrenocorticotrophic hormone i.e. ACTH; corticosterone) and cytokines (interleukin i.e. IL-I, IL-X; tumor necrosis factor α i.e. TNF α). Enzyme-linked immunosorbent assays are used to quantify those hormones in the blood plasma and serum. Body weight is monitored with minimal disturbance to the animal. It appears to be a reasonably sensitive indicator of stress, especially chronic stress, and therefore it is strongly recommended that animals which may be stressed should weighed regularly and their body weights compared with those of the sham exposed group. Daily observations of the rats' behaviour are part of the protocol.

3.2 The exposure itself

In a first series of experiments the *Wistar albino* rats are exposed in groups of 32 in an exposure unit (1.11 m x 0.60 m x 0.71 m), from the open end of a wave guide. This method constitutes an innovating element [5]. In most of the other studies indeed, rats are kept separately in plexiglass cylinders during exposure, where space to move is limited. Such narrow housing causes an enormous stress response in the rat [6]. This stressor creates a supplementary variable, which is susceptible to mask secretion of certain corticosteroids [7]. We use four-month old rats with a body weight of 300-350 grams. Four-month old rats are at the beginning of maturity and therefore ideal as a model for our experiments. We choose only male rats because of their constant metabolism compared to the variations in the female physiology. Animals are kept in normal vivarium conditions, and are made accustomed to experimental procedures, environment and handling two months prior to the beginning of the experiments. Daylight conditions start at 0700 *a.m.* and darkness begins at 0900 *p.m.* The *Wistar albino* rats are exposed to weak microwave doses as described above. It is important to run the experiment always on the same period of the day because of the influence of the circadian rhythm on the secretion of corticosteroids, for example corticosterone. Corticosterone is the most abundantly secreted glucocorticoid in the rat and helps the body to deal with stress. It acts as a negative feedback mechanism controlling the release of ACTH. It is therefore obviously important to sample glucocorticoids at the same time of the day if repeated measurements are to be made on different days. The peak in hormone secretion occurs towards the end of the light period. During the first months, the rats were already accustomed to manipulations and some blood samples were taken to assess a possible impact of a changing environment to the animal physiology. Handling, presumably acting as a mild stressor, during early life significantly reduced the glucocorticoid response to stress in adulthood [8].

4 Materials

The exposure unit is a self-made cage with the antenna – an open ended waveguide – on top (Figure 1). Its basis consists of a custom made box of polyethylene covered at the outside with microwave absorbing materials, themselves covered with wood (multiplex 15 mm) to prevent any artefacts arising from objects introduced in the microwave field.

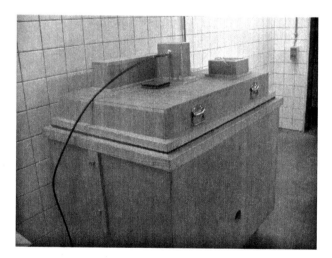

Figure 1:   Collective exposure unit for rats.

The microwave generator used is a sweep oscillator Hewlett Packard 8620A. The cover of the box is also self-constructed and its height is 0.12 m to be sure that the rats are exposed to the far field of the antenna. A rectangular aperture is made, covered by a fine-meshed gauze, on which is fitted the armature of a fluorescent lamp. Furthermore, a fan is built in to improve the internal ventilation of the exposure unit.

5 Rat marking

To identity the rats during the whole experiment (one and a half year) in general and during blood sampling in particular, an unmistakable permanent method to distinguish one rat from another has been thought out. The ear of the rat is pierced following a formerly established pattern of figures. This procedure is carried out under total anaesthesia for one minute on the basis of sevoflurane.

6 An appropriate exposure level

Based on ICNIRP [9] recommendations, an exposure level is derived related to both frequencies to which the *Wistar albino* rats are submitted. The deposition of radio frequency energy in the human body tends to increase the body temperature. During exercise, the metabolic heat production can reach levels of 3-5 W/kg. In normal thermal environments, a specific absorption rate (SAR) of 1-4 W/kg for 30 minutes produces average body temperature increases of less than 1 °C for healthy adults. Thus an occupational radio frequency guideline of 0.4 W/kg SAR leaves a margin of protection against complications to the thermally unfavourable environmental conditions. For the general population, which includes sensitive subpopulations, such as children and elderly, a SAR of 0.08 W/kg would provide a further margin of safety against adverse thermal effects from radio frequency fields. That is why one has defined basic restrictions based on observed biological effects. Assuming that the ratio in size between a human and a rat equals 10, one has to 'adapt' the ICNIRP recommendations, valuable for a human being, to the size of the rat by multiplying by 10 the key frequencies. This means that the exposure of a rat of 1 GHz corresponds to a human exposure of 100 MHz. In other words, an exposure of 1 GHz for a rat is equivalent of a 100 MHz exposure for man. The basis restriction value for man at 100 MHz is 2 W/m². This means that a power density of 200 µW/cm² is suitable in relationship with the exposure of rats. Following an identical reasoning leads us to the fact that a 1 GHz exposure for man corresponds to a 10 GHz exposure for rats. ICNIRP recommendations stipulate a basic restriction, expressed in power density, of f/200 (f = frequency), i.e. 1000 MHz/200 or 5 W/m² (500 µW/cm²). In the far field, 200 µW/cm² corresponds to an electric field strength of 27 V/m. That's the reason why we focus on this value in the next paragraph.

7 Results of the field uniformity measurements at 1 GHz

The evaluation of the field uniformity is carried out by means of an electric field measurement, using the Isotropic Field Monitor of the Company Amplifier Research.

Table 1:   Measured electric field E and power density P.

Square nr.	E[V/m]	P[μW/cm²]	Square nr.	E[V/m]	P[μW/cm²]
A1	26.5	186.3	D7	27.2	196.2
A2	25.4	171.1	D8	21.5	122.6
A3	24.0	151.0	D9	23.5	146.5
A4	20.2	108.2	D10	32.4	278.5
A5	29.0	223.1	D11	18.7	92.7
A6	32.3	276.7	E1	31.4	261.5
A7	25.2	168.4	E2	19.4	99.8
A8	34.0	306.6	E3	26.7	189.1
A9	36.3	349.5	E4	28.5	215.5
A10	30.2	241.9	E5	8.8	20.5
A11	24.2	155.3	E6	31.4	261.5
B1	32.8	285.4	E7	25.2	168.4
B2	27.2	196.2	E8	22.2	130.7
B3	14.4	55.0	E9	28.7	217.0
B4	22.2	130.7	E10	36.0	343.8
B5	25.4	171.1	E11	20.9	115.9
B6	35.6	336.2	F1	34.8	321.2
B7	28.4	213.9	F2	25.5	172.5
B8	37.3	369.0	F3	17.7	83.1
B9	49.2	642.1	F4	21.8	126.1
B10	34.0	306.5	F5	13.6	49.1
B11	43.0	490.5	F6	33.6	299.5
C1	32.4	278.5	F7	29.5	230.8
C2	24.6	160.5	F8	31.2	258.2
C3	8.2	17.8	F9	35.4	332.4
C4	20.7	113.7	F10	36.8	359.3
C5	13.6	49.1	F11	38.6	395.2
C6	29.7	234.0	G1	30.6	248.4
C7	26.7	189.1	G2	22.8	137.9
C8	21.0	117.0	G3	25.9	177.9
C9	36.6	355.3	G4	23.2	142.8
C10	34.9	323.1	G5	29.3	227.7
C11	23.0	140.3	G6	41.8	463.5
D1	35.8	340.0	G7	32.8	285.4
D2	44.8	532.4	G8	30.4	245.1
D3	25.4	171.1	G9	32.2	275.0
D4	21.4	212.5	G10	23.0	140.3
D5	12.0	38.2	G11	25.0	165.8
D6	28.5	215.4			

	E[V/m]	P[μW/cm²]
Mean	27.2	201.2
SD	7.4	114.6

This instrument measures the electric field E in space along three axes. Afterwards, the corresponding power density values were derived from these data. The bottom of the exposure unit is first subdivided in 77 squares of 10 cm². In a following step the probe is placed successively in the center of each square and the electric field strength is recorded. The squares are denominated from [A-G][1-11]. The mean value of the electric field strength is 27 V/m (standard deviation 10 V/m). In order to make the electric field more uniform some PVC constructions are build at the inside of the exposure unit. We started from the rough data of the measurement series and plotted them in a scheme of the exposure unit. Afterwards we focused on the squares were the value of the electric field is less than 27 V/m. Empirically, we constructed on the bottom of the exposure unit a PVC platform-like shape, to uniformize the electric field followed by an analogous measurement session as mentioned above. These constructions also reduce the stress level of the rats. The results are shown in Table 1.

8 Results

Base line determination blood samples have been collected early March. In the meantime, statistical analysis of 10 000 blood parameters is in progress.
Preliminary results will be presented at the Environmental Health Risk 2005 Conference.

References

[1] M. Repacholi, Low-level exposure to radio frequency electromagnetic fields: health effects and research needs, Bioelectromagnetics, 19 (1), pp. 1-19, 1998.

[2] A. Laurence et al. Biological effects of electromagnetic fields-mechanisms for the effects of pulsed microwave radiation on protein conformation, J. Ther. Biol., 206, pp. 291-298, 2000.

[3] A.G. Johnson Liakouris, Radiofrequency (RF) sickness in the Lelienfield study: an effect of modulated microwaves?, Arch. Environm. Health, 53(3), pp. 236-238, May-June 1998.

[4] H. Yoav, The potential carcinogenic hazards of electromagnetic radiation: a review, Cancer Detection and Prevention, 19(3), pp. 244-249, 1959.

[5] D. Adang, Study on the long-term athermal biological effects of radar radiation in rats, Proceedings of URSI Forum 2003, Brussels, December, 2003.

[6] K. Gärtner et al., Stress response of rats to handling and experimental procedures, Lab. Anim., 14, pp. 267-274, 1980.

[7] C.E. Manser, The assessment of stress in laboratory animals, Royal Society for the Prevention of Cruelty to Animals, RSPCA, London, UK, pp. 30-32, 1992.

[8] A. Armario, J.L. Montero, J. Balash, Sensitivity of corticosterone and some metabolic variables to graded levels of low intensity stresses in adult male rats, Phys. Behav., 37, pp. 595-561, 1986.

[9] ICNIRP Guidelines, Guidelines for limiting exposure to time-varying electric, magnetic and electromagnetic fields (up to 300 GHz), Health Physics, vol. 74, pp. 494-522, April 1998.

Section 7
Housing and health

The built environment in poor urban communities on the outskirts of Beirut, Lebanon

R. R. Habib, S. H. Basma, J. S. Yeretzian & D. Aybout
P1 Faculty of Health Sciences, American University of Beirut, Lebanon

Abstract

This research examined the association between the existing built environment in poor urban communities in Lebanon and the presence of illnesses among household members. Data were collected in poor urban communities in the outskirts of Beirut, Lebanon on 2797 households using a face-to-face interview with a household member. A structured questionnaire comprising several sections on the built environment and socio-demographic characteristics was used. Association between the presence of illness among household members and four built environment indices, namely housing conditions, infrastructure and services, crowding, and the availability of durable goods in the household, was determined using odds ratios from binary logistic regression models. Covariates such as education of head of household and total monthly household income were taken into account. Poor housing conditions were significantly associated with the presence of illness among household members in the studied sample. Households indicating six or more problems relating to housing conditions, mainly poor ventilation, infestation with rodents and cockroaches, cracks in ceiling and walls and others, were twice more likely to report the presence of illness among household members when compared to households with one or no problems [OR=2.10; 95 % CI=(1.68, 2.63)]. This line of research contributes to the understanding of the general context of the built environment and its influence on the health of residents in poor urban communities in developing countries.
Keywords: built environment, poor housing conditions, outskirts of Beirut.

1   Introduction

The literature on the built environment in underserved urban communities is vast and growing. Communities residing in urban areas, are more likely to reside in poor built environment, with outdoor air pollutant mainly from fumes of industrial zones, insecure tenure and poverty (Galea and Vlahov [10]; Northridge *et al.* [21]; Curtis *et al.* [5]; Kahlemeier *et al.* [15]). To date, a number of studies have investigated the impact of the built environment namely infrastructure and services, housing conditions, indoor air quality, and crowding on the health of individuals (Al-Khatib *et al.* [1]; Bierman-Lytle [2]; Dunn [6]; Jackson [13]; Krieger and Higgins [16]; Kumie and Berhane [17]; Lawrence [18]; Northridge *et al.* [21]; Perdue *et al.* [22]; Sharfstein and Sander [24]; Samet and Spengler [23]; Sirinivasan *et al.* [25]; Wallerstien *et al.* [28]; Xavier *et al.* [30]). A comprehensive review of studies in the literature indicates an association between poor housing conditions and presence of ill health namely dizziness, headache, irritation of eyes and skin, upper respiratory tract infection and increase in the prevalence of cardiovascular diseases (Al-Khatib *et al.* [1]; Chiaverini *et al.* [3]; Jones [14]; Krieger and Higgins [16]; Lowry [19]; Sirinivasan *et al.* [25]; Xavier *et al.* [30]). This research examined the association between the existing built environment in poor urban communities in Lebanon and the presence of illnesses among household members.

2   Methods

2.1 Study area

Densely populated urban communities were selected based on poverty conditions, inadequate services and infrastructure, rural-urban influx, war displaced populations and proximity to metropolitan Beirut. The studied communities are located within the eastern and southern suburbs of Beirut.

2.2 Data and survey instrument

Data were collected using face-to-face interviews with a proxy respondent in a cross-sectional survey based on a two-stage probability sample of 2,797 households conducted in 2002 by the Faculty of Health Sciences at the American University of Beirut. Prior to data collection, the University Review Board approved the questionnaire. All respondents were informed of the objective of the study and oral consent was obtained. The overall response rate was 88.3%. Data included demographic, health and socio-economic factors as well as information on the built environment indices concerning housing conditions, infrastructure and services, crowding conditions and durable goods.

2.3 Formulation of the measures in the study

The educational attainment of the head of the household and total monthly household income was used in the analysis of this study. The total household monthly income, measured in thousands Lebanese pounds, was categorized into three levels: low (less than 460,000 LBP) medium to low (460,000 to 700,000 LBP) and medium (700,000 LBP) based on the frequency distribution. Completed years of education for head of household were also categorized into three levels: none-elementary, primary-intermediate, and secondary and above (Table 1).

Table 1: Characteristics of households in poor urban communities in Beirut, Lebanon Urban Health Survey 2003.

	Frequency (n)	Percentage (%)
Household Characteristics		
Households (n)	2797	100.0
Type of Household		
One individual	117	4.2
Nuclear	2236	79.9
Extended	444	15.9
Size of household (number of individuals)		
1-3	885	31.6
4-6	1476	52.8
>6	436	15.6
Head of household highest educational level (completed number of schooling years)		
None-elementary	1006	37.0
Primary-Intermediate	950	34.8
Intermediate-Secondary	768	28.2
Total monthly income of household. (In 1000 Lebanese Pounds)		
<460	1058	37.8
460-700	614	21.9
>700,000	827	29.5
Occupation of head of household (ILO Classification)		
Economically active	2071	74.0
Economically inactive	671	24.0
Presence of illness		
Yes Only one reported illness	564	32.7
More than one	1158	67.2
Total	1722	61.5
No	1075	38.4

* Total observations per variable differ due to missing data.

Four built environment indices were used namely housing conditions, infrastructure and services, crowding and durable goods (Table 2).

Table 2:   Built environment indices and presence of illnesses among household members in poor urban communities (n=2797) in the outskirts of Beirut, Lebanon.

Housing Conditions	Unadjusted OR (95 % CI)	Adjusted OR (95 % CI)
0-4 problems	1	1
5-7 problems	1.41 (1.18-1.69)	1.40 (1.14-1.69)
8-15 problems	2.36 (1.94-2.88)	2.10 (1.68-2.62)
Measures of Housing Conditions	N	%
Lack adequate lighting in living room	1038	37.1
Lack adequate lighting in bedroom	1140	40.8
Poor ventilation	2420	86.5
Presence of humidity	1682	60.1
Presence of cracks in walls	1369	48.9
Presence of cracks in ceiling	945	33.8
Presence of seepage in walls	1799	64.3
Presence of seepage in ceilings	1370	49.0
Presence of main source of heating	1962	70.1
Presence of broken windows	703	25.1
Presence of exposed electrical wires	447	16.0
Mice infestation	645	23.1
Rats infestation	405	14.5
Insects infestation	2136	76.4
Water overflow from drains	1064	38.0
Infrastructure and Services	Unadjusted OR (95 % CI)	Adjusted OR (95 % CI)
0-1 problem	1	1
2-3 problems	1.27 (1.05-1.54)	1.10 (0.89-1.37)
4-9 problems	1.32 (1.06-1.64)	1.11 (0.87-1.41)
Measures of Infrastructure and Services	N	%
Availability of drinking water	2797	100
Adequacy of drinking water	2784	99.5
Problems in timing of garbage	382	13.7
collection	2106	75.3
Problems in garbage collection	141	5.0
Problems in sewage disposal	931	33.2
Cuts in electrical power for more than	912	32.6
4 hours/ day	393	14.1
Problems with the reliability of	84	2.0
electrical power	78	2.8
Rain water flooding	-	-
Evacuation due to rainwater flooding	-	-
River water over flooding		
Crowding Index	Unadjusted OR (95 % CI)	Adjusted OR (95 % CI)
U≤ U 2 persons/room	1	1
> 2 persons/room	0.97 (0.83-1.14)	0.94 (0.78-1.13)

Table 2 continued.

Education of Head of Household		
None- Elementary	1	1
Primary- Intermediate	0.52 (0.44-0.63)	0.57 (0.46-0.70)
Intermediate-Secondary+	0.38 (0.32-0.47)	0.44 (0.35-0.55)
Total Monthly Income of Household		
Low	1	1
Medium	0.69 (0.56-0.84)	0.82 (0.67-1.02)
High	0.65 (0.54-0.80)	0.44 (0.70-1.12)
Durable Goods		
0-8 items	1	1
9-10 items	0.69 (0.56-0.84)	0.57 (0.73-1.12)
11-22 items	0.65 (0.54-0.80)	0.44 (0.68-1.08)

2.3.1 Housing conditions index

Data on housing conditions consisted of 15 indicator variables measuring the absence of adequate lighting in both living rooms and bedrooms, the absence of a source of heating; the presence of poor ventilation, humidity, cracks in walls and ceilings, leakage in walls and ceilings, broken windows, exposed electrical wires, infestation due to mice, rats and cockroaches and water overflow from drains.

2.3.2 Infrastructure and services index

The infrastructure and services indicators comprised 10 items including the availability of a source of drinking water, adequacy of drinking water, problems in garbage disposal related mainly to (method of collection, timing and frequency of collection), problems in sewage disposal, cuts in electrical power for more than 4 hours per day, reliability of the electrical power (low or high volt), floods due to rain water, house evacuation due to rainwater flooding and river water over flooding.

Indicators used in the calculations of these built environment indicators were dichotomized into 0 for the "absence" or 1 for the "presence" of the problem. The numbers were then summed to form a score ranging from 0 to 15 problems for housing conditions, and 0 to 10 problems for infrastructure and services. The more numerous the reported problems, the poorer the quality.

2.3.3 Durable goods

The total number of durable goods present per household out of 22 items including: refrigerator, electrical appliances, tele-communication equipment and other items was used as a measure of the level of comfort in the household.

2.3.4 Crowding index

The crowding index was based the number of persons per room (Lowry [19]). Crowding was defined as the ratio of the number of people in the household to the number of rooms in the household excluding the kitchen, unclosed balconies, bathrooms and garage. The crowding index was categorized into two levels: less than or equal to two persons / room and more than two persons/room (Table 2).

The housing, infrastructure and durable goods indices were divided into 3 categories based on the tertiles of their respective frequency distributions as follows: (0-4; 5-7; 8-15 problems) for the housing conditions index, (0-1; 2-3; 4-10 problems) for the infrastructure and services index, and (0-8; 9-10; 11-22 items) for durable goods (Table 2).

2.3.5 Outcome measure

Presence of illnesses among household members was the outcome of interest. It was dichotomized into 0 indicating the absence of illness among all household members and 1 indicating the presence of any illness among one or more household members. Reported illnesses were classified according to the 10th revised edition of the International statistical classification of diseases and related health problems (ICD-10) (WHO 1992).

2.4 Statistical analysis

To determine the association between the built environment and the health status of members of the household, a logistic regression was done. Adjusted odds ratios and 95 % confidence intervals (CI) were computed using the Statistical Package for Social Sciences (SPSS) 11.0 software.

3   Results

The majority of the households (79.9 %) were nuclear with an average size of 5 persons per household (Table 1). 37.0 percent of household heads did not complete an elementary educational level, and 34.8 percent attained a primary to intermediate level education or more. The majority of the heads of household (74.0 %) were economically active. 37.8 percent of the households reported an income of less than 460,000 Lebanese pounds per months (around 300 US Dollars). Results showed that 61.5% of households reported the presence of illness among household members and of these, 67.2 % reported two or more types of illness (Table 2).

Adjusted odds ratios for the presence of illnesses among household members were calculated using binary logistic regression models (Table 2). The findings of the study indicated that a significant positive association exists between the presence of illness and housing conditions. No significant association was found with other built environment indices including infrastructure and services, crowding conditions and durable goods.

A significant education gradient was also apparent for the presence of illnesses in this population; the higher the educational level attained by the head of the household, the lower was the prevalence of illnesses among household members [OR=0.57, 95% CI= (0.46-0.70 for primary-intermediate; OR=0.44, 95% CI= (0.35-0.55) for intermediate-secondary].

4 Discussion

Our findings indicated that inadequate housing conditions were associated with the presence of illnesses among household members residing in underprivileged urban communities. Poor ventilation, excess humidity, inadequate lighting, cracks and leakage in walls and ceilings, and cockroach and rodent infestation prevailed in a large proportion of households. The positive association between poor housing conditions and ill health has been previously established in the literature (Chiaverini *et al.* [3]; Samet and Spengler, [23]; Sirinivasan *et al.* [25]; Krieger and Higgins [16]; Hynes *et al.* [12]). Empirical evidence links the prevalence of respiratory diseases, cardiovascular diseases, skin diseases, cancer, psychosocial distress, and reported mental health problems to poor housing conditions which characterize urban squatters in developing cities (Chiaverini *et al.* [3]; Jackson, [13]; Samet and Spengler, [23]; Sirinivasan *et al.* [25]; Evans *et al.* [8]; Krieger and Higgins [16]; Jones [14]; Al-Khatib *et al.* [1]; Cardoso *et al.* [4]. Our findings did not show an association between existing infrastructure and services and ill health among household members. It is worth noting that the studied areas have access to basic services and sanitation mostly provided by formal and informal networks and community associations (Fawaz [9]). Contrary to some published studies (US Census of Bureau [27]; Evans *et al.* [8]; Evans and Kantrowitz [7]; Gray [11]; Kumie and Berhane [17]) we did not find an association between crowding conditions and ill health although a large proportion of the population resides in crowded dwellings. The literature on this association has been inconclusive due to the confounding effect of hygiene practices and access to health care (Gray [11]; Myers *et al.* [20]). These indicators were not taken into account in our analysis due to lack of data.

In conclusion, poor housing conditions were a significant predictor of self-reported illnesses by household members living in poor urban communities in the outskirts of Beirut. Our results add to the understanding of the built environment, a recurrent and global issue. Further studies should focus on issues relating to self- satisfaction with housing conditions, housing tenure and their association with social health.

References

[1]   Al-Khatib, I., Juba, A., Kamal, N., Hamed, N., Hmeidan, N. & Massad, S. Impact of housing conditions on the health of the people at al-Ama'ri refugee camp in the West Bank of Palestine. *Int. J. Environ. Health. Res.* 13 (4), pp. 315-326, 2003.

[2]   Bierman-Lytle, P. Creating a healthy home: environmental building materials-what are they? Where are they*?. Environ. Health. Perspect.* 103(6), pp. 67 – 70. 1995.

[3]   Chiaverini, L., Hesser, J. & Fulton, P. Damp Housing Conditions and Asthma in Rhode Island. Office of Health Statistics: Department of Health in Rhode Island. 5 (5), 2003.

[4]   Cardoso, M.R.A., Cousens, S.N., Alves, F.M., Ribeiro, M.M.M. & Abreu Nato, B.P. Diagnosis and prognosis of wheezing disorders in young children in the city of Sao Paulo, Southeast Brazil. *Acta Paediatr*, 89, pp1484-1489, 2000.

[5]   Curtis, C., Cave B & Coutts A. Is urban regeneration good for health? Perceptions and theories of the health impacts of urban changes. *Environ.Plann.C: Gov Policy*: 20, pp-517-534, 2002.

[6]   Dunn, J.R. Housing and inequalities in health: a study of socioeconomic dimensions of housing and self reported health from a survey of Vancouver residents. *J. Epidemiol. Community. Health.* 56, pp 671-681, 2002.

[7]   Evans G., & Kantrowitz E.. Socio economic status and health: the potential role of environmental risk exposure. *Annal of .Review of Public. Health* 23: 303-31, 2002

[8]   Evans G, Lercher P & Kofler W. Crowding and Children's Mental Health: The Role of House Type. Journal of Environmental Psychology.. 22: 221-31, . 2002.

[9]   Fawaz, M. *Strategizing for Housing: An investigation of the production and reulation of low-income housing in the suburbs of Beirut.* Unpublished Dissertation, MIT, USA, 2004.

[10]   Galea, S & Vlahov, D. Urban health: evidence, challenges and directions. *Ann. Rev. Public. Health* 26: pp. 1-25, 2005.

[11]   Gray, A. Definitions of crowding and the effects of crowding on health: a literature review. Ministry of Social Policy, New Zealand, 2001.

[12]   Hynes, P., Brugg, D., Watts, J., & Lally, J. Public health and the physical environment in Boston Public Housing: A community-based survey and action agenda. *J. Plann. Pract. Res.* 15,(1/2): 31-49, 2000.

[13]   Jackson, M. The Impact of the Built Environment on Health: An Emerging Field. *Am. J. Public. Health.* 93: pp. 1382-1384 , 2003.

[14]   Jones, A.P. Asthma and domestic air quality. *Soc. Sci Med.* 47(6), 755-764, 1998.

[15]   Kahlmeier, S., Schindler, C., Grize, L. & Braun-Fahrlander, C. Perceived environmental housing quality and wellbeing of movers. *J Epidemiol Community Health.* 55: pp. 708-715, 2001.

[16]   Krieger, J & Higgins, D.L. Housing and Health: Time Again for Public Health Action. *Am. J. Public. Health.* 92(5), pp 758-768, 2002.

[17]   Kumie A, & Berhane Y. Crowding in a traditional rural housing ("Tukul") in Ethiopia. *Ethiop. J. Health Dev.* 16(3), 303-309, 2002.

[18]   Lawrence, R.J Housing and Health. World Health. March/April, 44 (2), 21, 1991.

[19]   Lowry, S. *Housing and Health*, London: British Medical Journal, 1991.

[20]   Myers D, Baer W & Choi, SY. The changing problem of overcrowded housing. *J. Am. Plann Association* 62 (5): 66-84, 1996.

[21]   Northridge, M., Sclar, E & Biswas, P. Sorting out the connection between the built environment and health: A conceptual framework for navigating

pathways and planning health cities. J. *Urban Health: Bulletin of New York Academic of Medicine.* 80 (4:12), pp. 556-567, 2003.

[22] Perdue, W.C., Stone, L & Gostin. L.O The Built Environment and Its Relationship to the Public's Health: The Legal Framework. *Am J Public Health* 93, 1390-1394, 2003.

[23] Samet, J & Spengler, JD Indoor Environments and Health: Moving Into the 21st Century". *Am. J. Public. Health.* 93(9), pp. 1489-1493, 2003.

[24] Sharfstein, J & Sander, M Inadequate housing. *J. Housing and Community Development,* 55 (4), pp. 14-24, 1998.

[25] Sirnivasan, S., O'Fallon, L.& Dearry, A. Creating healthy communities, health homes, healthy people: Initiating a research agenda on the built environment and public health. *Am. J. Public. Health.* 93 (9): pp1446-1450, 2003.

[26] Thomson, H., Petticrew, M and Morrison, D. Health effects of housing improvement: systematic review of intervention studies. *BMJ* 323,187-190, 2003.

[27] United States Census of Bureau Census 2000: The American Housing Survey. United States of America, 2000.

[28] Wallerstein, N, Duran, B.M., Aguilar, J., Lorendo, J., Loretto, F., Toya, A., Yepa-Waquie, H., Padilla, R and Shendo, K. Jemez Pueblo: Built and Social-Cultural Environments and Health Within a Rural American Indian Community in the Southwest. *Am. J. Public. Health* 93, pp. 1517-1518, 2003.

[29] WHO World Health Organization. International Statistical Classification of Diseases and Related Health Problems (10th Edition). WHO, Geneva, 1992.

[30] Xavier, R., Braubach, M., Moissoner. B., Monolbaev, K & Robbel, N Housing and health in Europe: Preliminary Results of a Pan-European Study. *Am. J. Public. Health.* 93 (9), 1559-1563, 2003.

Development of a comprehensive indoor environment indicator for green building labelling in Taiwan

C.-M. Lai
Department of Construction Technology, Leader University, Taiwan

Abstract

This paper presents the methodology for developing a comprehensive indicator for indoor environment assessment. It intends to provide the occupants with the measures of Indoor Environment Quality (IEQ). These indicators were drawn up by a literature review based on the practicability, economic and feasible aspects. The categories we considered included acoustics, vibrations, illumination, thermal comfort, indoor air quality, water quality, greens and electromagnetic fields. The AHP (Analytic Hierarchy Process) method was used to carry out the weighting among the categories and these indicators in the same category respectively. The consistency ratio was also calculated to filter out the null questionnaire. Finally, a comprehensive indicator, $IEI_{(AHP)}$ (Indoor Environment Indicator), composed of the filtered indicators, is proposed to assess the indoor environment in built buildings.
Keywords: indoor environment, AHP, green building.

1 Introduction

It is a common consensus within the "green building" activities that indoor-environment issue has to be an essential part of the global sustainability. There is a worldwide trend to develop a system that can provide comprehensive performance-assessments of buildings in different environmental scales: global, local and indoor issue. The government of Taiwan is toward this trend. One of the main areas of an environmental assessment method under development is the impact of the indoor environment on occupants' health.

Chen *et al.* [1] mentioned that indoor environment is important for people's health and welfare, because up to 90% of a typical person's time is spent indoors.

Their productivity is also highly related to the indoor environment. Arthur Rosenfeld, a senior advisor at the U.S. Department of Energy (1998), cited a cost/benefit analysis of high-efficiency filtration in an office building. The costs are $23 a person for filters and $1 a person for energy. The benefits are $39 a person from a 10% decrease in respiratory disease; $70 a person from a 1% increase in productivity among the 20% of workers who are allergic; and $90 a person by decreasing the productivity loss from building-related illness from 1% to 0.75%. Those show a strong relationship between IAQ and productivity, and serious initiatives to improve indoor environment have a tremendous return.

Chiang *et al.* [2,3] pointed out that occupants in a built-environment (illumination, acoustics, air quality, diet, thermal comfort and social environment) reflect the situation, which surrounds them by their physiological and mental sensations (sight, hearing, smell, taste, touch and mentality). The indoor environment is complex and made up of many factors. It's necessary to take various aspects of those environmental factors into consideration, when dealing with the influence of built-environment on occupants.

2 Method

This study describes the method of the indoor environment assessment on existing buildings in Taiwan, and intends to draft indoor-environment preservation indicators from eight categories respectively, including acoustics, vibration, illumination, thermal comfort, indoor air quality (IAQ), water quality, greens and electromagnetic fields (EMF).

2.1 Structure of the indoor environment assessment

In the similar manner of risk assessment, presented by references [4, 5], we propose a comprehensive index, indoor environment index ($IEI_{(AHP)}$), to evaluate the indoor environment. It is assumed that there is an integrated effect accumulated from every category of physical-environment impact on occupants' health. Therefore, the index $IEI_{(AHP)}$ shown in Equation 1 is based on the summation of Sx, the evaluated score of the physical-environment category x, multiplied by Wx, the weighting of the physical-environment category x.

$$IEI_{(AHP)} = \sum S_x \cdot W_x \qquad (1)$$

In addition, there is not less than one indicator in the physical-environment category. The evaluated score of the i_{th} indicator in the category x, Sxi, is evaluated on a score-grade of 20, 40, 60, 80 and 100, which corresponded to the risk values on the occupants' health. When the score of Sxi exceeds 60, it means no sanitary risk is incurred. The Sx is based on the scores consisted of Sxi. If there exists $Sxi<60$, then the score of Sx is the minimum of Sxi in order to emphasize the worst conditions of indoor environment; if for all $Sxi \square 60$, it means that no one is reached sanitary risk, we give Sx the arithmetic mean of Sxi, that's:

$$if, \exists i, S_{xi} < 60, then : S_x = \min(S_{xi}), else, S_x = \frac{1}{n}\sum_{i=1}^{n}S_{xi} \qquad (2)$$

2.2 Weighting

The analytic hierarchy process (AHP) method, which was developed by Thomas L. Saaty (1971) [6], is carried out to do the weighting, Wx, among those indicators in the same category respectively. Expertise with respect to every professional field was involved in the process of deciding the relevant weight. To begin with, the literature review, group brainstorming and Delphi method were used for selecting the proposed indicators. These indicators, then, were classified into the independent categories to set up the hierarchy. The nominal-ratio scale of pairwise comparison among the indicators represented as the score from 1 to 9 was adopted, which was filled in a positive reciprocal matrix to calculate the eigenvector and maximum eigenvalue. The consistency ratio was obtained to filter out the null questionnaire when the value of the consistency index (C.I.) was greater than 0.1. For each category, the weighting value was obtained by the geometric mean of experts' questionnaires.

2.3 Physical indicators

According to the literature review and the authors' knowledge, the indoor physical- environment performance and quality was consisted of eight physical-environment categories. Each category is then expressed in its relevant indicators for field measurement as illustrated in Table 1. There are 48 items of the total indicators as the precise version, then, due to the consideration of the practicable, economic and acceptable aspects, we select 24 items of those significant indicators for simplifying the assessment process as the practical version. These items and their weightings of the physical categories and indicators are determined by the experts' consultation using the AHP analysis.

3 Determination of the essential category and the weighting

From Equation 1, there are two processes of the assessment procedure on the indoor physical-environment. Presented in first process is to determine the essential physical-categories and their relative weighting by the experts' questionnaire. Presented in second process is to define the relationship transferred the physical magnitude of each indicator respectively into the score represented from 20 to 100.

The original weighting is listed in sequencing: "IAQ" (0.221), "Thermal comfort" (0.159), "Acoustics" (0.155), "Illumination" (0.125), "EMF" (0.103), "Greens" (0.070), "Vibration" (0.054) and "Water quality" (0.051). This occurrence reflects the opinions from the experts on the practical aspects of the recent period and the domestic situation. According to the economic sense, the minor categories whose weighting were less than 0.1 were filtered out. It means that the influence ratio of each minor category is less than 10% of whole benefit for the recent environment. Figure 2 shows the results after the adjustment, there are five categories left, and the adjusted weighting is listed in sequencing: "IAQ" (0.290), "Thermal comfort" (0.208), "Acoustics" (0.203), "Illumination" (0.164) and "EMF" (0.135). Substituting the adjusted weighting into Equation 1, we get:

Table 1:   Lists of the indoor physical-environment indicators.

Physical category	Indicators for assessment	Precise version		Practical version	
		general dwelling	office building	general dwelling	office building
Acoustics	$TNEL_{30}$	□	□		
	$TNEL_{30}'$	□	□	□	□
	Equalized sound pressure level in morning time ($L_{eq}M$)	□			
	Equalized sound pressure level in daytime ($L_{eq}D$)		□		◎
	Equalized sound pressure level in night time ($L_{eq}N$)	□	□		
	Equalized sound pressure level in 24 hours ($L_{eq}24H$)	□	□	◎	
	L_{10}	□	□		
	L_{50}	□	□		
	L_{90}	□			
	NR curve	□	□		
	NC curve	□	□		
Illumination	Average illuminance at the targeted face	□		□	
	Average artificial illuminance at the targeted face	□		□	
	Uniformity ratio of illuminance at the targeted face	□		□	
	Uniformity ratio of artificial illuminance at the targeted face	□		□	
	Ratio of daylight-use	□		◎	
	Direct glare at the window face	□			
	Discomfort glare of lamps	□			
	Color temperature of lamps	□			
	Color rendering index	□			
Thermal comfort	Indoor temperature	□		□	
	Indoor humidity	□		□	
	Indoor air velocity	□		□	
	PMV	□		□	
	Temperature difference in altitude	□			
	Solar heat gain	□			
	Outdoor temperature	□			
	Outdoor humidity	□			
	Outdoor air velocity	□			
Indoor air quality	Suspended particle, $PM_{2.5}$	□			
	Suspended particle, PM_{10}	□		□	
	Carbon monoxide (CO)	□		□	
	Carbon dioxide (CO_2)	□		□	
	Formaldehyde (HCHO)	□		□	
	Volatile organic compounds (VOCs)	□		□	
	Ozone (O_3)	□			
	Radon (Rn-222)	□			
	Bacteria	□			
	Fungus	□			
	Endotoxin	□			
	Allergen	□			
	Ventilation rate	□		□	
	Locally average air age	□		□	
Water quality	Tap water quality	□		□	
Greens	Greens covered rate	□		□	
Vibration	Whole body vibration exposure factor	□		□	
Electromagnetic fields	ELF electric field intensity	□		□	
	ELF magnetic flux	□		□	

Table 2:   Scale of the evaluated score corresponded to field-measured value.

Advised indicators Through literature review and experts' consultation	Units	Evaluated score corresponded to the field-measured value				
		20	40	60	80	100
■ "Acoustics" Category						
For dwellings, Equalized SPL in 24 hours (L_{eq}24H)	dB(A)		>55≧	>50≧	>45≧	>40≧
For offices, Equalized SPL in daytime (L_{eq}D)	dB(A)		>59≧	>56≧	>53≧	>50≧
■ "Illumination" category						
Average illuminance of the ambiance	lx		<70≦	<150 ≦	<300 ≦	<500≦
Average illuminance at the operated face in offices	lx		<500≦	<750 ≦	<1000 ≦	<1500≦
Uniformity ratio of illuminance at the targeted face	%		<0.5≦	<0.6≦	<0.7≦	<0.8≦
Ratio of daylight-use	%		<0.5≦	<0.7≦	<1.0≦	<2.0≦
■ "Thermal Comfort" category						
Indoor temperature, summer season	℃		>29≧ <21≦	>28≧ <22≦	>27≧ <23≦	>26≧ <24≦
Indoor temperature, spring & autumn season	℃		>28≧ <20≦	>27≧ <21≦	>26≧ <22≦	>25≧ <23≦
Indoor temperature, winter season	℃		>27≧ <19≦	>26≧ <18≦	>25≧ <17≦	>24≧ <16≦
Indoor Relative Humidity	%		>90≧ <30≦	>80≧ <35≦	>70≧ <40≦	>60≧ <45≦
Indoor air velocity	m/sec		>0.45≧	>0.35 ≧	>0.25 ≧	>0.15≧
PMV	--		>2.0≧ <-2.0≦	>1.5≧ <-1.5≦	>1.0≧ <-1.0≦	>0.5≧ <-0.5≦
■ "Indoor Air Quality" category						
Suspended particulate matter (PM_{10}), 24 hr	mg/m³		>350≧	>150 ≧	>50≧	>25≧
Carbon monoxide (CO), 8 hr	ppm		>15≧	>9≧	>4.5≧	>2≧
Carbon dioxide (CO_2), 8 hr	ppm		>2500≧	>1000 ≧	>800 ≧	>600≧
Formaldehyde (HCHO), 8 hr	ppb		>1000≧	>100 ≧	>16≧	>8≧
Volatile organic compounds (VOCs), 8hr	mg/m³		>3≧	>0.3≧	>0.1≧	>0.5≧
■ "Electromagnetic Fields" category						
Electric field intensity of extremely low frequency (ELF)	kV/m		>25≧	>19≧	>12≧	>5≧
Magnetic flux of extremely low frequency (ELF)	μ tesla		>1600≧	>1100 ≧	>600 ≧	>100≧

$$IEI_{(AHP)} = 0.203 \cdot S_{Acoustics} + 0.164 \cdot S_{Illumination} \tag{3}$$
$$+ 0.208 \cdot S_{ThermalComfort} + 0.290 \cdot S_{IAQ} + 0.135 \cdot S_{EMF}$$

The scale being used to transmit the value of the field-measurement to a grade is the score of 20, 40, 60, 80 and 100. Table 2 shows the relationship of the evaluated score corresponded to the field-measurement magnitude. These indicators consisted from the five categories were advised through literature review and experts' consultation on the practicable and essential aspects. The manner of score-evaluation was represented a five-interval scale, divided from the physical magnitude, and used a set of references as the benchmarks for determining the scores of 20, 40, 60, 80 and 100. Here, the references corresponded to the score 60 were referred to the criteria of the regulation adopted widely for human-health protection. It means evaluated score of any indicator is less than 60, respectively.

In "Acoustics" category, two indicators, the equalized sound pressure Leq24H for dwellings and LeqD for offices, were included. In "Illumination" category, four indicators, including the intensity of illuminance for the ambiance and the operated face, uniformity ratio and daylight-use ratio, were used for assessment. In "Thermal Comfort" category, there were six indicators for assessment, including indoor temperature in various season, relative humidity, air velocity and PMV. In "IAQ" category, five common indoor air pollutants were appointed as the characteristic compounds. In "EMF" category, the electric-field intensity and the magnetic flux on the extremely low frequency (50/60 Hz) were used.

4 Conclusion

The presented results, announced a set of physical indicators, the weightings of various physical categories and evaluated scales corresponded to the field-measured values, are feasible for the assessment on the built environment to benefit the occupants' health. The experts' opinions, based on the recent situation and the domestic environment, were applied.

The project is now proposed to continue with the field measurement and occupants' questionnaire to make up the assessment system, especially on identifying the weightings and the evaluated scales. Also, for a planned building, the project is proposing to develop the assessment method, which suit to the planned building. The same structure will be used, but the input will be taken the place of the data obtained from the checklists, including the quality assurance system, drawings, and descriptions of a building. From many aspects, it is more difficult to predict future.

Acknowledgement

The authors would like to thank the National Science Council of the Republic of China for financially supporting this research under Contract No. NSC 89-2621-Z-006-019.

References

[1]   Chen, Q., Yuan, X.X. *et al.*, Detailed Experimental Data of Room Airflow with Displacement Ventilation. *Proceedings of 6th International Conference on Air Distribution in Rooms, ROOMVENT '98*, Stockholm (Sweden), 1998, Vol. 1, pp. 133-140.

[2]   Chiang, C.M. *et al.*, Empirical Study on post-occupancy evaluation of housing indoor air environment in Taiwan. *Journal of Housing Studies*, 1994, No. 2, Jan. RESEARCH, pp.107-132 (in Chinese).

[3]   Chiang, C.M., Chou, P.C. *et al.*, A Study of the Impacts of Outdoor Air and Living Behavior Pattern on Indoor Air Quality - Case Studies of Apartments in Taiwan. *Proceedings of Indoor Air '96*, Nagoya (Japan), 1996, Vol. 3, pp. 735-740.

[4]   Anderson, E. L. and Albert, R. E., *Risk Assessment and Indoor Air Quality*, Lewis Publishers.

[5]   Hult, M., Assessment of Indoor Environment in Existing Buildings. *Proceedings of Green Building Challenge '98*, Vancouver (Canada), 1998, Vol. 2, pp. 139-146.

[6]   Saaty, T.L., Erdener, E., A new approach to performance measurement the analytic hierarchy process. *Design Methods and Theories*, 1979, Vol. 13, No. 2.

Section 8
Remediation

Biodegradation of carbaryl and phthalate isomers by soil microorganisms

P. S. Phale
Biotechnology, School of Biosciences and Bioengineering,
Indian Institute of Technology-Bombay, Powai, Mumbai-400 076, India

Abstract

Pseudomonas sp. strain PP4 and C5 utilize phthalate isomers (*o-, m-* and *p-*) and carbaryl as carbon source, respectively. Degradative pathways were elucidated by isolating and characterizing metabolites, whole-cell O_2 uptake and enzyme activity studies. Metabolic studies suggest that phthalate isomer degrading pathways converge at 3,4-dihydroxybenzoic acid. Phthalate dioxygenases responsible for the degradation of the respective phthalate isomers are induced specifically, suggesting that probably there are three different phthalate dioxygenases. This was supported by whole-cell O_2 uptake studies and cells grown on glucose failed to show the activity of phthalate pathway enzymes. Glucose-grown cells lost the phthalate degradation property indicating probable involvement of plasmid, which is expressed and maintained selectively in the presence of phthalate isomers. The metabolic studies with *Pseudomonas* sp. strain C5 suggest that carbaryl is first hydrolyzed to 1-naphthol by carbaryl hydrolase. Generated 1-naphthol is metabolized *via* 1,2-dihydroxynaphahtlane, salicylate and gentisic acid to TCA cycle intermediates, thus serving as the sole source of carbon and energy. The ability to utilize phthalates (0.3%) and carbaryl (1%) at high concentrations make these strains suitable candidates for bioremediation. Detailed understanding of metabolic pathways and genetic make-up will enable one to modify these strains by genetic engineering tools for suitable application in bioremediation.
Keywords: Phthalate degradation, Carbaryl metabolism, oxygenases, bioremediation, pseudomonas.

1 Introduction

Aromatic hydrocarbons are used heavily in various industries, which found their way in to soil, water and air thus polluting the environment. Due to the persistence of these toxic and carcinogenic compounds in nature, microbes have evolved with novel metabolic pathways to release the 'Locked Carbon'. Phthalate isomers (*o*-, *m*- and *p*-) and their esters are major industrial pollutants, used heavily in plastic, textile, paint, pesticide carrier, munition, and cosmetic industries. The majority of them are recalcitrant and toxic causing teratogenic, reproductive and neuromuscular disorders [1]. The microbial metabolism of *o*-phthalate is well studied. Many *Pseudomonas* sp. have been reported to degrade *o*-phthalate and phthalate esters to 4,5-dihydroxyphthalate, which enters into the TCA cycle *via* 3,4-dihydroxybenzoate [2]. However very little is known about the degradation of tere- and iso-phthalate. So far there are no reports on a single bacterial strain degrading all three phthalate isomers as the sole carbon source. Besides an environmental pollutant, isophthalate is known to be a competitive inhibitor of glutamate dehydrogenase (GDH) responsible for conversion of α-ketoglutarate to glutamate [3].

Carbamate insecticides, such as carbaryl (1-naphthyl-*N*-methylcarbamate), are highly toxic with a wide range of activities and are used heavily in agricultural industry. Carbamates are competitive inhibitors of neuronal nicotinic acetylcholine receptors and acetylcholinesterase [4]. *N*-Nitrosocarbamates and 1-naphthol generated are potent mutagens, more toxic and recalcitrant than carbaryl itself [5, 6]. Microbial metabolic studies have indicated that the first step in degradation is hydrolysis of carbaryl to 1-naphthol by hydrolase. Depending on the strain, 1-naphthol is metabolized *via* salicylate to either gentisate or catechol [7-10], however the steps and enzymes responsible for the conversion of 1-naphthol to salicylate have not been demonstrated so far.

We have isolated two soil bacterial strains capable of utilizing phthalate isomers and carbaryl. Here we are presenting the metabolic pathway and inhibition of GDH by isophthalate in strain PP4. Based on the metabolic studies, we propose the carbaryl degradation *via* 1,2-dihydroxynaphthalene (1,2-DHN) in *Pseudomonas* sp. strain C5.

2 Materials and methods

2.1 Organism and growth

Pseudomonas sp. strain PP4 and C5 were isolated by an enrichment culture technique from soil contaminated with petroleum products. Strains were grown on Minimal Salt Medium [11] at 30°C with appropriate carbon source.

2.2 Metabolite isolation, bio-transformation and whole-cell O$_2$ uptake studies

To isolate and identify carbaryl metabolites, a late-log phase spent medium was acidified to pH 2 with 2N HCl and extracted with equal volume of ethyl acetate, dried over anhydrous sodium sulfate, concentrated and analyzed by TLC using Hexane:Chloroform:Acetic acid 8:2:1 (v/v/v). Metabolites were identified by TLC (R_f and UV-fluorescence), GC-MS and UV-Visible spectroscopy. GC-MS analysis was carried out on Hewlett-Packard G1800A mass spectrometer attached to a gas chromatograph as described [12]. Whole-cell O_2 uptake rates were monitored as described [13], using an Oxygraph (Hansatech, UK) fitted with Clark's type O_2 electrode. Rates were corrected for endogenous O_2 consumption and expressed as nmol of O_2 consumed min^{-1} (mg wet cells)$^{-1}$.

2.3 Preparation of cell-free extracts, enzyme assays and activity staining

PP4 cells were harvested, washed and suspended in buffer HEPES (20 mM, pH 8.5), EDTA (1 mM) and NaCl (100 mM) and disrupted by sonication using an Ultrasonic processor (model GE130, USA) at 4°C. The cell homogenate was centrifuged and the supernatant was used as the source of enzyme. GDH was assayed spectrophotometrically and activity staining was performed as described [14]. Pseudomonas C5 cells were suspended in K-phosphate buffer (50 mM, pH 7.5, K-PO$_4$ buffer) and disrupted by sonication at 4°C, 4 cycles of 15 pulses each, out-put 11 watt. Cell homogenate was centrifuged at 40,000 g for 30 min at 4°C. The clear membrane-free supernatant obtained was referred to as cell-free extract and used as enzyme source. Carbaryl hydrolase (CH) was monitored spectrophotometrically by measuring the rate of increase in absorbance at 322 nm due to formation of 1-naphthol. The reaction mixture (1 ml) contained substrate (100 µM), an appropriate amount of enzyme and K-PO$_4$ buffer. The activity was calculated by using molar extinction coefficient of 1-naphthol ε_{322nm} 2200 in K-PO$_4$ buffer. 1-Naphthol hydroxylase (1-NH) was monitored by the oxygraph method. The reaction mixture (2 ml) contained K-PO$_4$ buffer, substrate (100 µM), FAD (6.25 µM) and NADH (100 µM). Reaction was started by addition of an appropriate amount of enzyme. 1,2-Dihydroxynaphthalene dioxygenase (12DHNO, 15), gentisate dioxygenase (GDO, 16), protocatechuate dioxygenase (PDO, 17) and catechol dioxygenase (CO, 18) were monitored as described. The specific activities are reported as $nmol.min^{-1}.mg^{-1}$ of protein. Protein estimation was carried out as described [19].

3 Results and discussion

3.1 Metabolism of phthalate isomers by Pseudomonas strain PP4

Pseudomonas strain PP4 has the ability to utilize all three-phthalate isomers as the sole source of carbon. Cell respiration studies are summarized in Table 1. Cells grown on isophthalate showed good respiration on isophthalate and 3,4-DHB and similar results were observed for other phthalate isomers. The cells failed to respire on 2,3-DHB and 2,5-DHB (Table 1). These results suggest that specific phthalate isomer induces respective phthalate dioxygenase responsible for the initial ring hydroxylation, which is further metabolized to TCA cycle intermediate *via* 3,4-DHB. Glucose-grown cells failed to show O_2 uptake suggesting that the enzymes are inducible. Based on these results the proposed pathway is as shown in Fig.1.

Table 1:   Whole-cell O_2 uptake rates by strain PP4 grown on different carbon sources (Iso, Isophthalate; Pht, Phtalate; Tere, Terephthalate; Glc, Glucose; DHB, dihydroxybenzoate; nd, not detected; tr, O_2 uptake < 0.5 nmol min^{-1} mg^{-1}).

Carbon	Cell respiration on intermediates, nmol O_2 consumed min^{-1} mg^{-1}					
	Iso	Pht	Tere	3,4-DHB	2,3-DHB	2,5-DHB
Iso	1.6	nd	nd	2.6	tr	tr
Pht	nd	3.5	nd	2.7	tr	1.2
Tere	nd	nd	3.5	1.9	nd	tr
Glc	tr	tr	tr	tr	tr	tr

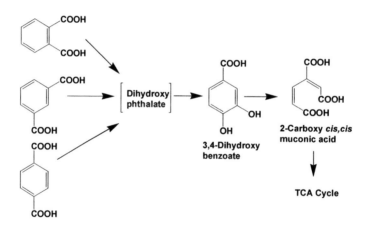

Figure 1:   Proposed pathway for the degradation of three phthalate isomers by strain PP4.

The metabolic pathway for phthalate is studied in detail for various enzymes involved, gene regulation and role of plasmids. However, not much information is available on the degradation of iso- and tere-phthalates. Strain PP4 is unique and utilizes all phthalate isomers and converges metabolic pathway into 3,4-DHB. Generated 3,4DHB is ring cleaved to 2-carboxy-*cis,cis*-muconic acid which enters TCA cycle, thus serving as the sole source of carbon and energy. When grown on simple carbon source like glucose, the cells lost their ability to degrade phthalate isomers, suggesting that probably the degradation phenotype is unstable in the absence of specific carbon source and probably genes are located on the plasmid.

3.2 Isophthalate as GDH inhibitor

GDH catalyzes reversible reaction, and equilibrium favors glutamate synthesis. In microorganisms, the biosynthetic reaction of GDH (ammonia assimilating) is catalyzed by NADP-GDH while the oxidative deamination reaction is catalyzed by NAD-GDH. Strain PP4 has NADP-GDH when grown on isophthalate. Glutamate-grown cells had high NAD-GDH activity compared to glucose-grown cells (Table 2). Inhibition of GDH by isophthalate (1mM) is shown in Table 2. GDH from glucose grown PP4 is more sensitive (66%) to isophthalate inhibition compared to GDH from isophthalate grown cells (28%).

Table 2: Specific activity of GDH and its inhibition by isophthalate (1 mM). (Glc, glucose; Glu, glutamate; nd, no activity detected; values in bracket are % inhibition).

Growth on	Amination reaction		
	NADH	NADPH	NADPH+Iso
Iso	nd	231	166 (28)
Glc	28	184	63 (66)
Glu	108	41	22 (47)

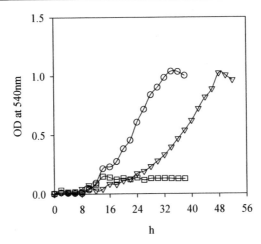

Figure 2: Effect of glutamate on the growth profile of strain PP4 on isophthalate (∇); iosphthalate + glutamate ($\bigcirc$) and glutamate ($\square$).

Strain PP4 when grown on isophthalate showed a lag phase of ~ 20 h and reached a stationary phase by 48 h. When supplemented with 1mM glutamate, cells grew faster with short lag phase (12 h) and reached a stationary phase around 34 h (Fig. 2). In the initial phase of the growth, glutamate is taken up by the cells, which might be helping to overcome the inhibition by isophthalate and hence the culture is growing faster with small lag phase. NADP-GDH activity staining was done with crude extracts from PP4 grown on different carbon sources. The staining pattern for PP4 on isophthalate showed a staining band of lower mobility compared to glucose grown cells. These results suggest that in strain PP4 two GDH isozymes are present and induced depending on the carbon source.

Rapid growth on isophthalate in the presence of glutamate and carbon source dependent changes in the isozyme pattern suggests inhibition of GDH by isophthalate *in vivo*. Probably, isophthalate is acting as a metabolic inhibitor.

3.3 Metabolism of Carbaryl by *Pseudomonas* sp. strain C5

To elucidate the carbaryl degradative pathway, metabolites were extracted and resolved by TLC. Four major spots with R_f, UV fluorescence and GCMS properties similar to authentic carbaryl, 1-naphthol, salicylate and gentisate were identified (Table 3). The analysis failed to detect spots corresponding to 1,4-naphthoquinone and catechol.   To elucidate the metabolic sequence, biotransformation experiments were performed using carbaryl, 1,4-naphthoquinone and salicylaldehyde. When cells were supplemented with carbaryl, TLC showed metabolite spots similar to authentic carbaryl, 1-naphthol, salicylate and gentisate. With salicylaldehyde, two major metabolites salicylate and gentisate were detected. However no metabolites with 1,4-naphthoquinone were observed.

Table 3:   Identification of carbaryl metabolites from the spent media.

TLC		UV-Vis (nm)	MS analysis {m/z (% relative intensity) [molecular ion]}	Inference
R_f	UV-Fluo			
0.62	Dark blue	280, 312, 318	201(4)[M^+], 144(100), 127(3), 115(52), 89(10), 77(2)	Carbaryl
0.73	Brown black	298, 308, 323	144(100)[M^+], 115(77), 88(10), 77(2)	1-Naphthol
0.77	Sky blue	306	--	Salicylate
0.15	Blue-green	338	154(37)[M^+], 136(100), 108(10), 77(1)	Gentisate

To elucidate steps involved in the conversion of 1-naphthol to salicylaldehyde, whole-cell O_2 uptake rates, enzyme activities in the cell-free extracts and products of bulk enzyme reactions were monitored. Cells showed good O_2 uptake on carbaryl, 1-naphthol, 1,2-DHN, salicylate and gentisate (Table 4). Salicylate grown cells showed O_2 uptake on salicylate and gentisate but significantly low respiration on carbaryl, 1-naphthol, 1,2-DHN and salicylaldehyde. However, glucose grown cells showed very low respiration (Table 4).

Table 4: Whole-cell O_2 uptake rates for cells grown on various carbon sources.

	O_2 uptake* (nmol of O_2 consumed $min^{-1}.mg^{-1}$ cells), cells grown on		
	Carbaryl	Salicylate	Glucose
Carbaryl	3.8	tr	tr
1-Naphthol	7.8	tr	tr
1,2-DHN	1.0	tr	tr
1,4-Naphthoquinone	tr[#]	tr	tr
Salicylaldehyde	4.4	0.4	tr
Salicylate	1.2	0.7	tr
Gentisic acid	1.7	1.0	tr
Catechol	tr	tr	tr

* Values corrected for endogenous O_2 uptake; # tr, uptake rates < 0.3 nmol.

Table 5: Various enzyme activities from the cell-free.

Enzyme	Specific activity, $nmol.min^{-1}.mg^{-1}$ protein		
	Carbaryl	Salicylate	Glucose
CH	71	1.1	1.1
1-NH	270	4	2
1,2-DHNO	52	32	29
GDO	425	601	1
CO	56	55	39

Specific activities of CH, 1-NH, 1,2-DHNO and GDO are summarized in Table 5. Salicylate cultures showed a comparable activity of GDO and a significantly low activity of CH and 1-NH. All enzyme activities from glucose grown cells were significantly low (Table 5). The enzyme activities and whole-cell O_2 uptake rates from carbaryl and glucose grown cells suggest that the enzymes are inducible. Involvement of 1-naphthol and salicylate in carbaryl metabolism is reported earlier. Here we demonstrate, for the first time, the presence of 1-NH and 1,2-DHNO activities in the cell-free extract of carbaryl degrading strains. 1-NH was studied for its cofactor and O_2 requirement. Under aerobic conditions the cell-free extract showed conversion of 1-naphthol to salicylate in the presence of NADH and FAD. However under anaerobic conditions, we failed to detect salicylate. These results suggest that the enzyme is oxygenase type and requires O_2 for its optimum activity. The enzyme showed good activity with FAD and NADH. When NADPH and FAD were used as cofactors, 20-30% increase in activity was observed.

Based on metabolite studies, we propose a degradative pathway for carbaryl in strain C5 as shown in Fig. 3.

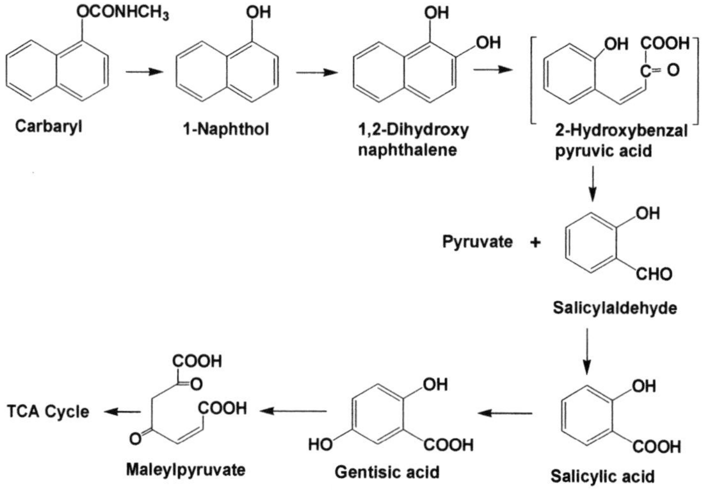

Figure 3: Proposed pathway for the degradation of carbaryl in *Pseudomonas* sp. strain C5.

It has been proposed that prior to ring cleavage, 1-naphthol is hydroxylated either to 4-hydroxy-1-tetralone [21], 3,4-dihydro-dihydroxy-1(2H)-naphthalenone [22] or 1,4-naphthoquinone [23]. Detection of 1-NH, and 1,2-DHNO activity and whole cell O_2 uptake on 1-naphthol and 1,2-DHN strongly suggests 1,2-DHN as intermediate in the pathway. The pathway from 1,2-DHN onward is similar to the naphthalene metabolic pathway, however strain C5 failed to utilize naphthalene.

In conclusion, strains PP4 and C5 are unique, degrade phthalate isomers and carbaryl at higher concentrations, respectively. These strains are isolated from the environment and are very efficient in degradation of compounds of interest. Further characterization and genetic engineering of these strains helps in the degradation of a wide range of aromatic hydrocarbons efficiently. Development of such a metabolically engineered strain has an advantage and will help in effective bioremediation and environmental pollution clean up processes.

Acknowledgement

We thank DBT, Govt. of India for the Research grant.

References

[1] Lovecamp, S.T. & Davis, B.J., Mechanism of phthalate ester toxicity in the female reproductive system. *Environmental Health Perspectives,* **111**, pp. 139-146, 2003.

[2] Ribbons, D.W., Keyser, P., Kunz, D.A., Taylor, B.F., Eaton, R.W. & Anderson, B.N., Microbial degradation of Phthalates. In: Gibson, D. T.,

(ed) Microbial degradation of organic compounds. Marcel Dekker, Inc. New York and Basel. pp. 371-398, 1984.

[3] Caughey, W.S., Smiley, D.J. & Hellerman, L., L-Glutamic acid dehydrogenase: Structural requirements for substrate competition: effect of Thyroxine. *J. Biol. Chem.*, **224**, pp. 591-607,1957.

[4] Smulders, C.J., Bueters, T.J., Van Kleef, R.G. & Vijverberg, H.P., Selective effects of carbamate pesticides on rat neuronal nicotinic acetylcholine receptors and rat brain acetylcholinesterase. *Toxicol. Appl. Pharmacol.*, **193**, pp. 139-146, 2003.

[5] Elespuru R., Lijinsky, W. & Setlow, J.K., Nitrosocarbaryl as a potent mutagen of environmental significance. *Nature,* **247**, pp. 386-387, 1974.

[6] Wilson, G.D., d'Arcy Doherty, M. & Cohen, G.M., Selective toxicity of 1-naphthol to human colorectal tumor tissue. *Br. J. Cancer*, **51**, pp. 853-63, 1985.

[7] Chapalamadugu, S. & Chaudhry, G.R.. Hydrolysis of carbaryl by *Pseudomonas* sp. and construction of a microbial consortium that completely metabolizes carbaryl. *Appl. Environ. Microbiol.*, **57**, pp. 744-750, 1991.

[8] Doddamani, H.P. & Ninnekar, H.Z., Biodegradation of carbaryl by a *Micrococcus* species. *Curr. Microbiol.*, **43**, pp. 69-73, 2001.

[9] Hayatsu, M., Hirano, M. & Nagata, T., Involvement of two plasmids in the degradation of carbaryl by *Arthrobacter* sp. strain RC100. *Appl. Environ. Microbiol.,* **65**, pp. 1015-1019, 1999.

[10] Larkin, M.J. & Day, M.J., The metabolism of carbaryl by three bacterial isolates, *Pseudomonas* sp. (NCIB 12042 & 12043) and *Rhodococcus* sp. (NCIB 12038) from garden soil. *J. Bacteriol.*, **60**, pp. 233-242, 1986.

[11] Mahajan, M.C., Phale, P.S. & Vaidyanathan C.S., Evidence for the involvement of multiple pathways in the biodegradation of 1- and 2-methylnaphthalene by *Pseudomonas putida* CSV86. *Arch. Microbiol.,* **161**, pp. 425-433, 1994.

[12] Basu, A., Dixit, S.S. & Phale, P.S., Metabolism of benzyl alcohol via catechol *ortho*-pathway in methylnaphthalene-degrading *Pseudomonas putida* CSV86. *Appl. Microbiol. Biotechnol.,* **62**, pp. 579-585, 2003.

[13] Phale, P.S., Mahajan, M.C. & Vaidyanathan, C.S., A pathway for biodegradation of 1-napthoic acid by *Pseudomonas maltophilia* CSV 89. *Arch. Microbiol.,* **163**, pp. 42-47, 1995.

[14] Bellion, E. & Tan, F., NADP-dependent glutamate dehydrogenase from a facultative methylotroph, *Pseudomonas* sp. strain AM1. *J. Bacteriol.,* **157**, pp. 435-439, 1984.

[15] Patel, T.R. & Barnsley, E.A., Naphthalene metabolism by Pseudomonads: purification and properties of 1,2-dihydroxynaphthalene oxygenase. *J. Bacteriol.*, **143**, pp. 668-673, 1980.

[16] Suarez, M., Ferrer, E. & Martin, M., Purification and biochemical characterization of gentisate 1,2-dioxygenase from *Klebsiella pneumoniae* M5a1. *FEMS Microbiol. Lett.*, **143**, pp. 89-95, 1996.

[17]   Whittaker, J.W., Orville, A.M. & Lipscomb, J.D., Protocatechuate 3,4-dioxygenase from *Brevibacterium fuscum. Meth. Enzymol.,* **188**, pp. 82-88, 1990.

[18]   Kojima, Y., Fujisawa, H., Nakazawa, A., Nakazawa, T., Kanetsuna, F., Taniuchi, H., Nozaki, M. & Hayashi, O., Studies on pyrocatechase: Purification and spectral properties. *J. Biol. Chem.,* **242**, pp. 3270-3278, 1967.

[19]   Lowry, O.H., Rosebrough, N.J., Farr, A.L. & Randall, R.J., Protein measurement with the folin phenol reagent *J. Biol. Chem.,* **193**, pp. 265-275, 1951.

[20]   Wang, Y.Z., Zhou, Y. & Zylstra, G.J., Molecular analysis of Isophthalate and Terephthalate degradation by *Comamonas testetosteroni.* YZW-D *Environmental Health Perspectives,* **103**, pp. 9-12, 1995.

[21]   Bollag, J.M., Czaplicki, E.J. & Minard, R.D., Bacterial metabolism of 1-naphthol. *J. Agr. Food. Chem.,* **23**, pp. 85-90, 1975.

[22]   Walker, N., Janes, N.F., Spokes, J.R. & Van Berkum, P., Degradation of 1-naphthol by a soil Pseudomonad. *J. Appl. Bacteriol.,* **39**, pp. 281-286, 1975.

[23]   Rajgopal, B.S., Rao, V.R., Nagendraappa, G. & Sethunathan, N., Metabolism of carbaryl and carbofuran by soil enrichment and bacterial cultures. *Can. J. Microbiol.,* **30**, pp. 1458-1466, 1984.

Environmental pollutants and human diseases: diagnosis and treatment

G. Passerini[1], R. Cocci Grifoni[1] & M. M. Mariani[2]
[1]*Dipartimento di Energetica, Università Politecnica delle Marche, Italy*
[2]*SITEC, Società Italiana Terapia Chelante, Italy*

Abstract

Environmental factors play a central role in the processes of human development, health, and disease. Human exposure to hazardous agents in the air, water, soil, and food and to physical hazards in the environment is a major contributor to increased morbidity and mortality. Hazardous substances that originally are discharged as air pollutants may find their pathway to human exposure through multiple routes, including ingestion and dermal contact, as well as direct inhalation. The mechanisms for modeling and understanding the fate of air pollutants through atmospheric transport, deposition into water and soil, bioaccumulation, and ultimate uptake to receptor organs and systems in the human body are complex. A single contaminant source often may represent only a fraction of a total body pollutant burden. The EDTA chelation therapy enables the removal of toxic metals and excess calcium from the body.

In this study we present results related to the detoxification treatment through continuous intravenous infusion of EDTA of 78 patients with cardiovascular problems and chronic fatigue syndrome. A comparison between toxic metals found in urine before and after the chelation-therapy treatment has been carried out. EDTA has been administered before urine collection, and a wide range of toxic metals (mercury, lead, arsenic, cadmium, nickel, and others) has been measured with reference to urine creatinine.

1 Introduction

Health effects originated by air pollutants range from subtle biochemical and physiological changes to difficult breathing, wheezing, coughing and aggravation of existing respiratory and cardiac pathologies. Many health effects are directly associated with breathing of polluted air, but air also transports pollutants and deposits them onto soils or surface waters, where they can potentially affect plants, crops, property, and animals. Toxic substances in plants and animals can move through the food chain and pose potential risks to human health.

Through eating, breathing and skin absorption, some contaminants (namely Aluminium, Mercury, Iron, Lead, Cadmium) can be accumulated into the body and become a source of excess free radicals. Natural detoxification pathways of the body cannot eliminate them and the build-up can eventually reach toxic and dangerous levels. Too much Iron can give rise to heart problems and high levels of Lead and Cadmium can trigger high blood pressure. In addition high levels of toxic metals can lead to chronic fatigue and multiple chemical sensitivity (MCS) syndrome also known as environmental illness.

EDTA is well recognized as a therapy for Lead toxicity. EDTA also removes other toxic heavy metals such as Iron, which promote cancer, by catalyzing free radical pathology.

The intravenous infusion of Ethylene Diamine Tetra-Acetic Acid (EDTA), together with certain minerals and vitamins in measured dosages, is the main part of the chelation therapy treatment. A slow-drip method is used to administer such infusion, which flows through the bloodstream and, in the process, flushes out toxic metals. EDTA, the main component of chelation therapy has the capacity to bind with toxic heavy metals, such as Lead, Cadmium, Aluminium, and Mercury, and pull them out of the body in the urine, through the kidneys.

Large amounts of oral and intravenous antioxidants are given with chelation therapy, especially E and C vitamins. Treatment is aimed at removing accumulation in the body of harmful levels of Aluminium, Iron, Copper, and toxic heavy metals, all of which enhance free radical damage. Treatment objectives also include the removal of metastatic calcium from soft tissues, enhancement of the levels of ionic magnesium at cellular level, and reduction of pathologically enhanced clotting mechanisms, especially platelet adhesiveness. These mechanisms of action were described in the extensive review article by Cranton and Frackelton [1].

Chelation therapy protocol is a multifarious procedure that combines intravenous EDTA, nutrition therapies, and lifestyle changes.

Increased urinary Lead excretion after injection of EDTA is a recognized test for heavy metals accumulation in the body. Urinary toxic metals excretion was measured before and after EDTA infusion in 78 patients and, in each case, a substantial increase in heavy metals excretion was measured.

The purpose of this study is to determine more precisely and to statistically analyze the reduction of some pollutant elements after treatment with EDTA.

2 Human health and heavy metal exposure

Metals, a major category of globally distributed pollutants, are natural elements that have been extracted from the earth and harnessed for human activities and products for millennia.

Metals are notable for their wide environmental dispersion from such activity, their tendency to accumulate in select tissues of the human body, and their overall toxicity even at relatively minor levels of exposure.

Some metals, such as Copper and Iron, are essential to life and play irreplaceable roles, for example, in the functioning of critical enzyme systems. Other metals are xenobiotics, i.e. they have no useful role in human physiology (and that of most other living organisms) and may be toxic even at trace levels of exposure as for Lead and Mercury. Even those metals that are essential, however, have the potential to turn harmful at very high levels of exposure.

Exposure to metals can occur through a variety of routes. Metals may be inhaled as dust or fume (tiny particulate matter, such as the Lead Oxide particles produced by the combustion of leaded gasoline). Some metals can be vaporized (e.g., Mercury vapor in the manufacture of fluorescent lamps) and inhaled. Metals may also be ingested involuntarily through food and drink. The amount that is actually absorbed from the digestive tract can vary widely, depending on the chemical form of the metal and on the age and nutritional status of the individual. Once a metal is absorbed, it distributes in tissues and organs. Excretion typically occurs primarily through the kidneys and digestive tract, but metals tend to persist in some storage sites, like liver, bones, and kidneys, for years or decades.

The toxicity of metals most commonly involves the brain and the kidney, but other manifestations occur, and some metals, such as Arsenic, are clearly capable of causing cancer. An individual, even under high-dose and/or acute metal toxicity, typically has very general symptoms, such as weakness or headache. This makes the diagnosis of toxicity of metals, in a clinical setting, very difficult unless a clinician has the knowledge and training to suspect the diagnosis and is able to order the correct diagnostic test. Chronic exposure to metals at a high enough level to cause chronic toxicity effects (such as hypertension in individuals exposed to Lead and renal toxicity in individuals exposed to Cadmium) can also occur in individuals who have no symptoms. Much about metals toxicity, such as the genetic factors that may render some individuals especially vulnerable to metals toxicity, remains a subject of intense investigation. Perhaps, low-level exposure to metals could contribute to the causation of chronic diseases and impaired functioning much more than previously thought.

3   EDTA Chelation therapy

Heavy metals such as Lead, Mercury, Cadmium, Arsenic, Nickel, and Antimony have been shown to relentlessly accumulate in human tissue over a lifetime. These poisonous metals disrupt the normal biochemical processes. They insinuate themselves into the active sites of enzymes thereby altering such enzymes' activities, and they initiate "free radical reactions", which produce noxious chemicals that damage cellular structures such as proteins, cell membranes and DNA. The results at the level of the whole organism are the development of degenerative diseases, arteriosclerosis, arthritis and cancers. The removal of these poisonous metals with Chelation Therapy is probably a major means by which Chelation normalizes biochemical activity thereby improving circulation and energy.

The word "chelation" derives from the Greek word chele, which is the claw of a crab or lobsters. Chelation is thus the natural process of a pincer-like binding of metallic ions to the chelating substance. In the case of Chelation Therapy, a chelating agent does the grasping and a metal atom is the grasped object. This chelating agent forms a very stable chemical complex with a mineral or metal ion known as a "heterocyclic ring structure". There are many examples of chelates in nature such as magnesium in the chlorophyll molecule in plants, iron in the hemoglobin of blood cells in man and other higher organisms and the incorporation of cobalt in the vitamin B-12 molecule.

Chelation is a process whereby the metals are held and positioned by body chemicals so as to facilitate chemical reactions, which are essential to life. Intravenous Chelation Therapy is the introduction by slow infusion of naturally occurring or synthetic organic chemicals into the human body in order to facilitate chemical reactions, which lead to the discharge of poisonous metals from the body and the rearrangement of essential metals in the body for the promotion of life's chemical reactions.

The synthetic chelator, intravenous EDTA (Ethylene Diamine Tetra-acetic Acid, an amino acid) is used in this study as chelating agent (Fig.1).

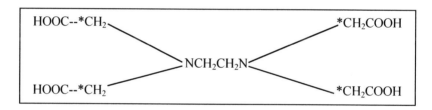

Figure 1:   EDTA molecular structure.

The EDTA drags abnormal metal ions out of the body, reducing the production of free radicals. A free radical is an oxygen molecule with an odd number of electrons in an outer orbital ring of one of its atoms. This characteristic makes the free radical violently reactive with almost any and every cell structure, leading to damage and eventually to degenerative disease processes such as arteriosclerosis. By significantly reducing these reactions, chelation therapy allows the body to heal itself and reverse the disease processes.

In addition, chelation also mobilizes calcium from the bones and other tissues. This actually stimulates additional bone deposition, improving bone density. Calcification of tissues is generally caused when free radical damage upsets cell membranes. This leads to tissue and organ malfunction and eventually to death. Thus the reversal of this process by EDTA chelation therapy can be seen as a true longevity treatment.

Free radicals can damage DNA, which in turn can lead to the development of cancer. A study has shown [2] that EDTA chelation therapy has a protective effect on the development of pollution diseases.

3.1 Mechanism of EDTA

EDTA was synthesized in Germany in 1935, and first patented in the US in 1941. Its first uses were in industry as a chelating agent, as an anticoagulant for clinical laboratory use, and as a treatment for lead poisoning. In 1955, Dr. Norman Clarke, then Director of Research of Providence Hospital in Detroit, Michigan, reported on his use of intravenous EDTA to dissolve what he referred to as "metastatic calcium". Metastatic calcium is calcium that has been deposited where it is not wanted, as in arteries (atherosclerosis), joints (arthritis), kidneys (kidney stones), and the bony ossicular system in the ears (otosclerosis), with generally unfavorable results. Since 1955, hundreds of papers have been published on the effects of chelation therapy in a variety of chronic diseases, the vast majority reporting favorable results.

The first, and probably most widely held belief is that the benefits are due to EDTA's ability to bind with ionic calcium in the blood. This temporarily lowers the blood calcium level, which stimulates the parathyroid gland to release parathyroid hormone (PTH). PTH, in turn, stimulates osteoclastic and osteoblastic activity of the bone, mobilizing calcium from unwanted parts of the body (i.e., arteries, joints, etc).

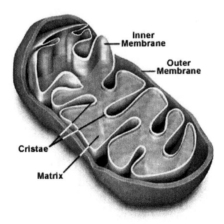

Figure 2:   Mitochondria.

One more significant mechanisms of intravenous EDTA may be that of its ability to "restore mitochondria". Mitochondria are the "power plants" of every cell in the body (Fig. 2). Within the mitochondria the process of oxidative phosphorylation takes place to generate energy by producing ATP without which life could not exist. Loss of mitochondrial function has long been considered as one of the primary causes of the aging process [3-5]. Recently, the role of impaired mitochondrial function in the pathogenesis of many diseases has been reported [6-8]. EDTA was recognized ever since the 50's to have the ability to stabilize mitochondria [9].

The one issue that all chelating physicians overwhelmingly agree on is the great benefits that can be obtained in a variety of degenerative, age-related conditions, using this safe and non-invasive therapy.

3.2 Free Radical theory

In the normal course of metabolism, our body produces small high-energy particles that are known as free radicals. These are unstable molecules with free electrons that can be used for energy production and numerous other physiological functions. In some cells they may be used as the weapons to kill viruses and bacteria. Unfortunately, because of their extremely high energy, they can also be damaging to normal tissues if too many of them are produced.

Free radicals disrupt the normal generation of DNA and alter the lipids (fats) in cell membranes. They also affect the blood vessels and the production of prostaglandins. Prostaglandins regulate many physiological functions. Free radicals are also found in the environment. There are many sources of excess free radicals, including certain metals (such as excess iron), cigarette smoke, air pollution, drugs, poisons, highly processed foods and food additives, ultraviolet sunlight and radiation

According to the free radical theory, perhaps 80-90% of all disease process is an excess of free radical activity [6-9].

Every oxygen factor also has an antioxidant factor in our physiological systems. In other words, we are normally capable of neutralizing the harmful effects of atoms and molecules that have a high affinity with other elements and chemicals, and would otherwise damage tissue and cells in attaching to cellular components.

Whenever one side or the other of this oxidation/anti-oxidation free radical system becomes unbalanced, damage accrues. This damage leads to diseases of the circulatory system, malignancies, inflammatory conditions and immunologic disorders [9].

EDTA chelation therapy removes metals that act as catalysts for the production of excessive free radical reactions, thus the disease process and/ or repairing the damage. The body, to prevent the damage due to free radicals, uses compounds known as antioxidants.

4 Data analysis

A group of 78 adults was considered in this analysis. All patients resided in two Italian cities, namely Bologna [10] and Ascoli Piceno. The treated group consisted of 43 women and 35 men.

The study patients received slow infusion of EDTA plus vitamin C, vitamin B6, vitamin B12, Potassium, Magnesium, Pantothenic Acid, Taurine, Glutathione and B complex. The purposes of the vitamin and mineral cocktails are:

- to replace the minerals lost due to the action of the coupling agents;
- to re-supply the minerals identified to be in inadequate quantities in the bodily stores;

- to supply antioxidant protection before or after detoxicant program;
- to alkalize the body fluids, which promote better enzymatic and immune functions;
- to supply in large pharmacological doses the Krebs cycle enzyme cofactors and other enzyme systems, which force cellular uptake, thus providing energy, enhanced detoxification and repair;
- to supply the nutrients to prevent the formation of Homocystiene, a potent oxidizer, which damages the lining of the blood vessels causing atheriosclerosis.

Increased urinary lead excretion after injection of EDTA (i.v. EDTA) is a recognized test for heavy metals accumulation in the body. Urinary excretion of heavy metals, namely lead, Aluminium, Mercury, was measured before and after EDTA infusion in all patients. The normal range of metal values is 0-20 mcg/l for lead and aluminium and 0-15 mcg/l for mercury.

The results of this analysis are summarized in Tables 1, 2 and 3 where a comparison between toxic metals found in urine before and after the chelation-therapy treatment has been illustrated.

Table 1: Lead found in urine before and after the intravenous EDTA treatment.

Measured Pb values before i.v EDTA (μg/l)	Number of Patients	Measured Pb values after i.v. EDTA (μg/l)	Number of Patients
0-20	74 (94.9%)	0-20	37 (47.4%)
21-30	4 (5.1%)	21-88	32 (41.0%)
		89-155	4 (5.1%)
		156-223	5 (6.5%)

Table 2: Aluminum found in urine before and after the intravenous EDTA treatment.

Measured Al values before i.v EDTA (μg/l)	Number of Patients	Measured Al values after i.v. EDTA (μg/l)	Number of Patients
0-20	38 (48.7%)	0-20	16 (20.5%)
21-50	26 (33.3%)	21-88	40 (51.3%)
59-95	7 (9.0%)	89-155	15 (19.2%)
95-132	7 (9.0%)	156-223	7 (9.0%)

Table 3: Mercury found in urine before and after the intravenous EDTA treatment.

Measured Hg values before i.v EDTA (µg/l)	Number of Patients	Measured Hg values after i.v. EDTA (µg/l)	Number of Patients
0-15	78 (100%)	0-15	46 (59.0%)
		16-26	22 (28.2%)
		27-37	7 (8.9%)
		38-69	3 (3.9%)

In each case, a substantial increase in metals excretion was measured after the intravenous EDTA treatment.

5 Discussion

It is clear from the Tables 1, 2 and 3 that before chelation treatment 94.9% of the patients had Lead values within normal range (0-20 mcg/l); after EDTA chelation treatment only 47.4% had normal lead levels and some patients presented lead levels ten times the normal values.

Regarding Aluminium levels, we can observe that before chelation treatment 48.7% of the patients had lead values within normal range (0-20 mcg/l) while after EDTA chelation treatment only 20.5% had normal aluminium levels.

100% of the patients did not present alarming urinary Mercury excretion before injection of EDTA (over 15 mcg/l); after intravenous EDTA only 59% had values within normal range.

These results demonstrate that increased urinary heavy metal excretion after intravenous EDTA chelation can be considered the recognized test for the accumulation of heavy metals in the body. Consequentially, chelation therapy benefits may still however be primarily the result of the obvious heavy metal detoxification.

6 Conclusions

Through eating, breathing, skin absorption, and everyday exposure to limitless products and chemicals made and used by humans, contaminants find their ways into the body.

Over time these heavy metals, toxic chemicals, plaques and other unnatural intruders continue to slowly accumulate. Whenever the body's natural detoxification pathways cannot eliminate them faster that they enter the body, the buildup can, eventually, reach toxic and dangerous levels. Urinary toxic metals excretion after intravenous EDTA infusion has demonstrated that patients excreted a large quantity of lead, aluminium and mercury reducing the "toxic metal deposits".

Chelation Therapy can be used as the primary treatment for heavy metal intoxication by lead, cadmium, aluminum, mercury, arsenic, and even iron.

The Chelation therapy consists of the intravenous infusion of a solution containing Ethylene Diamine Tetra-acetic Acid (EDTA), along with vitamins, minerals, and other substances. Because this therapy involves the vascular system, and because blood flow affects every cell in the body, it is not surprising to find a wide ranging set of lack-of-health conditions improved or outright cured after its use.

Acknowledgement

The authors are extremely grateful to Dr. F. Verzella and Dr. S. Zanella for providing data to carry out their work.

References

[1]   Cranton EM, Frackelton., Free radical pathology in age-associated diseases; treatment with EDTA chelation, nutrition and antioxidants, *J. Hol. Med.*;**6**, pp 6-37, 1984.

[2]   Blumer, W. & Cranton, EM, *Journal of Advancement in Medicine,*; **2,** (1/2), 1989.

[3]   Harman, D. The biologic clock: The mitochondria? *J Am Geriatr. Soc.*, **20**,pp 145-147, 1972.

[4]   Miquel, J., Economos, A.C., Fleming, J., and Johnson, J.E. Mitochondrial role in cell aging. *Exp Gerontol*, **15**, pp 575-591, 1980.

[5]   Miquel, J. An update on the mitochondrial-DNA mutation hypothesis of cell aging, *J. Mutation Research*, **275**, pp. 209-216, 1992.

[6]   Wallace, D.C., Mitochondrial genetics: a paradigm for aging and degenerative diseases? *Science*, **256**, pp.1063-1064, 1992.

[7]   Shoffner, J.M. and Wallace, D.C. Oxidative phosphorylation diseases and mitochondrial DNA mutations: diagnosis and treatment, *Ann Rev. Nutr,* **14**, pp. 535-568, 1994.

[8]   Flier, J.S. and Underhill, L.H. Mitochondria, DNA and disease, *New England J of Medicine*, **233**, pp. 638-644, 1995.

[9]   Gallagher, C.H. Aging of mitochondria. *Nature*, **187**, pp.566-568, 1960.

[10]   Verzella, F., *Nutrizione Comportamento & Salute*, Editai Srl, 2002.

Engineering *Pseudomonas putida* to minimize clogging during biostimulation

A. Matin, D. Hahm & D. F. Ackerley
Department of Microbiology and Immunology, Stanford University, USA

Abstract

Bacterial bioremediation is a safe and inexpensive means of decontaminating environmental pollution. However, low nutrient concentrations at polluted sites frequently limit bioremediating activity. Biostimulation by exogenous application of nutrients does not always promote effective transformation of pollutants, and the high levels of biomass that result can cause clogging around feeding ports, further constraining this strategy. To overcome these limitations we propose the application of starvation promoters to selectively express genes that are useful in bioremediation at maximal levels in nutrient-limited cells. Here we show that placing toluene monoxygenase (TMO) genes under control of the Pstarv1 starvation promoter in *Pseudomonas putida* MK1 brought about an 8-fold increase in the rate of phenol degradation by stationary-phase cells over exponentially growing cells. Under nutrient-limiting conditions these cells were also able to transform trichloroethylene with a conversion efficiency approximately 64-fold greater than unmodified cells, which only express appreciable levels of TMO in exponential phase. We also mapped and characterized the native promoter of *chrR*, a *P. putida* gene encoding a chromate-reducing enzyme, and show that it is likely to be under the transcriptional control of sigma 32, a heat shock and starvation regulated sigma factor. Consistent with this observation, *P. putida* cells grown at different dilution rates in a chemostat exhibited maximal chromate-reducing activity at low growth rates. These results are promising for maximizing the expression of chrR under field conditions for chromate bioremediation.
Keywords: *bioremediation,   biostimulation,   phenol,   trichloroethylene, hexavalent chromium, toluene monoxygenase, chromate reductase, starvation promoter.*

WIT Transactions on Biomedicine and Health, Vol 9, © 2005 WIT Press
www.witpress.com, ISSN 1743-3525 (on-line)

1   Introduction

Environmental pollution is a serious problem world-wide. While current remedial solutions such as excavation, incineration, pump and treat, and entombment, are viable approaches, they nonetheless have considerable disadvantages, such as exposure of workers to potential hazards, increased inputs to waste repositories, and high expense. Bioremediation has the advantage of being able to restore damaged environments at lower cost, more rapidly and with lower human risk. There are, however, several technical barriers to the effective application of this technology to environmental cleanup. In the first place, most of the environmental pollutants that are harmful to humans are toxic also to the bacteria that can remediate them, greatly impeding their beneficial activity. Second, polluted sites generally possess a mixture of different toxic compounds. At the Department of Energy waste sites in the United States, for example, which span over 2,800 square miles, heavy metals, radionuclides, complexing agents, chlorinated and fuel hydrocarbons, organic solvents, parachlorobiphenyls (PCEs), and ketones co-exist in different combinations at different sites; Riley and Zachara [1]. This mixed waste can be lethal to indigenous microorganisms required to detoxify individual contaminants: solvents can kill metal-resistant microbes; metals, the solvent-resistant ones; and radionuclides, the radiation-sensitive bacteria.

Another hurdle facing effective bioremediation by bacteria is that most polluted sites possess low nutrient concentrations, making microbial growth so slow that their remediating activities cannot be effectively expressed. A solution to this problem is provided by the process of "biostimulation," in which nutrients are added to the environment to stimulate the growth of indigenous bacteria, thus enhancing their transforming activity. However, biostimulation of natural populations can result in large bacterial biomass formation and nutrient consumption. Many reactions useful in bioremediation are fortuitous ("co-metabolic") processes from which the remediating bacterium derives no benefit. Only small proportions of the available nutrients (typically no more than 0.005 - 1.6% of the available electrons) are consumed on these processes since bacteria would rather grow than remediate. Estimates are that dehalogenation of 16.3 kg of PCE (a typical amount per m^3 of a contaminated soil) would require 970 kg of lactate and result in 140 kg of bacterial biomass; Bouwer [2]. Such biomass formation can cause clogging around the feeding port, confining effective remediation to a narrow zone; McCarty and Semprini [3].

For all these reasons, there is growing recognition that the powerful tools of genetic and molecular engineering can provide a solution to these complex problems. These approaches can likely permit generation of bacteria that can survive and remediate multiple contaminants, and are able to function under the low nutrient conditions of the polluted sites. However, such approaches have so far been sparingly applied to addressing bioremediation problems, and their potential for bioremediation remains largely to be demonstrated. This demonstration will go a long way in mitigating public concerns about the use of "artificial" life forms in environmental cleanup, especially when information is also provided on the excellent means that are available for controlling the spread of engineered microbes, should the need arise; Lewis [4].

We have been using molecular approaches to address both of the problems mentioned above. Thus, we have identified and cloned genes encoding bacterial enzymes that detoxify chromate in a way that is least harmful to the remediating bacterium. Three such "safe" enzymes have been characterized, two in *Escherichia coli* (YieF and NfsA), and one in *Pseudomonas putida* (ChrR); Ackerley et al [5, 6]. We have shown that recombinant bacteria overproducing these types of enzymes exhibit decreased chromate toxicity making them more effective agents of chromate bioremediation; and are currently using DNA shuffling technology to increase the efficacy of these enzymes for chromate reduction and to amplify their range, so they can remediate additional contaminants.

For the clogging problem associated with biostimulation, we have made use of special regulatory elements of *Escherichia coli* to selectively express high levels of different enzymatic activities in metabolically sluggish cells; Kim et al [7]; Matin [8]. These regulatory elements (the starvation promoters) were derived from starvation genes, which are selectively switched on in slowly growing cells. While the expression of most other genes is greatly attenuated, starvation genes exhibit a high level of expression in this state; Blum et al [9]; Matin et al [10]; McCann et al [11]; Tunner et al [12]. Using a variety of approaches, we demonstrated that starvation promoters permit induction and sustained expression of desired enzyme activities in slowly growing cells, so that marked transformations can be achieved with much reduced biomass production; Tunner et al [12].

In a "proof-of-concept" study, we examined TCE and phenol degradation in recombinant *E. coli* strains. These strains contained plasmids in which the expression of the toluene monooxygenase enzyme complex (TMO) was controlled by starvation promoters; Matin et al [13]. TMO is encoded by the *tmoABCDEF* operon, and is a mixed function oxygenase cloned originally from *Pseudomonas mendocina*; Yen et al [14]. Its physiological role is to enable *P. mendocina* to use toluene as a growth substrate. But it can, co-metabolically, also degrade phenol and TCE to products that can be readily attacked and mineralized by other bacteria. Recombinant *E. coli* bearing starvation promoters (e.g., P*groEL* or P*cstC*; Kim et al [7]) spliced to the *tmo* genes degraded phenol and TCE with a high conversion efficiency (i.e. the amount of contaminant degraded per unit amount of biomass synthesized and growth substrate consumed). This efficiency was over a hundred-fold greater than of the natural populations; Matin et al [13].

Since *E. coli* is not indigenous to polluted environments, we have applied the same principle to constructing recombinant *P. putida* strains, which are almost universally present in polluted sites. Our previously characterized and cloned *P. putida* starvation promoter (P*starv1*; Kim et al [7]) was spliced to the *tmo* gene cluster. P*starv1* is expressed at a significant level during exponential growth, but is markedly induced in the post-exponential phase. We report here the TCE and phenol conversion efficiency and other characteristics of *P. putida* containing a P*starv1-tmo* construct. In addition, we describe characterization of the regulatory elements that control the expression of the *chrR* gene in wild type *P. putida*. These findings will facilitate construction of a strain capable of expressing an improved safe chromate reductase in low-nutrient environments.

2 Materials and methods

2.1 Bacterial strains, plasmids, culture condition and chemicals

All strains and plasmids used in this study are listed in Table 1. Cells were grown in glucose-M9 medium. Cell growth was determined by measuring A_{660}; glucose by the Glucose [HK] 10 enzyme kit (Sigma); and total cell protein by the Bio-Rad DC protein assay kit. Indole and indigo were purchased from Sigma.

All plasmid manipulations were performed in *E. coli* DH5α or JM109. Plasmid transfer from *E. coli* to *Pseudomonas* strains was accomplished by triparental mating in the presence of the helper plasmid pRK600, as described previously; Kim et al [7]. The donor, recipient and helper cells (1:2:1, respectively) were collected on a 0.2 μm syringe filter (Nalgene). The filters were placed on LB agar plates and after allowing growth for 8 h at 30 °C, the mating mixture was suspended in 0.1% phosphate buffer and streaked on *Pseudomonas* Isolation Agar (Difco). Carbenicillin was used to select the *Pseudomonas* transformants.

Table 1:   Strains and plasmids.

Bacterial strain or plasmid	Relevant characteristics	Reference
Strains		
E. coli		
DH5α	*hsdRl7*($r_K^- m_K^-$) *supE44 thi-1 recA1 relA1 gryA (lacIZYA-argF)*	NEB
JM109	JM107 *recA1*	NEB
P. putida		
MK1	Derivative of ATCC12633: Rif^r	7
AMS1001	MK1 with pAM103	This study
AMS1002	MK1 with pAM104	This study
P. mendocina		
KR1	The strain from which *tmoABCDEF* was cloned	14
Plasmids		
pRK600	Cm^r *ori* ColE1 RK2-Mob$^+$ RK2-Tra$^+$	7
pGEM7Zf(+)	T7/SP6 cloning and transcription vector	Promega
pMMB67HE	Tac expression cloning vector with cloning sites of pUC18; Ap^r	ATCC
pMMB67HES	pMMB67HE with *PvuII-HindIII* fragment deleted; Ap^r	This study
pMKU101	pUC19with 0.65kb0CSP; Ap^r	7
pMKY341	pT7-5 with *tmoABCEDF*	14, 16
pAM101	pGEM7Xf(+) with *tmoABCEDF*	This study
pAM102	pMKU101 with *tmoABCEDF*	This study
pAM103	pMMB67HES with P*starv1*-*tmoABCEDF* construct	This study
pAM104	As pAM103 but without P*starv1*	This study

2.2 Construction of plasmids with the *tmo* operon under the control of the P*starv1* promoter

The *tmo* gene cluster was amplified from plasmid pMKY341 (Table 1) by PCR as previously described; Matin et al [13]. The resulting product was flanked by *Apa* I and *Eco* RI restriction sites, enabling it to be cloned downstream of the T7 promoter of pGEM7Zf(+), generating plasmid pAM101 (Table 1).   Upon addition of IPTG, the *E. coli* strains (Table 1) bearing this plasmid produced blue-colored colonies on LB agar plates, indicating the successful cloning of the *tmo* operon (the tryptophanase of *E. coli* converts tryptophan present in the LB medium into indole, which in the presence of TMO is converted into deep blue colored indigo).

The *tmo* operon was then excised from pAM101 by *Apa* I and *Eco* RI digestion and cloned into the corresponding sites of pMKU101, which contains the *starv1* promoter; Kim et al [7]. The resulting plasmid, designated pAM102, has the *tmo* gene cluster immediately downstream of the *starv1* promoter. To transfer the P*starv1-tmo* construct to a broad host range plasmid for expression in *P. putida*, we used the plasmid pMMB67HE. Deletion of a ca. 1.5 kb *Pvu* II-*Eco* RI fragment generated the plasmid pMMB67HES, lacking the *tac* promoter and the *lacI^q* gene. The P*starv1-tmo* construct was excised from pAM102 by *Sph* I and *Eco* RI digestion and transferred to pMMB67HES digested with the same enzymes, generating the plasmid pAM103 (Table 1).

The plasmid pAM103 was transformed into *P. putida* MK1 by triparental mating, as described above, generating strain AMS1001. AMS1001 turned blue upon starvation in glucose-M9 solid or liquid media; since *Pseudomonas* species lack tryptophanase, 1 mM indole was added to these media.

2.3 Northern analysis and transcript mapping

A 283 bp PCR product internal to the *chrR* gene was amplified using the primers CGATGTGGGTTCGCGTCCTTAC and TCAGACCGCCCTGTTCAACTTC, labeled with α-^{32}P ATP (Perkin Elmer) by nick translation, and used to probe total RNA isolated from an early stationary phase culture of *P. putida* KT2440 grown with 0.4 mM chromate.

Transcript mapping was performed using the Promega Primer Extension System (AMV reverse transcriptase) and a Thermo Sequenase Radiolabeled Terminator Cycle Sequencing Kit from USB. RNA for transcript mapping was isolated from early stationary phase cultures grown with or without 0.4 mM chromate. The primer GATGACCGTTCTCCTGTG, complementary to a region 53 bases upstream of the translational start site of the *chrR* gene, was used to localize the *chrR* promoter.

2.4 Analytical techniques

TMO assay relied on the ability of TMO to convert indole into indigo, which has a deep blue color; Ensley et al [15]. At indicated intervals, 1 ml aliquots of growing cell culture were removed. Indigo was extracted by treatment with an equal volume of ethyl acetate. Following centrifugation to separate the organic and aqueous phases, the absorbance of the ethyl acetate fraction was measured at 600 nm. The concentration of indigo was determined with reference to a standard curve of indigo dissolved in ethyl acetate; Ensley et al [15].

Crude extracts were prepared as described previously; Ackerley et al [5]. Reaction mixtures contained: 250 μM FeSO$_4$, 2.7 μM FAD, 1 mM NADH, and 400 μM phenol. Appropriate amounts of extract protein were added to the mixture. Reactions were started by the addition of phenol, and incubated at 30 °C; aliquots were removed at 1 min intervals and analyzed for residual phenol by the antipyrene dye method as described previously; Whited and Gibson [16].

Phenol consumption during growth was also monitored by the antipyrene dye method. TCE degradation and chromate reduction were measured as described by Matin et al [13] and Ackerley et al [5], respectively.

3 Results and discussion

3.1 AMS1001 degrades phenol and TCE in postexponential growth phase with high conversion efficiencies

The presence of 33 mg/L phenol did not affect the growth pattern of the strain AMS1001 (containing the *tmo* operon under control of the P*starv1* starvation promoter): the generation time remained ca. 2 h, and neither the time of entry into different phases nor the final yield were altered. Measurements showed that the exhaustion of glucose from the medium coincided with the end of the exponential phase (data not shown). There was minimal degradation of phenol (ca. 4 mg/L) in the exponential phase; based upon the total growth observed during this transformation, this corresponds to a conversion efficiency of 125 g cell mass generated per mg phenol transformed.

More rapid degradation occurred in the post-exponential phase, resulting in virtually complete conversion of the added phenol (Fig. 1). The highest rate attained was 400 μg phenol degraded/h/g cell dry-weight; ca. 29 mg/L phenol were degraded in this phase. The amount of phenol converted per unit biomass synthesized (the conversion efficiency) was calculated on the assumption that the total growth in the post-exponential phase corresponded to ca. 0.1 mg cell dry wt. Thus, in contrast to the exponential phase, only 3×10^{-5} g cell material was generated per mg phenol transformed.

TCE inhibits bacterial growth; McCarty and Samprini [3]; Whited and Gibson [16]. Therefore, in determining TCE degradation by AMS1001, this compound, at a concentration of 1 mg/L, was added at the onset of the post-exponential phase rather than from the start of the culture. The highest rate attained was ca. 110 μg TCE converted/h/g cell dry wt, and a total of 910 μg TCE were transformed. Thus, the conversion efficiency, calculated on the above assumption of biomass synthesis in this phase, was 110 mg cell material generated per mg TCE transformed. With natural populations, the corresponding value is 7 g cell material per mg TCE transformed; Hopkins et al [17]. AMS1004, which bears the plasmid pAM104 (containing the *tmo* operon, but not

P*starv1*), did not exhibit the above conversions, confirming that the expression of TMO in AMS1001 was indeed driven by the starvation promoter, P*starv1*.

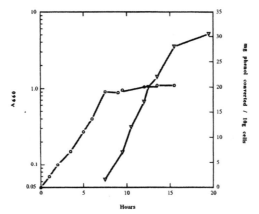

Figure 1:   Phenol degradation by AMS1001 in different growth phases in 0.1% glucose-M9 medium.   Symbols: (o) A_{660}, (▼) phenol degradation rate.

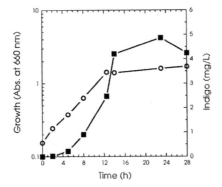

Figure 2:   *tmo* expression during exponential and stationary growth phases of *P. mendocina* KR1 in 0.15% glucose M9-medium plus 1 mM indole. Symbols: (o) A_{660}, (■) Indigo.

For comparative purposes, the pattern of TMO expression in *P. mendocina* KR1 in the various growth phases was examined.   TMO is apparently an inducible enzyme in this bacterium and phenol can serve as a growth substrate; Yen et al [14].   We therefore examined this pattern in 0.15% glucose-M9 medium supplemented with 1mM indole.   The latter can induce TMO but cannot serve as growth substrate.   Conversion of indole to indigo in this experiment began with a lag, peaked at the end of the exponential growth and then leveled off (Fig. 2).   The results strongly suggest that the native inducible promoter of the *tmo* operon in *P. mendocina* requires rapid exponential growth for expression and is not appreciably expressed in the post-exponential phase.

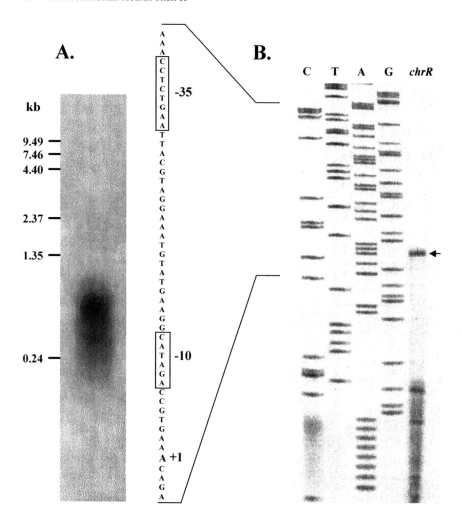

Figure 3: **A.** Detection of the *chrR* transcript by Northern hybridization. Total RNA was isolated from *P. putida* grown to early stationary phase in the presence of 400 μM Cr(VI) and probed with DNA internal to the *chrR* gene. The transcript size was estimated by comparison with ethidium bromide-stained RNA standards. **B.** Mapping of the transcriptional start point of *chrR* by primer extension. Lanes C, T, A, and G show the dideoxy-sequencing ladder obtained with the same oligo used for extension analysis (lane *chrR*). The extension product and corresponding base in the sequencing gel are indicated by an arrow. The nt sequence of the promoter region is shown to the left of the figure, with the proposed -35, -10, and +1 regions highlighted.

3.2 The transcriptional start site and promoter of *chrR*

By Western analysis, we previously showed that ChrR protein attains maximum levels in the stationary phase *P. putida*. This suggests that the native promoter of this gene in this bacterium is a starvation type promoter. If so, the task of improving the native promoter for high level expression during slow growth would be greatly facilitated.

Northern analysis showed that the *chrR* gene transcript was 650 – 750 bases long (Fig. 3A), indicating that this gene is not part of an operon. Twenty three base direct repeats, indicating a strong transcriptional terminator, were identified immediately downstream of the translational stop codon. From these data it was inferred that the transcriptional start site was likely to be located 100-200 bases upstream of the 561 bp *chrR* gene.

The precise transcriptional start site of the *chrR* gene was determined by primer extension analysis (Fig. 3B). The -10 and -35 regions of the *chrR* promoter are similar to the sigma 32 consensus; CATAGA cf CATNTA, and CCTCTGAA cf CCCTTGAA, respectively. It is possible that there is a second transcriptional product, initiated 22 bp downstream of the major transcriptional start site (Fig 3B); however the -10 and -35 regions of this site bear no homology to any known promoters, and the smearing around it suggests that this product is an artifact of primer extension. Transcript mapping of RNA isolated from cells exposed to chromate indicated that there is no alternative promoter activated by chromate challenge (data not shown). Thus, the major promoter regulating *chrR* expression appears to be regulated by sigma 32. The latter is both a heat shock and starvation responsive sigma factor; Jenkins et al [18].

3.3 ChrR activity in low growth rate *P. putida* cell extracts

To obtain more reliable information on *chrR* regulation, we compared chromate reductase activity of rapidly growing cells and those grown at submaximal rates. *P. putida* was grown at different dilution (growth) rates in a chemostat. Steady state cultures were harvested and their total chromate reductase activity measured in cell-free extracts. There was increased activity at low growth rates, the activity being 100 nmoles/min/mg protein at D=0.64 h^{-1}, but increased to 200 nmoles/min/mg protein at D=0.05 h^{-1}. These findings are consistent with *chrR* expression being controlled by a starvation promoter.

Studies currently underway are aimed at further analysis of the promoter region and a search for ancillary factors that may have a role in the regulation of these promoters.

4   Conclusions

1. Genes encoding enzymes that are active in bioremediation may be bioengineered to be under control of starvation promoters; this greatly reduces the amount of biomass formed per unit pollutant transformed. Thus, less nutrients will be required for biostimulation, and clogging will be minimized.

2. The *chrR* gene appears to be expressed from a native starvation promoter, which is highly promising for application of this gene in *in situ* chromate bioremediation.

References

[1]   Riley, R.G. and J.M. Zachara. Chemical Contaminants on DOE Lands and Selection of Contaminant Mixtures for Subsurface Science Research: U.S. Department of Energy Report. 1992.

[2]   Bouwer, E.J.   Bioremediation of chlorinated solvents using alternate electron acceptors. *In Handbook of Bioremediation*, Norris et al (Eds), Lewis Publishers, CRC Press, Inc, Boca Raton, Florida, pp. 149-175. 1994.

[3]   McCarty, P.L. and L. Semprini. Ground-water treatment for chlorinated solvents. *In Handbook of Bioremediation*, Norris et al (Eds), Lewis Publishers, CRC Press, Inc, Boca Raton, FL, pp. 87-116. 1994.

[4]   Lewis, K. Programmed death in bacteria. *Microbiol Mol Biol Rev* **64**: 503-514. 2000.

[5]   Ackerley D.F., C. F. Gonzalez, C. H. Park, R. Blake, M. Keyhan, and A. Matin. Chromate-reducing properties of soluble flavoproteins from *Pseudomonas putida* and *Escherichia coli*. *Appl Environ Microbiol* **70**: 873-882. 2004.

[6]   Ackerley D.F., C.F. Gonzalez, M. Keyhan, R. Blake, and A. Matin. Mechanism of chromate reduction by the *Escherichia coli* protein, NfsA, and the role of different chromate reductases in minimizing oxidative stress during chromate reduction. *Environ Microbiol* **6**: 851-860. 2004.

[7]   Kim, Y., L.S. Watrud and A. Matin. A carbon starvation survival gene of *Pseudomonas putida* is regulated by sigma-54. *J Bacteriol* **177**:1850-1859. 1995.

[8]   Matin, A. Recombinant DNA Technology II. *Annal NY Acad Sci* **721**: 277-291. 1994.

[9]   Blum P.H., S.B. Jovanovich, M.P. McCann, et al. Cloning and *in vivo* and *in vitro* regulation of cyclic AMP dependent carbon starvation genes from *Escherichia coli*. *J Bacteriol* **172**: 3813-3820. 1990.

[10]   Matin A., E.A. Auger, P.H. Blum, J.E. Schultz. Genetic basis of starvation survival in nondifferentiating bacteria. *Ann Rev Microbiol* **43**: 293-316. 1989.

[11]   McCann, M.P., J.P. Kidwell, and A. Matin. The putative sigma factor KatF has a central role in development of starvation-mediated general resistance in *Escherichia coli*. *J Bacteriol* **173**: 4188-4194. 1991.

[12]   Tunner J.R., C.R. Robertson, S. Schippa, and A. Matin. Use of glucose starvation to limit growth and induce protein production in *Escherichia coli*. Biotechnol Bioeng **40**: 271-279. 1992.

[13]   Matin, A., C.D. Little, C.D. Fraley, and M. Keyhan. Use of starvation promoters to limit growth and select for trichloroethylene and phenol

transformation activity in recombinant *Escherichia coli*. *Appl Environ Microbiol* **61**: 3323-3328. 1995.

[14]   Yen, K.M., M.R. Karl, L.M. Blatt, et al. Cloning and characterization of a *Pseudomonas mendocina* KR1 gene cluster encoding toluene-4-monooxygenase. *J Bacteriol* **173**: 5315-5327. 1991.

[15]   Ensley, B.D., B.J. Ratzkin, T.D. Osslund, M.J. Simon, L.P. Wackett, and D.T. Gibson. Expression of naphthalene oxidation genes in *Escherichia coli* results in the biosynthesis of indigo. Science **222**:167-169. 1983.

[16]   Whited, M.W., and D.T. Gibson. Toluene-4-monooxygenase, a three-component enzyme system that catalyzes the oxidation of toluene to *p*-cresol in *Pseudomonas mendocina* KR1. *J Bacteriol* **173**: 3010-3016. 1991.

[17]   Hopkins, G.D., J. Munakat, L. Semprini, and P.L. McCarty. Trichloroethylene concentration effects on pilot fields-scale *in-situ* groundwater bioremediation by phenol-oxidizing microorganisms. *Environ Sci Technol* **27**: 2542-2547. 1993.

[18]   Jenkins D.E., E.A. Auger and A. Matin. Role of RpoH, a heat shock regulator protein, in *Escherichia coli* carbon starvation protein synthesis and survival. *J Bacteriol* **173**: 1992-1996. 1991.

Environment management and health risks of soil erosion gullies in São Luís (Brazil) and their potential remediation using palm-leaf geotextiles

A. Guerra[1], M. Marcal[1], H. Polivanov[1], R. Sathler[1], J. Mendonça[1], T. Guerra[1], F. Bezerra[1], M. Furtado[2], N. Lima[2], U. Souza[2], A. Feitosa[2], K. Davies[3], M. A. Fullen[3] & C. A. Booth[3]

[1]*Geography Department., Federal University of Rio de Janeiro, Brazil*
[2]*Federal University of Maranhao, São Luís, Brazil*
[3]*Research Institute in Advanced Technologies (RIATec), The University of Wolverhampton, U.K.*

Abstract

Urban soil gully erosion in São Luís, Brazil, has resulted in loss of lives and properties. Environmental conditions (soil properties/use, rain regime, slope characteristics) associated with deforestation, brought on by irregular, unplanned and unauthorized urban settlement expansion (without basic urban infrastructure, especially sanitation, rain pipes and paved roads), has promoted land degradation and initiated gully formation. Therefore, understanding the factors that generate erosive processes, as well as the application of control measures and prevention, are fundamental actions for public safety. A novel control approach is the application of palm-mat geotextiles. These offer considerable potential to contribute to soil conservation, through sustainable and environmentally friendly palm agriculture. Ongoing field and laboratory research, in Europe, South America, Africa and SE Asia, is investigating geotextile mats manufactured from palm-leaves to evaluate their long-term effectiveness in controlling soil erosion and to assess their sustainability and economic viability. Palm-leaf geotextiles are novel and offer new bioengineering solutions to environmental problems, as temporary application of geotextiles allows sufficient time for plant communities to stabilize engineered slopes. Initial investigations suggest palm geotextiles are an effective, cheap and economically-viable soil conservation method, with tremendous potential. Palm geotextiles offer enormous multi-faceted environmental and socio-economic benefits, which include environmental education and local community involvement in reclamation and environmental-improvement programmes that reduce local community health risks.
Keywords: urban settlement, soil erosion, soil properties, deforestation.

1 Introduction

Water erosion can contribute to landslides, endangering life and property [1]. Inappropriate land management, including the lack of maintenance of vegetation cover, is one of the causes of gully erosion [2]. By removing vegetation cover the erosion-resisting capacity of soil becomes disturbed. The kinetic energy of raindrop splash increases, resulting in increased soil detachment. Hydraulic surface flow increases with the lack of vegetation cover, which also increases soil susceptibility to erosion, by reducing cohesion and shear strength [3].

Urban soil erosion, particularly in Brazil, is attributed to both environmental and socio-economic conditions, principally unauthorized and/or inefficient urban development and planning [4]. In that sense, the occurrence of erosive processes is generally associated with irregular population settlement, that is, those areas where there are usually no formal urban design or planning regulations instigated. For instance, in São Luís City and surrounding areas (State of Maranhão) in northeastern Brazil (Figure 1), deforestation has paved the way for accelerated urban expansion, which has promoted very severe soil erosion and, in doing so, aided gully formation [5]. These are large-scale erosion features, which can cause homes and lives to be at risk (Plate 1). Between 1997-2003, soil gully erosion was responsible for five deaths and the destruction of 350 homes in São Luís City alone.

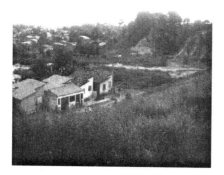 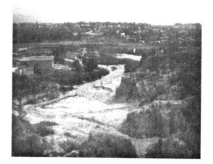

Plate 1: Soil erosion gullies bordering houses in São Luís City.

This work presents an insight into (i) the factors associated with soil erosion gully formation and (ii) the innovative approach of remediating gullies by the application of palm-mat geotextiles as a soil conservation technique and the widespread community based initiative to educate and safeguard the lives and properties of local populations in São Luís, Brazil.

2 Soil gully erosion

A gully (or large rill) is defined as "a channel or miniature valley cut by concentrated runoff but through which water commonly flows only during or immediately after heavy rains" [6, 7]. Meanwhile, gully erosion is defined as the process whereby runoff water accumulates and often recurs in narrow channels and, over short periods, removes the soil from this narrow area to considerable depths [8]. That said, natural slope failure is mainly associated with human intervention either for urbanization or for other development activities. A small initial movement in an unstable slope can trigger further soil water movement, resulting in soil erosion and consequent landslides. The degree of stability of a given slope can vary widely depending on the conditions existing at a given time [9].

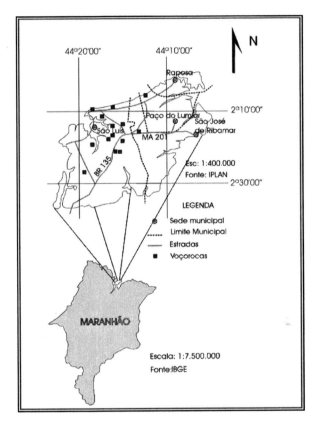

Figure 1:   Location map of the research area around the City of São Luís, on the Island of Maranhão, at the north of the State of Maranhão, along the northeastern Brazil coastline. For reference: Legenda – captions; Sede municipal – Municipal centre; Limite municipal – Municipal border; Fonte: Source; Escala – scale; Estradas – Roads; Voçorocas – Gullies.

Gullies mainly form on freshly exposed soils when the vegetation cover is very sparse. At such times, concentrated runoff, generated by rainstorms, erodes the (sealed) top soil layer when the flow shear stress exceeds a critical value

[10]. In general, rainfall intensity, catchment size, runoff coefficient, surface roughness and slope morphology collectively determine flow width. Flow discharge and surface slope together determine flow intensity. Soil moisture, soil structure and soil profile characteristics determine soil resistance to detachment and transport [7].

Poesen et al. [8] stated that once gullies develop, they often trigger other soil degradation processes, such as piping, soil fall or soil topple (driven by gravity) after tension crack development and undercutting. Furthermore, gully channels enhance the export of sediment produced on the intergully areas (sheet and rill erosion) by increasing the connectivity in the landscape, which leads to an increased risk of sediment deposition downslope. If no gully control measures are taken, gully growth rates usually decline exponentially.

Vegetation cover, because of its thinness, is often undervalued in terms of its control over landscape incision and evolution. Its resistance to erosion may be of the same order of magnitude as the underlying bedrock [8, 11]. In Brazil, deforestation, amongst others, is identified as one of the primary factors responsible for initiating gullying [12]. In that sense, the environmental landscape observed in São Luís is prone to gullying. The bedrock is very susceptible to weathering and erosion [13]. The annual rain regime is rather irregular, being marked by two different periods: a rainy one with moderate to high rain surpluses and another one with rain deficiency [5]. The soils are clay deficient, with low organic matter contents, which promotes their susceptibility to erosion. Consequently, where gullies have formed, the original vegetation cover has been felled and cleared for urban expansion, so soil erosion is common [13]. Therefore, depending on severity and timing, sudden mass movements of erodible materials within soil erosion gullies present environmental risks to both homes and the health of local communities.

3   Management and remediation of soil erosion gullies

In principle, gully prevention can be achieved by either preventing runoff from flowing, by increasing soil infiltrability (e.g. improving topsoil structure), or by increasing the resistance of the top layer of soil to concentrated flow erosion (e.g. soil compaction, no-tillage or establishing grassed waterways) [7]. Where possible, natural vegetation with well-developed root mats can be (re)established in disturbed concentrated flow zones affected by gully erosion. In doing so, soil loss and sediment production will be reduced [8]. Natural vegetation for sustainable erosion control and slope protection is a proven choice of soil conservation [9]. Those constructed from organic materials are highly effective [14].

Several slope protection/remediation techniques are currently employed to stabilize slopes. Application of geotextiles is especially beneficial for complex engineering problems, as temporary application of geotextiles allows sufficient time for plant communities to grow and stabilize slopes by intertwining of roots, which maximizes seepage of runoff into soil by intercepting rainfall and retarding runoff velocity [15]. Furthermore, if constructed from indigenous materials, such as palm-leaves, geotextiles can be effective, affordable and compatible with sustainable land management strategies. The ability of natural fibres to absorb water and degrade into the soil with time are prime properties, which offer an improvement over synthetic geotextiles for slope stability applications.

4   Application of palm-leaf geotextiles

4.1 Environmental and socio-economic rewards of palm-mat geotextiles

Preliminary investigations suggest palm-mat geotextiles could be an effective and cheap soil conservation method, with enormous global potential. The strategic impact of palm-leaf geotextiles involves the promotion of sustainable and environmentally friendly palm-agriculture, which will discourage deforestation, promote both reforestation and agroforestry and offer a potentially profitable technique to augment the income of financially deprived communities. Thus, construction of palm geotextiles could develop into a rural, labour-intensive industry, particularly encouraging the employment of socially-disadvantaged groups, such as women, disabled and elderly people (i.e. hand-work performed sitting down). Moreover, export of completed palm geotextiles will earn hard currency and promote development, based on the principles of fair trade.

Palm-leaf geotextiles can improve the socio-economic foundation for sustainable development in developing countries. Potential benefits include poverty alleviation, engagement of disadvantaged groups as stakeholders, employment for disadvantaged groups, SME development, export of geotextiles earning hard currency, environmental education and local community involvement in reclamation and environmental-improvement programmes. Education programmes are necessary to actively inform the public of the importance of soil as an essential resource. These schemes should particularly encourage 'land literacy' among participants so that society recognizes broader benefits of effective soil conservation, such as its potential contribution to habitat creation, biodiversity and carbon sequestration [16].

4.2 Geotextile palm-mat manufacture

A small workshop was established in Brazil, to harvest and manufacture palm mats (Plate 2). Fronds were cut and sun-dried over several weeks. The thick central spines, which give the leaf their fan-like appearance, were stripped and the vegetation cut into lengths ranging from 1-1.5 m length and 2 cm width. These were then soaked in water to make the material pliable and then using a 2,500 cm^2 wooden template, woven into 50 x 50 cm (2,500 cm^2) squares, where the outer edge of the mat was sewn using fibre from the leaf waste. Strips were then woven into a grid pattern, vertically and horizontally, using a slipknot at 5 cm intervals. Then every strip was wrapped around, working from one edge to the other, using the prepared material.

(a)   (b)   (c)

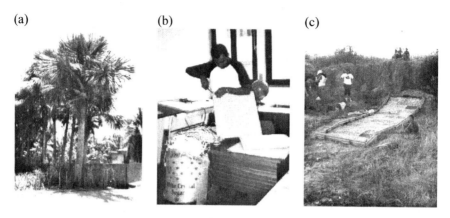

Plate 2: (a) Brazilian Buriti palms; (b) Palm-mat geotextile production and (c) A field erosion test plot covered with palm-mats.

4.3 Field application of palm-mat geotextiles: U.K. pilot study results

A pilot study is in progress, evaluating palm-mat effects on runoff and erosion rates from established runoff plots, based at the University of Wolverhampton's Hilton Experimental Site (52.0°033'5.7''N, 2.0°19'18.3''W). Eight runoff plots, situated on a 15° south-west facing slope, numbered D1-D8 and measuring 10 x 1 m, are used for the field study.

The runoff investigation consisted of 35 observations over 98 weeks, with the first six observations used as a calibration period (showing reasonable bare soil comparability: data not presented). Total plot data for the period 25/03/2002–09/02/2004 (precipitation total 1118.4 mm) is shown in Table 1. Runoff volumes from both grassed plots were similar. In contrast, runoff volume from the buffer zone plots and geotextile plots show noticeable differences. Comparatively, runoff from the geotextile covered plots was higher than the bare plots by a mean of 121.2%, while runoff from the buffer zone plots was lower than the bare plots by a mean of 60.5%. Total runoff as a % of the precipitation for the bare plots (0.59%) was notably higher than both the grassed (0.44%) and buffer (0.36%) treatments, but not the geotextile-covered plots (0.71%).

Erosion from the treated plots was noticeably lower than from the bare plots during the same period. Sediment yields from the buffer zone plots were similar. In contrast, there are notable differences in sediment yields from the bare, grassed, geotextile-covered and buffer zone plots. Hence, mean total soil loss equates to 0.81 t ha^{-1} from the bare plots, 0.30 t ha^{-1} from both the covered plots, 0.29 t ha^{-1} from the buffer zone plots and 0.12 t ha^{-1} from the grass plots. Since erosion from buffer strip plots approximately equals those from mat-covered plots, this indicates buffer strips are very effective in reducing erosion.

Pilot study data suggest palm-mat geotextiles are effective in reducing runoff when used as a buffer zone. However, it remains to be shown if the mats can reduce runoff compared to bare soil. While these results were obtained in a humid temperate climate, further experiments will verify their applicability in the humid tropics of Brazil.

Table 1:   Runoff and erosion plot data at the Hilton Experimental Site. Note - using random selection, plots D2 and D8 were completely covered with palm-mats, D4 and D5 had 1 m buffer zones of palm-mats at the plot lower end, D1 and D6 are the bare soil (control) plots and D3 and D7 are grassed plots.

Plot	Total runoff (l)			Total sediment yield (g)		
(n = 29)	Total	Mean	S.D.	Total	Mean	S.D.
D1	24.5	0.8	0.9	71.9	2.6	3.4
D2	22.8	0.8	1.0	41.9	1.5	1.8
D3	20.9	0.7	0.9	15.0	0.5	0.4
D4	12.8	0.4	0.7	29.4	1.0	1.4
D5	27.1	0.9	0.7	30.2	1.1	1.2
D6	41.1	1.4	1.3	89.6	3.2	5.4
D7	27.9	1.0	1.1	9.4	0.3	0.4
D8	56.6	2.0	1.9	15.1	0.5	0.4

5   Ongoing and proposed further work

A research team, based in Europe, South America, Africa and South-East Asia, funded by the EU for three-years (Project 'BORASSUS': Contract Number 510745), has recently commenced the first complete scientific and socio-economic evaluation of the potential of palm-leaf geotextiles. Full geotechnical evaluations of these geotextiles are an integral part of the work. Therefore, as part of the established information dissemination strategy, the team will publish manufacturing and production protocols and standards. These will be broadly disseminated and thus available for SMEs to adopt and adapt. These standards will contribute to the global production of high-quality palm-mat geotextiles suitable for multiple and complex applications [16].

5.1 South American (Brazilian) research work-package

Based on field studies at an established research site in São Luís, the work-package aims to: (i) understand where, how and at what rates gully erosion occurs; (ii) measure and assess urban gully erosion and identify the primary controlling factors; (iii) compare areas under palm mats protection with areas with no protection against erosion; (iv) examine the relation between gully erosion and environmental and socio-economic factors, and recuperate as many gullies as reasonably possible; (v) educate and assist local authorities and non-governmental organizations, in terms of alternative geotextile technology to recuperate urban gullies and (vi) engage with communities affected by these potentially life-threatening features, by initiating an environmental-awareness programme to inform and educate them on gully erosion and control.

6 Conclusions

Environmental and socio-economic conditions have attributed to urban soil erosion in Brazil, which has lead to the initiation and formation of gullies. The severity and sudden impact of these features has caused the loss of lives and homes. As part of an international research project (Borassus, funded by the EU for 3-years), a field site (São Luís) in NE Brazil is evaluating palm-leaf geotextile mats as a possible remediation technology.

Preliminary results indicate that geotextiles constructed from palm-leaves have potential as a biotechnical soil conservation method and effectively reduced soil erosion. If harvested correctly, palm leaves are highly sustainable and readily available in most semi-arid and sub-humid bioclimatic regions. They are biodegradable, providing organic content matter to stabilize the soil and their permeability makes them suitable for use with cohesive soils. There are no high-energy production procedures in the manufacturing process and, when used in their natural environment, they may provide a cost-effective method of conserving soil in developing countries, where land remediation techniques are scaled to low levels of disposable income. That said, ultimately, and more importantly, they might even save lives and properties of Brazilian communities

Acknowledgements

This work is dedicated to the memory of Dr Kathy Davies, to whom we acknowledge as the initiator and inspiration for palm-leaf geotextile research. All authors would like to gratefully acknowledge and thank the technical and support staff at each university.

References

[1] Hudson, N.W., *A study of the reasons for success and failures of soil conservation projects*. FAO Soils Bulletin No. 64. Soil Resources Management and Conservation Service, FAO Land and Water Development Division, Silsoe Agricultural Associates, Bedford, U.K., 2001.

[2] Casal, J., Lopez. J.J. & Giraldez, J.V., Ephemeral gully erosion in southern Navarra (Spain). *Catena*, **36**, pp. 65-84, 1999.

[3] Rickson, J., The best is yet to come. *Ground Engineering*, 34, pp. 13-14, 2001.

[4] Sobreira, F.G., A ocupação desordenada nas encostas de Ouro Preto, *MG. Revista Escola de Minas*, **42**, pp. 12-16, 1989.

[5] Mendonca, J.K.S., Relatório Final: *Diagnóstico da erosão urbana no município de São Luis-MA*. Relatório 03-2002/02. São Luis: UFMA, 2003.

[6] Soil Conservation Society of America, *Resource Conservation Glossary*. Soil Conservation Society of America, Ankeny (USA), 1982.

[7]   Poesen, J. & Govers, G., Gully erosion in the loam belt of Belgium: typology and control measures. In: *Soil Erosion on Agricultural Land*, Eds. J. Boardman, I.D.L. Foster, & J.A. Dearing, John Wiley & Sons: Chichester (UK), pp. 513-530, 1990.

[8]   Poesen, J., Nachtergaele, J., Verstraeten, G. & Valentin, C., Gully erosion and environmental change: importance and research needs. *Catena*, **50**, pp. 91-133, 2003.

[9]   Lekha, K.R., Field instrumentation and monitoring of soil erosion in coir geotextiles stabilised slopes – A case study. *Geotextiles & Geomembranes*, **22**, pp. 399-413, 2004.

[10]   Rauws, G. & Govers, G., Hydraulic and soil mechanical aspects of rill generation on agricultural soils. *Journal of Soil Science*, **39**, pp. 111-124, 1988.

[11]   Howard, A.D., Simulation of gully erosion and bistable landforms. In: *Proceedings of the Conference on Management of Landscapes Disturbed by Channel Incision*, Eds. S.S.Y. Wang, E.J. Langendoen & F.D. Shields, Center for Computational Hydroscience & Engineering, The University of Mississippi, Oxford MS, pp. 516-521, 1997.

[12]   Guerra, A.J.T., Processos erosivos nas encostas. In: *Geomorfologia: exercícios, técnicas e aplicações*, Eds. Guerra, A.J.T. & Cunha, S.B., Bertrand: Rio de Janeiro (Brazil), pp. 139-155, 1996.

[13]   Guerra, A.J.T.; Mendonca, J.K.S.; Marcelo, R. & Alves, I.S., Gully erosion monitoring in São Luis city – Maranhão State – Brazil. In: *Gully Erosion Under Global Change*. Eds. Li, Y.; Poesen, J. & Valentin, C., Chengdu, China: Sichuan Science and Technology, 2004.

[14]   Ogbobe, O., Essien, K.S. & Adebayo, A., A study of biodegradable geotextiles used for erosion control. *Geosynthetics International*, **5**, pp. 545-553, 1998.

[15]   Ahn, T.B., Cho, S.D. & Yang, S.C., Stabilization of soil slope using geosynthetic mulching mat. *Geotextiles & Geomembranes*, **20**, 135-146, 2002.

[16]   Booth, C.A., Davies, K. & Fullen, M.A., Environmental and socio-economic contributions of palm-leaf geotextiles to sustainable development and soil conservation. In: *Ecosystems and Sustainable Development V*, Eds. E. Tiezzi, C.A. Brebbia, S.E. Jorgensen & D. Almorza Gomar, WIT Press: Southampton (UK), pp. 649-658, 2005.

Section 9
Social and economic issues

Accessibility and urban environment sustainability in Sydney (1991–2001)

M. R. Rahnama[1] & A. Lyth[2]
[1]Mashhad Ferdowsi University, Iran
[2]Graduate School of Environmental Planning, Macquarie University, Australia

Abstract

One of the most important issues for enhancing environmental quality, especially in the urban environment, is developing accessibility versus mobility. With regard to this, we calculated the accessibility indicator by a zonal opportunity gravity model (employed person) for 38 local government areas (zones) with GIS tools, and, in addition, the changes in accessibility measured during 1991–2001. In addition, the relationship between the accessibility index and six sub socio-eco-physical factors was calculated by multiple regressing. The result yielded from a map of accessibility changes shows that two scenarios had taken place simultaneously. One is a high positive change of accessibility value both in the central core, mostly strap pattern (concentration) and sub-urban areas (decentralization), the other is the low positive or negative change of accessibility value in the middle rings of Sydney. The results achieved by calculating the relationship between the accessibility index and the socio-economic variables show that zones that have low car usage to work have high accessibility value. In contrast, zones with low weekly income families, far from the city center, with a high percentage of car usage to work have a low accessibility value.
Keywords: accessibility, Local Government boundaries, urban environment, sustainability.

1 Introduction

Accessibility has been argued about for over half of century, especially from the publication of the Hansen quantity method about accessibility (Hansen, [17]). The predominance of extensive sub-urbanization after World War II (1939-45)

and the vast use of cars for commuting between work and housing locations in the urban region (Newman et al. [16]). The energy crisis in the 1970s (significant rise in oil price initially in 1973 (Anna V.Gollner, [18]) and environmental concerns changed opinions from mobility to accessibility in urban and transportation planning and design, for example in Australia the planning of cities in the late 1970s and early 1980s was largely driven by resource conservation issues and the growing concerns of social equity issues (Anna Gollner, [19]). Some of cities similar to Vancouver in Canada (Newman et al. [16]) have used the principles of accessibility planning in urban planning and design.

Accessibility is defined as "the freedom or ability of people to achieve their basic needs in order to sustain their quality of life" (Nil Pasaogullari et al. [21]). Accessibility is basically divided into two types, that is, "relative accessibility" and "integral accessibility" (R.C.W. Kwork & A.G.O. Yeh, [20]). Therefore accessibility can generally be defined as the ease in reaching a place that is considered attractive. This definition implies the common inclusion of two components in the measurements. They are the land-use pattern and performance of the transport system. For the land use pattern, the more opportunities within a region, the higher the accessibility (hence total employed persons in the region is the pull power of attraction). For the performance of a transport system, the less impedance distance (time travel, cost) between a given point and its opportunities, the higher the accessibility. Here the spatial distance between points (center of local government boundries-38 L.G.B) is calculated.

2   Purpose of research

1-To calculate accessibility and its changes in Sydney during 1991 to 2001, 2-Measuring the relationship between the accessibility index and 6 Socio-eco-physical sub groups (16 variables).

3   Research model (hypothesis)

Figure 1 shows the process of research (hypothesis) and interaction between socio-eco-physical variables and accessibility index and it's feedback.

4   Socio-eco-physical factors

For achieving this research 6 factors have been used, each of them including several variables as follow: Population variables, dwelling variables, income variables, employment variables, transportation variables, and geographical variables.

5   Research methodology

5.1   General formulation

The following model is selected with regard to the data available:

$$\sum_{j=1}^{N} T_{i1,2} = \sum Sj/_{di\,j^a}$$

$Ti_{1,2}$= is a relative measure of the accessibility of zone 1 to an activity located within zone 2

S_j= Size of activity at zone 2, e.g. the number of jobs, people, etc (here is the people employed in 1991 and 2001)

D_{ij}= is the travel time, distance or cost from zone i to zone j

a=parameter and equal 2

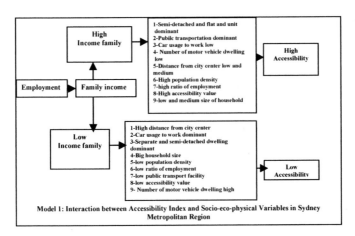

Figure 1.

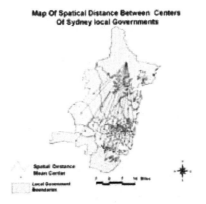

Figure 2.

5.2 Measuring interaction between zones

At the first distance among zones (d_{ij}) is calculated by using Arc.view (GIS) option means center. Then, for measuring the interaction among zones, the distance between zonal centers has been used (38×38 matrix of local government mean center). A sample point has it's distance calculated from other zones in figure 2. After calculating the distance between zones, the interaction between them should be measured, in this stage by using the above gravity equation and entering the total employed persons aged 15 years and over from ABS 1991 and 2001 (Australian Bureau statistics [1,2]) to the model as s_j and distance between zones as d_{ij}, the background for calculating interaction between zones and sum of each T_i provided.

6   Overview of Sydney

Sydney is located at latitude $35°$ south (Mike, [9]) and in New South Wales (NSW) state of Australia. This metropolitan had almost 63.7% total of the population (3997321 persons) of New South Wales 2001 (a.b.c2001). The population of Sydney changed from 3538314 in 1991 to 3997321 people in 2001. The percentage of change during this period was 13.1% and it is predicted that the population growth of this city will reach 5 million by 2022 (D.I.P, NSW, 2002). Mean household size of this city was 2.7 people in 2001. This city is the most important one in Australia and it has the biggest economy in the country, equivalent to Singapore and bigger than New Zealand (D.I.P.R, NSW, 2002). Labor force numbers in Sydney had changed from 1556448 people (89.7% employed of labor force) in 1991 to 1916223 person (93.9% employed of labor force) in 2001. The ratio of unemployed during this period reduced from 10.3% to 6.1%. The distribution of employment and population around the Sydney metropolitan region shows spatial difference. The ratio of employment in the central core and inner city is higher than the outer ring (from 70% to 35%). Therefore different travel modes to and from work are created in a metropolitan area. This situation produced more car travel to and from the work location; almost 70% of travel to work was by car, 15% train, 6% bus and 9% other in 1996 (Department of Urban Affairs and Planning, 2001).

Some of the differences in the stages of urban development include; pre and post-war II city development plans (Anna V. Gollner [18]), income family (range of income weekly family in Sydney varied from 500 to 1750 in 20001(a.b.c2001)), concentration of industries (factories), employment caused uneven and inequitable spatial urban morphology for Sydney, that many of researchers (Joan Vipond, et al, 1988) divided the city in three distinct zones: 1-inner Sydney: oldest city and 10 km distance from city center, 2 - middle Sydney located between 10 to 25 km from boundaries of inner Sydney and after World War II around rail road developed , 3 - Outer Sydney .

Urban Sprawl (approximately 12144.6 sq.km^2 and 3997321 persons population density 329.14 people /Esq.km^2) and 1356047 housing (2001) show that the Sydney metropolitan is one of the top 10 most sprawling world metro regions and low population density (Environmental Health [8]). Therefore this city has been faced with the problems of accessibility versus mobility. Also the value of community accessibility in Hong Kong was 99.3 compared with 36.8 in Sydney (William Ross Benvse, [22]). Because of overcoming problems resulting from mobility, this research was conducted to recognize accessibility and its changes during 1991 to 2001 in the Sydney metropolitan region, and analysis was carried out to determine the influence that factors had on accessibility as follows:

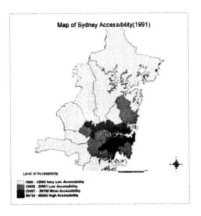

Figure 3.

7 Discussions

7.1 Measuring 1991 Accessibility Index

For measuring accessibility two variables were used. One is distance between the center of statistical trace (local government boundaries in 1991 and 2001), another is the number of employed persons as opportunity (d_j) meager in each zone during this period. The result of this measuring for 1991 accessibility is shown in figure 3.

The result of the analysis of accessibility in 1991 in Sydney showed that the central core and its fringes is the zone with high and medium accessibility index. The most remarkable feature of this region is the concentration of central business district (CBD) and civic infrastructure (rail, high way, bus, ferry and mono rail and so on). Therefore this precinct has the highest accessibility and especially with regard to public transportation facilities. From the center of the city towards the outskirts of Sydney the gradient of accessibility value decreases.

7.2 Accessibility Index in 2001

The result of this calculation is illustrated in figure 4. With the quartile option of Arc.view all of the zones from the accessibility index are classified in four sub groups 1 - very low (10 zones), 2 - low (10 zones) 3- medium (9 zones) and 4- high accessibility (9 zones). The central core and inner city rings have the highest rate of accessibility similar to 1991 ones. As a consequence accessibility value decreases by the increasing distance from the city center both in 1991 and 2001.

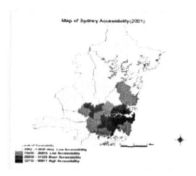

Figure 4.

7.3 Changes of Accessibility Index during 1991 to 2001

Figure 5 shows the result. The mean accessibility change index was 18%, with the minimum change 4% (Blacktown) and maximum change 61% (Strathfild). The related map shows that that two processes take place simultaneously in the Sydney metropolitan region. One is Decentralization of accessibility in suburban areas and the other is Concentration (Centralization of accessibility in central core but with strap pattern). A new question can be considered - why decentralization took place?

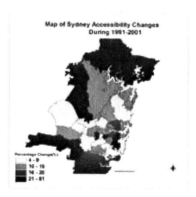

Figure 5.

8 Analysis relations between accessibility index and Socio-eco-physical variables

The coefficient correlation between accessibility indexes in 2001 and 14 variables have been calculated and the results are illustrates as follows:

8.1 Positive relation

This sub group has 4 variables (travel by train and bus to work, number of unit, flat and apartment dwellings, population density, semi detached dwellings). Relationships between these variables and accessibility are positive. That means, zones with a high value in the above-mentioned variables have a high value of accessibility. Therefore they are concentrated in and around the central core.

8.2 Negative relation

This sub group has 10 variables (distance from city center, travel to work by car, percentage separated and semi detached dwellings, mean household family, percentage separated dwellings, percentage of employment, income family, travel to work by train and travel to work by bus and train. The relationship between these variables and accessibility index is negative. That means these zones are located far from the central core in the sub-urban region of Sydney.

9 Conclusion

The results obtained from the application of this model indicate that Sydney from an accessibility standpoint is an un-equal environment, and the city can be divided in four sub-groups as follow:

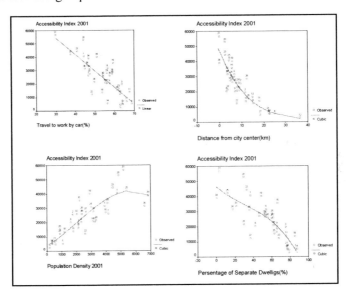

Figure 6: Relationship between Accessibility Index and socio-eco-physical variables in Sydney (2001).

9.1 Very low accessibility and low income family (more than 8 zones)

These zones are located at the outer fringe of metropolitan area of Sydney (far from the city center). They have a low population density, low ratio of employment, high car usage for traveling to work and other activities, priority of separated dwellings, low access to public transportation facilities, big household size and low rent dwelling are the important characteristic and remarkable of these zones.

9.2 Low accessibility and high income (more than 6 zones)

These zones have a large household size. Located far from the city center, high car usage, low access to public transportation, and high proportion of separate and semidetached dwelling. The important differences between theses regions with the very low sub group accessibility are that some are high-income families and are a little closer to the city center and have some access to public transportation.

9.3 Low income family and high accessibility (similar Auburn and etc- 7 zones)

More than half on these zones are located in the inner ring of Sydney. They have good potential for future development, but are faced with some problems including; the high rise ratio of unemployment in this region, high population density, low-income family, high usage of public transportation to work and low usage car to travel to work. Spatial distribution and proximity of these zones is low and somewhat dispersed.

9.4 High income family and high accessibility (more than ten zones)

For the most part these zones are located in the inner ring and central core of Sydney. The nucleus initial of urban development and historical concentration of business district in this region to the attendant of concentration of other facilities have caused this zone to become the most important in the city of Sydney. Therefore this region has the highest index of accessibility.

Finally, the initial hypothesis at the beginning of the discussion rejected the direct positive relation between high-income family status and high car usage for traveling to work and hence far from city core location dwelling and high accessibility. Because it was proved that zones with high-income families are not dispersed in the outer suburb of Sydney metropolitan. They are concentrated mostly in the inner ring of Sydney with a medium distance from the city center. Therefore they have good access to the public transportation mode of travel to work. Hence they use a low private mode of travel to work (mostly car usage). Also in the region with low accessibility and low income, many of the residents do not have access to public transport, therefore they prefer to have a car for meeting their needs. Using car in these zones has many advantages including:
1- to decrease transport cost, 2- Access to big house (separated dwelling) with low rent and big household size in the remote suburban areas. Owning a car to provide these direct advantages and to substitute costs of long distance. Therefore there is not direct relation between car usage and family income. Even

in this research after dividing income family groups into three subgroups (low 700-1030, medium 1000-1330 and high 1330-1700AU$) and calculating the relationship of these three groups with car usage by "One Way Analysis "had approved that there was significant difference between the percentage of car usage and sub income groups especially between the first group (low income group -68% car usage) as compared to the third group (high income group-56% car usage).

References

[1]   Australian Bureau of Statistic (ABS), 2001 Census of Population and Housing: Time Series Data.
[2]   Australian Bureau of Statistic (ABS), 1991 Census of Population and Housing: Time Series Data.
[3]   Conell Jhon (2000) The emergence of a world city, Sydney, Oxford, University Press.
[4]   Brodde Makri Maria (2004) Accessibility indices. A tool for comprehensive land use planning, division of traffic planning, department of technology and society, LUND University Sweden.
[5]   C.Y. Lau Joseph & C.H. Ciu Catherine (2003) Accessibility of low-income workers in Hong Kong, Cities, Vol.20, No.3, P.197-204.
[6]   Department of Infrastructure, planning and natural resources, NSW (2002) Planning for a better future, metropolitan strategy, Sydney grate metropolitan region, www.metrstrategy.
[7]   Department of Urban Affairs and Planning, NSW (2001) Integrating land use and transport, employment and journey to work patterns in the Greater Metropolitan Region.
[8]   Environmental Health, Focus (Smart Growth in Washington DC), Vol.112, No.11, 2004.
[9]   Gillen Mike, (2005) Urban governance and vulnerability: exploring the tensions in Sydney's response to bushfire threat, cities, Vol.22, No.1, p.55-64.
[10]   Gudmundsson Henrik, Hjer Mattias (1996), Sustainable Development Principles and Their Implications for Transport, Ecological Economics, No19, pp269-288.
[11]   Halden Derek (2002) Using accessibility measures to integrate land use and transport policy in Edinburgh and the Lothians, Transport Policy, No.9, pp313-324.
[12]   Hamentt Stephen and Robert Freestone (2000) The Australian Metropolis, Allen and Unwin Ltd.
[13]   Handy Susan L (1992) Regional versus Local Accessibility: Neo-Traditional Development and its Implications for Non-Work Travel, Built Environment, vol. 18, No. 4, pp.253-267.
[14]   Hay Alan (2005), The Transport Implications of Planning Policy Guidance on the Location of Superstores in England and Wales:

Simulation and Case Study, Journal of Transport Geography, No.13, pp13-22

[15] Hellemman Gerben, Wassenberg Frank (2004) The renewal of what was tomorrow's idealistic city, Amsterdam's Bijlmeree, cities.Vol.21, No1, P.3-17.

[16] Newman Peter, et al (1999) Sustainability and cities; overcoming automobile dependences, Island Press, USA.

[17] Hanson, W.G. (1959) How Accessibility Shapes Land-use, Journal of American Institute of Planner, 25.73-76.

[18] Anna V. Gollner (1994) Sub-urbanization, Sustainability & Climate Change Policy, A PHD thesis submitted to the department of geography, school of earth sciences, Macquarie University, Sydney, Australia

[19] Anna V. Gollner (1996) To Sprawl or Not TO Sprawl, A Journey to Work Perspective, Australian Planner, Vol. 33. No.3, p 138-141.

[20] Yeh A.G.O & Kwork R.C.W. (2000) The use of the model accessibility gap as an indicator for sustainable transport development, Urban Transport VI, L. Sucharov, so on Wit Press, UK. Pp 267-274.

[21] Nil Pasaogullari et al (2004) Measuring Accessibility and Utilization of Public Space in Famagusta, Cities, Vol.21. No.3, pp225-232

[22] William Ross Benvse (1999) personal mobility or community Accessibility; A planning choice with social, environmental and economic consequences, Doctoral thesis, Murdoch, University, AU.

Impact assessment and public outreach strategies of local governments

S. Conway[1], P. Washeba[2] & I. Navis[3]
[1]*Urban Environmental Research, LLC, U.S.A.*
[2]*Avnet, Inc., U.S.A.*
[3]*Clark County Department of Comprehensive Planning Nuclear Waste Division, U.S.A.*

Abstract

In 1987, Clark County was designated by the United States Congress and the U.S. Department of Energy as an "affected unit of local government" under the Nuclear Waste Policy Act, as amended. The Nuclear Waste Policy Act was designed to establish a location for a geologic high-level nuclear waste repository. Under the provisions of the Act, Clark County is permitted the opportunity to, among other things, conduct impact assessment studies and prepare reports to articulate the findings of those studies. Clark County staff and consultants have developed impact assessment studies and prepared reports in several key socioeconomic areas.

This paper summarizes the potential socio-economic impacts that have been identified as part of Clark County's Nuclear Waste program. These findings were incorporated into Clark County's Impact Assessment Report on the Yucca Mountain Program that was submitted to the Department of Energy. The Impact Assessment Report has been distributed in paper and compact disk format, as well as being placed on the Department of Comprehensive Planning Website.
Keywords: stigma, hazardous waste, nuclear, socio-economic, risk perception.

1 Introduction

The Nuclear Waste Policy Act (NWPA) was designed to establish a location for a geologic high-level nuclear waste repository. In 1987, Clark County was designated by the United States Congress and the U.S. Department of Energy as an "affected unit of local government" (AULG) under the Nuclear Waste Policy

Act, as amended (NWPAA). Under the provisions of the NWPAA, AULG's are authorized to conduct a broad range of activities in conjunction with DOE's site characterization activities at Yucca Mountain. These activities include reviewing and commenting on various U.S. Department of Energy (DOE) documents; independent socio-economic, environmental and technical impact analysis; and, public outreach and information dissemination.

This paper summarizes the results of the socio-economic impact assessment studies conducted by Clark County staff and consultants. The results that were incorporated into Clark County's Impact Report were submitted to the Secretary of Energy in 2001. It should be noted that this paper does not address the technical, environmental, and transportation findings that were also incorporated into the Impact Assessment Report. The paper begins with a brief summary of the bases for Clark County's activities. This is followed by an overview of the methodology and findings from the studies that have been conducted over the last fifteen years in the areas of:

- economic impacts;
- property value impacts;
- public safety impacts;
- other non-public safety governmental impacts: and
- public involvement.

1.1 Bases

Since 1983 Clark County has been recognized as an active participant in monitoring the DOE Yucca Mountain nuclear waste program efforts. In 1987, DOE officially designated Clark County as an "Affected Unit of Local Government (AULG)" under provisions of the NWPAA, when the search for a geologic repository study site was reduced to only one alternative: *Yucca Mountain.* The AULG designation was an acknowledgement by the federal government that activities associated with the Yucca Mountain Project could result in considerable impacts to our residents and community. In fact, the provisions under the Act enable Clark County to determine "any potential economic, social, public health and safety, and environmental impacts of a repository," 42 U.S.C. Section 10135(c)(1)(B)(i).

In addition to the NWPAA, applicable case law supports Clark County's efforts to fully identify potential impacts. In *County of Esmeralda v. Department of Energy*, 925 F.2d 1216 (9th Cir. 1991), the court stated: "Affected unit status is also meant to ensure that all potential harms from repository operation – whatever the current estimate of their probability—are sufficiently studied before Yucca Mountain is approved as a repository."

Further, under the National Environmental Policy Act (NEPA), the DOE is required to follow specific processes for identifying and assessing environmental impacts that may result from the operation of a nuclear waste repository at Yucca Mountain.

1.2 Economic impacts

Clark County, with a land area of over 7,900 square miles, is the fastest growing county in the United States. At the time of the decision to narrow the DOE's search for a suitable site to store high level radioactive nuclear waste (HLNW), Clark County's population was half what it is today, over 1.5 million. Over the next twenty years, the area's population is expected to reach 2.8 million. With more than 35 million visitors annually, the primary engine that drives economic growth is the gaming industry. Also key to Clark County's economic growth are service and construction-oriented businesses.

In a region where the concept of "perception is reality" is particularly marked, the stigma and perception of any danger associated with high level radioactive nuclear waste presents a very real and significant threat to Clark County residents, businesses, and visitors.

Thus, Clark County identified potential effects on the tourism industry of the DOE's proposal to ship high-level waste through Clark County to a repository at Yucca Mountain as a key area for study. In order to identify both the nature and the range of concerns of key tourism leaders, focused, confidential interviews were conducted with 14 gaming executives and a representative of one of their trade associations. The gaming executives represented 10 casinos that generate 95.5% of the *Earnings Before Interest, Taxes, Depreciation, and Amortization* (EBITDA) within Clark County's gaming industry.

According to the gaming executives, the current downturn in the U.S. economy was identified as a significant challenge that will likely contribute to slowing growth among this sector in the near term. Overall, however, most of the executives believe that despite short-term cyclical responses to national and worldwide economic conditions, the overall trend for the gaming industry in the absence of high level radioactive nuclear waste shipments is positive. Further, all of the gaming executives interviewed expressed concern that an accident, even a minor one along a route anywhere in Clark County, could have a devastating impact on their business. While some representatives were unsure of the scientific viability of the Yucca Mountain repository, all indicated that under no circumstance should trucks carrying high level radioactive nuclear waste come through Clark County. Several noted that just the transportation of high level radioactive nuclear waste coming from California through Clark County en route to Yucca Mountain, could significantly affect their business in an adverse manner. These industry representatives noted that congestion, particularly on weekends along the California/Nevada transportation corridor, has already proved problematic. They believe the addition of slow moving trucks containing such dangerous wastes will increase the likelihood and severity of an accident, discouraging some Californians from driving to Las Vegas. These representatives stated that Californians make up 30% of the visitors to Clark County. The increase in congestion along the California/Nevada corridor, combined with rising energy costs, is seen as a significant risk to gaming in Southern Nevada, especially for the Las Vegas downtown casinos.

According to the gaming industry executives the most serious risk is from the stigma that will result if there is a HLNW transportation accident of any kind involving the shipment of high level radioactive nuclear waste. These representatives referenced the media coverage that is likely to accompany any incident involving a vehicle transporting HLNW. Several stated that an accident anywhere in Clark County would be reported worldwide and would be linked to Las Vegas because it is the nearest media outlet.

In order to understand how the Yucca Mountain Project might influence visitation rates, a survey of 1,013 visitors was conducted in early December 2001. Among those surveyed, 25% indicated that just the shipment of high level radioactive nuclear waste through Clark County would affect their decision to visit Las Vegas in the future, even if there were no incidents of any type. Among the 25% who indicated that the shipments of high level radioactive nuclear waste would affect their decision to visit, 77% stated that they would reduce their visits and 12% stated that they would never visit Las Vegas again.

In the event of a HLNW transportation accident, even a minor accident, 37% of the visitors surveyed indicated that it would affect their decision to visit Las Vegas. Among these visitors, 49% stated that they would never visit Las Vegas again and 47% said that the frequency of their visits would decrease. If a serious accident resulting in a release of radiation were to occur, those surveyed indicated that the results would be devastating. Almost 80% noted that it would affect their decision and of those who stated that it would affect their decision, 62% stated that they would never visit Las Vegas again and 35% indicated that they would reduce the frequency of their visits.

1.3 Property value impacts

A scenario-based survey methodology of expert's, i.e., Clark County lenders and appraisers, was used to measure the nature and extent of any potential property value change that might occur as a result of the HLNW shipment campaign. The scenarios used in the property value study, are also used as part of the analysis of impacts on both public safety agencies and other governmental agencies within Clark County. These scenarios are described below. In addition, public opinion surveys were conducted to corroborate the findings of the technical experts.

1.4 Experts survey

The results of focused interviews with Clark County lenders and appraisers were applied to the assessed valuation data for three groups of land uses within Clark County. UER conducted a survey of 18 Clark County lenders and 35 certified appraisers in May 2000.

Under the first scenario, the appraisers and lenders were asked to evaluate whether there would be any changes in property values along the corridor if "no event" occurred, but there was adverse publicity, particularly, at the onset of the shipment campaign. This scenario was assigned to three discreet residential, commercial, and industrial properties that were characterized in terms of size, location, lease fees, and other factors. The lenders and appraisers were also asked to differentiate the level of impact, if any, that might be experienced at two varying distances along the corridor (within 1 mile of the shipment route and within 1 to 3 miles of shipment routes). A second scenario describes a HLNW shipment accident where no release of radiation occurs. The third scenario describes a serious HLNW shipment accident that is accompanied by a release of radiation.

Tables 1 and 2 summarize the results of the property value loss under each of the scenarios as estimated by the Clark County bankers and lenders. According to the lenders and appraisers, residential properties would lose the most value in percentage terms under each of the scenarios. For example, under Scenario 1, when the rates of property value diminution are applied to residential fair market value data at a distance of up to three miles from the Beltway route, the diminution ranges from $203.2 million to $462.5 million. From the I-15 route, the diminution ranges from $243.6 million to $549.6 million (Table 1).

What these tables suggest is that among those most experienced with estimating Clark County property values, there is a perception that significant adverse impacts will occur along either of the Clark County routes proposed, for all property types examined, even under the most benign scenario.

The findings also indicate that increasing the severity of events within the scenarios, as illustrated in Scenario 2 and 3, results in significantly larger rates of impact. Under Scenario 3, the most serious accident event evaluated, residential property diminution rises to $5.3 billion - $6.2 billion within 3 miles of the Beltway route and $6.2 billion - $7.3 billion within 3 miles of the I-15 route.

While, the many uncertainties surrounding the DOE's proposed HLNW shipment campaign make it impossible to estimate the nature and extent of any property value reductions, there is no doubt that it poses a significant threat to property values in Clark County.

Table 1: Property value diminutions under three scenarios within 3-mile distance of the proposed beltway route.

Groups	Residential	
	Lenders	Appraisers
Scenario 1	$203,219,474	$462,500,346
Scenario 2	$646,024,023	$1,175,472,314
Scenario 3	$5,269,739,823	$6,203,196,049
	Commercial	
Scenario 1	$5,615,300	$14,100,251
Scenario 2	$12,424,417	$33,873,129
Scenario 3	$171,414,257	$189,179,886
	Industrial	
Scenario 1	$5,919,186	$9,518,200
Scenario 2	$15,892,269	$27,680,400
Scenario 3	$125,658,343	$192,465,463

Table 2:   Property value diminutions under three scenarios within 3-miles of the I-15 shipment route, by professional group (Lenders and Appraisers).

Groups	Residential	
	Lenders	Appraisers
Scenario 1	$243,567,363	$549,526,426
Scenario 2	$772,643,577	$1,392,987,706
Scenario 3	$6,218,675,720	$7,318,862,089
	Commercial	
Scenario 1	$21,388,171	$72,531,494
Scenario 2	$76,137,260	$171,126,151
Scenario 3	$704,094,009	$926,894,417
	Industrial	
Scenario 1	$14,103,817	$25,012,894
Scenario 2	$54,535,563	$83,790,291
Scenario 3	$361,917,017	$507,543,183

Table 3:   Economic impacts based up property value estimates from years 2010 through 2035.

Economic Losses	Scenario 1	Scenario 3
	Minimum Impact	Maximum Impact
Population	11,294	90,718
Job	5,393	54,429
Gross Regional Product Annual Cumulative***	$182 million* $5.6 billion**	$1.4 billion* $68.1 billion**
Disposable Personal Income Annual Cumulative***	$136 million* $4.7 billion**	$686 million* $42.1 billion**

* Projected for 2010 in constant 1992 dollars.
** All dollars are in constant 1992 dollars due to the REMI model. Therefore, all dollars   represented are conservative estimates.
*** For period from 2010 through 2035; dollars are in constant 1992 dollars.

1.5 Economic losses based upon property values and population estimates

UNLV's CBER was requested to utilize the results from the lenders and appraisers survey as input into the Regional Economic Model, Inc. (REMI) and to compare these outputs to the normal REMI outputs. CBER estimated minimum and maximum impacts on employment, income, expenditures, and population. The REMI model utilizes 1992 dollars. Therefore, <u>all</u> dollars reflected in this section are in 1992 constant dollars. This results in estimates that are extremely conservative as shown in Table 3.

1.6 Minimum impacts (based upon scenario 1)

The impacts identified as minimum impacts within Scenario 1 (trucks utilizing the Clark County transportation system without incident) are as follows, Employment would be reduced by 5,393 jobs. Gross Regional Product (Spending) would be reduced by $185 million. This is a one-year figure and will be cumulative over the life of the project to $5.6 billion. Real Disposable Income would be reduced by $136 million for one year. Cumulatively, over the life of the project, losses of Real Disposable Income could exceed $4.7 billion. Population would be reduced by 11,294 people. This is an average population loss over the life of the project. Of interest to note is that over this last decade, the population within Clark County has <u>never</u> declined and in fact has grown, on average, 6.27% per year.

1.7 Maximum impacts (based upon scenario 3)

The impacts identified as maximum impacts within Scenario 3 (a serious accident including the release of radioactive materials involving the Clark County transportation system) are as follows. Employment would be reduced by 54,429 jobs. It should be noted that this is equivalent to increasing the current unemployment rate by approximately 6.5% (roughly 10 times the impact under Scenario 1) to more than 13%.

Gross Regional Product (Spending) would be reduced by $1.4 billion. This is a one-year figure and will be cumulative over the life of the project to $68.1 billion. This is equivalent to the expenditures made by over 30 major hotel properties. Real Disposable Income would be reduced by $686 million for one year. Cumulatively, over the life of the project, this figure rises to $42.1 billion. Population would be reduced by 90,718 people, more than 8 times the loss under Scenario 1. This is an average population loss over the life of the project. These estimates under Scenario 3 reflect an expected magnitude of impact. However, it is difficult to verify the duration and likelihood of this impact based upon the information provided by the DOE to date.

1.7.1 Residential survey

A random survey of 512 Clark County residents was conducted by the Canon Center at University of Nevada Las Vegas (UNLV) in August 2000. The purpose of the survey was to identify the attitudes, opinions, and perceptions of Clark County, Nevada residents regarding property values in Clark County, and to characterize their beliefs about the potential impacts of the proposed shipments on property values along the transportation corridor.

The survey found that over one-half of the residents of Clark County consider the risk of an accident from the transportation of radioactive wastes to be serious or very serious. Approximately 80% of the respondents indicated that they were familiar with the proposed Yucca Mountain Project, while 75% said that they knew about the DOE's plans to ship high level radioactive nuclear waste through Clark County.

Altogether almost 82% of the respondents stated that a nearby high level radioactive nuclear waste route would either "decrease a lot" or "decrease somewhat" their likelihood of purchasing a residential property. Seventy-eight percent of the respondents utilized negative terms to describe the effects of the proposed high level radioactive nuclear waste shipment campaign through Clark County.

Forty percent of the respondents indicated that commercial property would decrease with another 5.8% indicating generally "negative effects" on properties. Interestingly, 6.2% responding to this open-ended question suggested adverse effects on business operations located near these routes. In contrast to the general question on property values, 33.9% of responses to the question on commercial properties indicated that there would be "no effect" on these values. Almost three-fourths of the respondents declared that they would not consider purchasing property along the transportation routes under *any conditions*.

Eighty-two percent of the respondents believe such a property would sell for less, than an identical property that *is not near* such a route; 15% think it would not make a difference; and only the remaining 3% believe it would sell for more.

Of the 369 Clark County respondents who expect lower selling prices for homes near shipment routes, the mean expected drop in selling price in Clark County is estimated at approximately 25% compared to identical homes not near a highway that transports high-level radioactive nuclear waste.

1.8 Public safety impacts

The following fiscal impacts reflect an integrated view of impacts to all public safety agencies in Southern Nevada. The integrated impact study does not attempt to estimate the total costs to public safety agencies within Clark County government and its local jurisdictions from the Department of Energy's shipping of high level radioactive nuclear waste. Rather, only the incremental or additional costs to governmental entities that would be directly attributable to the siting of the repository at Yucca Mountain and the subsequent shipping campaign are projected. This fiscal impact study of public safety agencies uses a scenario based case study approach consistent with the survey of bankers and lenders. Public safety personnel were asked to describe how the events would impact their agency. Public safety personnel were then asked to compile a list of resources, training, personnel, equipment, and capital outlays necessary for them to be able to ensure the public health, safety, and welfare and to carry out their agency's mission for each of the three scenarios.

Because of the length of time between now and when shipments may actually begin, the ambiguities surrounding the actual shipment routes and the modal mix, the estimated fiscal projections are tentative.

Despite the high degree of professionalism and organization, none of the public safety agencies are currently adequately prepared, trained, or equipped to respond to any of the three high level radioactive nuclear waste shipping scenarios used in the study. This finding is consistent with the 1995 Public Safety Advisory Committee's report that examined public safety needs in Clark County.

The current County Emergency Operations Center that would be the focal point of the County's response to an incident involving high level radioactive nuclear waste is only adequate for a very short duration event.

Southern Nevada hospitals are not adequately equipped, nor are personnel properly trained to effectively manage a high level radioactive nuclear waste incident like that contained in Scenario 3. The hospital system is already strained under current needs, and the projected hospital needs for the area are daunting. This system will not be adequate to handle the events described in the scenarios in this study.

The total projected cost to just the public safety agencies examined in this study to be adequately prepared for a Scenario 3 event is $359,986,630 (Table 4).

Table 4:   Total projected costs by community/county.

	Cost
Clark County	$274,196,809
Las Vegas	$45,158,058
North Las Vegas	$23,340,046
Henderson	$1,386,929
Mesquite	$6,980,411
Boulder City	$404,880
Moapa	$8,519,497
Totals	$359,986,630

* Las Vegas Metro provides services to both Clark County and the City of Las Vegas
** Because of the projected distance to the high level radioactive nuclear waste shipment corridor, Boulder City estimated impacts only for the Police Department.
*** In Mesquite, Emergency Management is a function of the Fire Department and thus costs are combined under Fire.

The largest projected costs to these public safety agencies fall under the categories of facilities, equipment, personnel, and training. For police services, the projected fiscal cost is over $72.5 million for the communities examined in this study. The Fire Departments' projected fiscal costs total over $275.3 million, and the Offices of Emergency Management fiscal cost projections total over $12 million. These cost projections are for the agencies to be prepared for a Scenario 3 incident beginning in 2010. The projections do not include costs that will be recurring such as vehicle and equipment replacement costs or the dollar costs of training new employees after 2007. Hence, the fiscal cost projections in the report will tend to underestimate (are conservative) some of the fiscal impacts to the public safety agencies.

Additional Haz/Mat Radiological personnel, training, and equipment are viewed as critical needs among the public safety agencies. The hospitals lack sufficient decontamination facilities, equipment, and trained personnel.

Current planning activities are progressing, regional public safety organizations are beginning to grapple with the problems posed by high level radioactive nuclear waste shipments, and a Southern Nevada hospital system approach is developing with the help of the Clark County Health District. There is a critical need for a strong regional effort to ensure that the County, the municipalities, and the Moapa Band of Paiutes are prepared for high level radioactive nuclear waste shipments. Additional resources for the hospitals and the Health District are not projected in this study, only their training and equipment needs.

References

[1] Urban Environmental Research, Clark County Property Value Report on the Effects of DOE's Proposal to Ship High Level Radioactive Waste to a Repository at Yucca Mountain, (June 2001).
[2] Urban Environmental Research, Impacts to Clark County Public Safety Agencies Resulting from the Yucca Mountain Project (June 2001).
[3] Urban Environmental Research, Impacts to Clark County Non-Public Safety Governmental Agencies Resulting from the Yucca Mountain Repository, (June 2001).
[4] Urban Environmental Research, Gaming Industry Impacts Resulting from the DOE's Yucca Mountain Proposal (June 2001)

Application of the ISHTAR Suite for the assessment of the health effects of Rome environmental policy

E. Negrenti[1], A. Agostini[1], M. Lelli[1], P. Mudu[2], A. Parenti[3] & C. Lanciano[4]

[1]ENEA, Italy
[2]WHO-ECEH, Rome, Italy
[3]ASTRAN S.r.l.Viterbo, Italy
[4]G&O S.r.l.,Rome, Italy

Abstract

The ISHTAR Suite is an innovative software tool that integrates several models for the simulation of the effects of transport and land use policies on the urban environment, population health and artistic heritage. Starting from the simulation of the effects of the postulated measure on the citizens behaviour in terms of daily movements, the suite calculation path goes through the modelling of transport, vehicles safety and emissions of pollutants and noise, pollutants dispersion and noise propagation, exposure to pollutants, noise and accidents and related risk assessment, monuments degradation, up to the overall comparison of the alternative scenarios in terms of cost-benefit or multi criteria analysis. The software modules are integrated by a Suite Manager that controls the tools execution by means of dedicated software 'connectors', and is linked to a User Interface, a suite database and a commercial Geographic Information System. The ISHTAR Suite is now being tested in the seven cities involved in the FP5 EESD Programme ISHTAR Project: Athens, Bologna, Brussels, Graz, Grenoble, Paris and Rome, with the analysis of different measures and policies. In the Rome application the effects on health of a traffic banning policy were studied.
Keywords: integrated software, models suite, policies assessment, urban planning, transport systems impacts, traffic banning.

1 Introduction

Worldwide cities face common challenges concerning their quality of life: degradation of the urban environment, significant risks for citizens health, traffic congestion causing stress and economic inefficiency, progressive damage of the artistic and monumental heritage. Additional difficulties derive from the lack of integrated tools that allow cities to make balanced decisions on a wide range of issues. In this context the European Commission funded in 2001 the ISHTAR Project (Negrenti et al. [1]) aiming at building an Integrated Suite of software models for assessing the impacts of urban policies and actions on the quality of life of citizens, and in particular on traffic congestion, air quality, citizens health and conservation of monuments.

The ISHTAR Project (Negrenti et al. [2]) had several objectives:
• The integration of a large number of software tools and the creation of specific modules for the simulation of key processes such as transport behaviour and its direct impacts on the urban environment.
• The achievement of a high spatial and temporal flexibility in the use of the tool, for maximizing the possibilities of application from local short-term actions to widespread long-term policies.
• Development of specific modelling areas such as the representation of policies effects on citizens behaviour, the 24 hours simulation of traffic emissions, noise and safety, the analysis of air pollution effects on health and monuments.

2 Methodology

2.1 Integration of a relevant number of modelling tools

The ISHTAR Suite is based on a high number of software tools whose aim is the modelling of various aspects of the impact analysis of short-term actions and long-term policies. Standard models suites normally include only a few of those models. It also represents a strong enlargement of the applicability area, since with this kind of 'multi-impacts' suite the users are able to analyse in an integrated and 'coherent' way the various aspects of 'global' urban policies, without having to perform separate studies relying on different input data. The wide scope of applicability offers the potential of easing the cooperation between different departments in municipal authorities: in fact the tool will be of interest for planning and assessment work in the transport, environment, health and artistic heritage sectors.

2.2 Evolution of modelling techniques in crucial impact areas

The scientific core value of the Suite is largely linked to a few crucial modelling developments on which the accuracy and the significance of the results deriving from the Suite application strongly depend. These areas are:

a) prediction of the effects of citizens' reaction to postulated measures.

b) improvement of the modelling of vehicle emissions, particularly concerning the consideration of speed variability along the network links, and the spatial-temporal distribution of 'cold start emissions'.

c) development of an urban road safety model, which can take into account the variable flow levels in the network

d) disaggregated estimate of pollution effects on citizens' health based on the analysis of population groups' movements.

2.3 Realisation of integrated specific modules inside the suite

The ISHTAR Suite aims at the highest flexibility of use: this is reflected in some of the tools. The choice of building an 'Integrated Transport Module' which makes use of different models, having complementary characteristics in terms of applicability field, is of key significance. Also relevant is the consequence of this flexibility in transport modelling: the downstream models (emission, noise, safety, exposure models) will have to be flexible in their input characteristics in order to give the proper accuracy whichever transport model is used. This implies the use of 'advanced' emission, noise and safety models capable of treating flexible input data. Also the module dedicated to the overall evaluation of the policy scenarios includes parallel elements: in this case a Cost Benefit Analysis tool is complemented by a Multi criteria Analysis software.

2.4 Space and time flexibility

Among the crucial characteristics of the Suite, a large flexibility in space and time plays an essential role. The starting point for the achievement of this goal was the realization of the so called '24hours capability': traffic flows, vehicles speed, emissions, noise levels, pollution levels are calculated (when needed) hour by hour thanks to the characteristics of the citizens behaviour, transport, emission, noise and dispersion models that have been selected or developed. This flexibility greatly enhances the scope of applicability of the tool.

3   Project results

The ISHTAR Suite (Negrenti et al. [3]) was built over the following software modules including one or more software tool. The modules exchange a number of data, schematically represented in Figure 1.

3.1 The Cellular Transport Methodology

The Cellular Transport Methodology (CTM) is a new software tool developed by ISIS (Italy) that simulates the effects of policies and measures on the behaviour of citizens in terms of movements, thus producing the modified Origin-Destination matrices. This tool is considered as an 'ancillary element' of the suite because it is likely that the city teams wishing to use the ISHTAR software will already have a local 'mobility demand model' or alternative techniques for estimating the modification of the trip matrices.

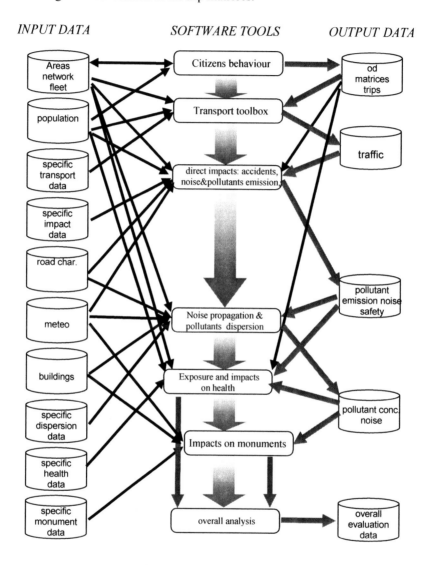

Figure 1: Main Data flows and Input-Output Data in ISHTAR Suite.

3.2 The transport toolbox

After an analysis of the available transport models, the new VISUPOLIS model has been selected as the best tool to integrate in the suite. This model has been developed by PTV (Germany) integrating the well-known VISUM model and the innovative tool 'METROPOLIS' by Prof. A. De Palma from the University of Clergy Pontoise (F). However the potential users are free to continue to use their own traffic model (as most of the cities participating in ISHTAR Project did). VISUPOLIS is now being tested in the Paris case study (the Car Free day).

3.3 The Transport Direct impacts module

The direct impacts model chosen for the suite is TEE2004, developed by ENEA and ASTRAN (Italy). This tool is particularly flexible in terms of space and time, includes advanced modelling of kinematics and cold start effects on the emissions, and feeds several downstream suite elements by calculating the emissions of pollutants and noise and the occurrence of accidents. The tool is compatible with most of the traffic models output. In facts the large number of options about the description of vehicle kinematics, the definition of the local fleet at link level and the approach for estimating the fraction of cold vehicles guarantees an easy coupling with the upstream used traffic model.

3.4 Noise propagation and pollutants dispersion module

The pollutants dispersion can be calculated with one of the two tools provided by ARIA Technologies depending on the spatial and time scale. For urban scale and long term analysis the suite will rely on ARIA Impacts, while for meso scale and short term events ARIA Regional will be the future reference, not yet fully integrated in the suite. For the noise propagation the Soundplan software (by Braunstein and Berndt GmbH - D) has been integrated. These software tools operate on a common and harmonised set of input data.

3.5 Exposure and Impacts on Health module

For assessing population exposure to pollutants and noise, a completely new software denominated TEX (Transport Exposure) has been developed by WHO (ECEH office in Rome). Such a tool provides exposure of population groups in their residential areas or along the trips in the city network. The evaluation of the health risk related to the exposure to pollutants, noise and accidents is run with the HIT software, also developed by WHO. This tool provides estimates of life years lost due to air pollution, noise annoyance and accidents effects.

3.6 Impacts on monuments

The air pollutants impact on monuments is simulated by a software developed by ENEA (I) and PHAOS (GR). This software named MODA (Monuments Damage) can assess the loss of material and the deposition of crust and the money needed for maintenance. The model provides estimates of damage for specific monuments or for types of monuments and buildings.

3.7 Overall scenarios analysis tool

For the overall analysis of the policy scenarios two methodologies and software pieces are available: the Cost-Benefit Analysis and the Multi-Criteria Analysis.

These tools gather the data from the upstream models and give the results of the comparison of the scenarios considered. In any case the MCA takes into account the results of the CBA. Both of them are developed by TRaC – LMU (UK).

3.8 Software integration

The integration of the modules is made by a Software Manager that launches the 'software connectors'. The connectors upload the data needed by the single tool in the appropriate format, launches the tool and then downloads the results of the run in the ISHTAR Suite Database making them available for other tools or for the output through the Geographic Information System (ARCGIS) used for managing geographic data. An overall scheme representing the integration architecture of the ISHTAR suite is reported in Figure 2.

3.9 Case studies

The suite is being tested with seven case studies involving the cities of ISHTAR project: Athens, Bologna, Brussels, Graz, Grenoble, Paris and Rome. These studies can be summarised as follows.

The Athens case study 'Attiki Odos' addresses the motorway, Attica Periphery Road, which is assessed in terms of traffic, toll strategy and pricing, and environmental impacts. The Bologna Provincial Authority case study concerns the evaluation of infrastructure scenarios for the city of Imola with reference to alternative road paths. The aim of the Belgian case study is to prepare the implementation of traffic banning measures in the Brussels area, according to the Plan Ozone of the Federal Government. In the Brussels case study the focus is on the population behaviour, the modelling of traffic flows and the effects of the measure on pollutant emissions. The Graz case study is based on the traffic and noise impact evaluation of a 600 m long new road tunnel causing a relevant local traffic rerouting. Grenoble case study is intended to monitor the effects of the installation of reserved lanes for public transportation and new traffic lights on boulevards with heavy traffic. The focus in this case is on traffic and emissions. Every September 22nd the city of Paris takes part in a car free day. This typical short-term event can be modelled with the ISHTAR suite of modules. The results include emissions of pollutants and air pollution. The Rome large-scale case study involves the HEAVEN FP5 Project area banning to the more polluting vehicles. In the northern part of the city centre a number of models of the suite have been used, from the locally available traffic model (Transcad) to the Overall Evaluation module.

4   Application to the Rome policies for environmental quality

The city of Rome has established various strategies to tackle traffic problems implementing a framework to rebalance the modal split towards public transport and promote alternative means of transport. An access restriction for non-catalysed vehicles has been implemented within the "Rail Ring". The "Rail Ring" area, which surrounds the historic centre, is densely populated with a high concentration of activities making it one of the key areas in the city for interventions to reduce emissions caused by vehicles. This measure had as main effect a change in the fleet composition and no major effects were expected on traffic flows. The measures impact on urban mobility has been performed by the Rome Agency for Mobility (STA) throughout the analysis of detected traffic flows on predefined road links carried out in four different campaigns (November 2001, February 2002, May 2002 and November 2002), one for each stage of the Rail Ring restriction policies implementation.

A simulation of the ISHTAR suite was prepared to test the input-output connections among different software of the suite, data exchange with external software, modelling factors, and clarity of output comprehension. The analysis carried on is based on a comparison between two simulated scenarios:

1) Do nothing scenario;
2) Actual scenario (based on the traffic measures described above).

Pollutants modelled both by the Emission and Dispersion modules were CO and PM10. CO was also modelled by the exposure module and PM10 by the Health effects module.

4.1 Area of investigation

The Rome case study involves the "Heaven" area within the internal rail-ring, excluding the Rome "ZTL" (Limited Traffic zone) that covers part of the historical centre. The laboratory area of ISHTAR Project (see Figure 2) has a surface of 16.35 square kilometres. This area represents a "bridge" between the historical Centre and the peripheral North areas. The socio-economic status of the population is here high and there is a big flow of traffic going through the area, mainly in the roman consular streets Nomentana and Salaria, but also through some primary streets. Green areas in this domain are Villa Borghese and Villa Ada (where there is an air quality monitoring station). The Origin-Destination Matrices (O/D) used in the traffic simulation phase, with the static assignment model TRANSCAD, are based on the data obtained by the National Statistical Institute (ISTAT) census. An update, with the aim of defining more realistic traffic values has been carried out by means of 40,000 telephone interviews and this made it possible the evaluation on the daily car and motorcycle O/D matrices. The fleet composition is defined in accordance with ACI (Italian Automobile Club).

Rome air monitoring network consists of 13 monitoring stations classified in four different types: A (located in areas not directly affected by traffic sources such as park or green areas), B (located in areas with heavy traffic conditions), C (located in residential areas) and D (located outside the urban area, almost in the countryside). The monitoring network acquires concentration data every hour. Data are sent to the regional environmental protection Agency (ARPA) for validation and delivered to the Environmental Department of the Municipality of Rome that is responsible for data collecting, storing and delivering. Moreover the

Municipality of Rome carries on campaigns with diffusion tubes. These campaigns last one week and are distributed on the whole urban area, during different periods of the year. Monitoring tubes are usually located in secondary streets, to give information on background pollution. Population data include:

· Registered residents in the area in the year 1999, split by gender and age;
· Registered residents in the area in the year 2000;
· Working people in the year 1991.

The population registers were used as source of population data

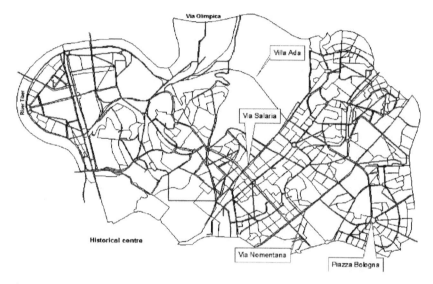

Figure 2:   The HEAVEN area considered for the application of the ISHTAR Suite.

4.2 Impacts of the measure

Taking into account the traffic data (flows and speeds along all the links) calculated by TRANSCAD, the direct impact model (TEE2004) software has been used for the calculation of CO and PM10 emissions. The aggregated results of TEE during the simulation day shows the reduction of CO of about 50%, in terms of emissions, confirms the validity of the adoption of the catalyst system regarding such kind of pollution. Regarding the Particulate Matter with diameter below 10 micrometer the emission reduction is about 18 percent. Pollutant concentrations, the 12th of November 2001, have been calculated for CO and PM10 with the Gaussian dispersion model ARIA IMPACT (by Aria Technologies) taking into account the emission data calculated by TEE, the measured meteorological data, the topography and the background measured by the Villa Ada monitoring station.

  The pollutant concentrations due to the emission within the Heaven area are low, as the area is quite small and surrounded by the city, in fact the concentration increase due to the calculated emissions coming from the road traffic, compared to the background is about 2,5 % for PM10 and 10 % for CO. In any case the difference in terms of concentration between the two scenarios is 0,33 % for PM10 and 4,76 % for CO.

After running the ARIA model in ISHTAR it is possible to calculate the exposure of people to a pollutant through software TEX (Traffic EXposure). The dispersion values considered for an exposure assessment cover the period of one day (the model refers to the 12th November 2001). The data, obtained from a Transcad output produced by STA, were considered as an hourly series from midnight to midnight. As expected, results indicate a stronger exposure of the people living and working on the main arterial network but also some area of high exposure of CO with low population concentration and some areas with lower level of exposure with high population concentrations (see Fig.3). While the exposure output, if all inputs are available, offer an evaluation of the relation between a spatial dispersion of a pollutant and the distribution of the population, the application of dose-response curves happens at a broader approximate level. In fact, as it is well-known to assess the effects of a particular pollutant, in our case of ambient PM10 pollution, over an exposed population, there are two assumptions to be done: the concentration consists of the average measured in the city or area where the population live, everyone is assumed to be exposed to the same average concentration. With this information it is possible to calculate the attributable risk as a proportion, while to obtain the absolute number of attributable cases it is necessary to know, in addition, the observed rates of disease or mortality occurrence in the population under study. Within the ISHTAR suite the HIT software is included to assess the impacts of different sources of traffic-generated pollutants.

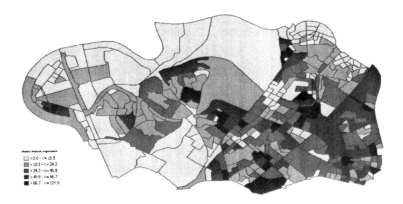

Figure 3:   Exposure simulation output.

The estimation of health impacts is possible by applying dose-response curves made available through the analysis of available literature. In the case under investigation the impact was simulated of the average value estimated for PM10 as it was a yearly average affecting the whole resident population. Total mortality was chosen as health end-point, both for the 'do nothing' and 'actual' scenarios. Concentrations of PM10 greater than 20 micrograms per cubic meter, considering an average of 30 produces a long term effect in terms of estimated number of excess cases of 337 (95% CI =110-558) and short term effects as 27 (95% CI = 23-32). Estimates are not only intended as "impact" on health, but ideally as "gains" that would be achieved by reducing average concentrations.

5   Conclusions

The ISHTAR Suite has the potential of becoming a reference tool for the future planning of urban policies in terms of traffic, environment, health, monuments protection (Negrenti [4]). The integrated tool will ease cooperation among planning departments of municipalities and will be of interest also for environmental agencies, consultants, transport companies, ministries. Project conclusion in May 2005 will be followed by a pre-commercialisation phase allowing the involved partners to transform a research project result into a marketable tool or a software system for running calculation services. Future users of the suite are expected in a fully international environment, having assessed the high interest by audiences worldwide (Negrenti [5] and Negrenti and Agostini [6]).

References

[1]   Negrenti, E. et al.: ISHTAR Project Proposal to EC DG RES (Issued by ENEA as Project Coordinator), p. 1-99, 2000.
[2]   Negrenti, E. et al.: ISHTAR Contract EVK4 CT-00034 (issued in Brussels by EC DG RES) p. 1-xx , 2001.
[3]   Negrenti E. et al.: ISHTAR web site: http://www.ishtar-fp5-eu.com, 2002.
[4]   Negrenti, E and Hoglund P. 'ISHTAR: an Integrated Models Suite for Sustainable Regional and Town Planning – Cities of Tomorrow Conference – Goteborg (S) – 23-24 August 2001.
[5]   Negrenti, E. 'ISHTAR Project: Building a Model Suite for Urban Sustainability - 21st ARRB/11th REAAA Conference 'TRANSPORT - our highway to a sustainable future' – Cairns – 18-23 May 2003.
[6]   Negrenti, E. Agostini, A. 'ISHTAR': 'integrated software for health, transport efficiency and artistic heritage recovery' 'Transport induced Air Pollution conference – Boulder (CO), September 2004.

Author Index

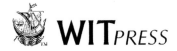

Environmental Exposure and Health

Editors: *M.M. ARAL, Georgia Institute of Technology, USA, C.A. BREBBIA, Wessex Institute of Technology, UK, M.L. MASLIA, ATSDR/CDC, USA and T. SINKS, NCEH, USA*

Featuring contributions from health specialists, social and physical scientists and engineers this volume evaluates current issues in exposure and epidemiology and highlights future directions and needs. Originally presented at the First International Conference on Environmental Exposure and Health, the papers included cover areas such as: METHODOLOGICAL TOPICS - Multipathway Exposure Analysis and Epidemiology; Statistical and Numerical Methods. SITE RELATED TOPICS - Work Place and Industrial Exposure; Air Pollution Exposure and Epidemiology. DATA COLLECTION TOPICS - Use of Remote Sensing and GIS; Data Mining and Applications in Epidemiology. SPECIAL TOPICS - Exposure Specific to the Developing World; Effects of Rapid Transportation in Epidemiology.
Series: The Sustainable World, Vol 14
ISBN: 1-84564-029-2   2005   apx 400pp
apx £140.00/US$224.00/€210.00

Environmental Health in Central Asia
The Present and Future

Editor: *D. FAYZIEVA, Academy of Sciences, Uzbekistan*

This book provides information on how environmental conditions in Central Asia have been affected by anthropogenic activity. It also reviews research carried out during the last decades on the impact of the environment on the health of the region's people.

Partial Contents: Air Quality and Population Health in Central Asia; Hydrosphere and Health of Population in the Aral Sea Basin;   Influence of Environmental Factors on Development of Non-Communicable Diseases; Environment and Infectious Diseases; Environment and Children's Health in Central Asia.
Series: Advances in Ecological Sciences, Vol 17
ISBN: 1-85312-945-3   2004   284pp
£84.00/US$134.00/€126.00

Safety and Security Engineering

Editors: *C.A. BREBBIA, Wessex Institute of Technology, UK, and T. BUCCIARELLI, F. GARZIA and M. GUARASCIO, University of Rome 'La Sapienza', Italy*

This book details recent developments in the theoretical and practical aspects of safety and security engineering. Originally presented at the first international conference on this topic, the contributions included highlight issues
including risk analysis, crisis management, security engineering, natural disasters and emergencies, terrorism, IT security, man-made hazards, and forensic studies.
The material provided will be of interest to engineers, scientists, field researchers, managers and other specialists involved in one or more aspects of safety and security.
ISBN: 1-84564-019-5   2005   944pp
£330.00/US$528.00/€495.00

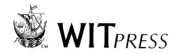
WITPRESS

Air Pollution XIII

Editor: **C.A. BREBBIA**, *Wessex Institute of Technology, UK*

Bringing together recent results and state-of-the-art contributions from researchers and practitioners active in the field of air contamination, this book contains papers from the Thirteenth International Conference on the Modelling, Monitoring and Management of Air Pollution. Experimental as well as computational techniques are featured in order to provide readers with a better understanding of the problems involved and potential solutions. The contributors cover topics including: Air Pollution Modelling; Air Quality Management; Atmospheric Chemistry; Urban Air Pollution; Transport Emissions; Monitoring and Laboratory Studies; Global and Regional Studies; Climatology; Indoor Pollution; Pollution Engineering; Aerosols and Particles; Health Effects; Remote Sensing; Biogenics, Agriculture and Landfill Emissions; and Acoustic Pollution.
Series: Advances in Air Pollution, Vol 15
ISBN: 1-85312-014-4   2005   696pp
£245.00/US$392.00/€367.50

Waste Management and the Environment II

Editors: **V. POPOV**, *Wessex Institute of Technology, UK,* **H. ITOH**, *University of Nagoya, Japan,* **C.A. BREBBIA**, *Wessex Institute of Technology, UK and* **A. KUNGOLOS**, *University of Thessaly, Greece,*

Highlighting present challenges and opportunities for progress, this book contains over 65 papers from the Second International Conference on Waste Management and the Environment. The topics discussed will be of interest to a wide readership including government officials, waste disposal experts, research scientists specialising in this area, and environmental engineers.
The contributions are divided under the following broad subject headings: Advanced Waste Treatment Technology; Hazardous Waste Management; Disposal of Hazardous Waste in Underground Mines; Biological Treatment of Waste; Biosolids, Composting and Agricultural Issues; Environmental Effects and Remediation; Waste Reduction and Recycling; Landfills, Design, Construction and Monitoring; Waste Management, Strategies and Planning; Waste Management in Greece; Waste and Wastewater Treatment; and Methodologies and Practices.
ISBN: 1-85312-738-8   2004   696pp
£245.00/US$392.00/€367.50

Human Exposure to Electromagnetic Fields

D. POLJAK, *University of Split, Croatia*

The first comprehensive text on the many aspects of interaction between human beings and electromagnetic fields.
Partial Contents: Electromagnetic and Thermal Modelling of the Human Body; Safety Standards and Exposure Limits.
Series: Advances in Electrical and Electronic Engineering, Vol 6
ISBN: 1-85312-997-6   2004   200pp
£81.00/US$129.00/€121.50

All prices correct at time of going to press but subject to change.
WIT Press books are available through your bookseller or direct from the publisher.

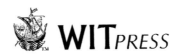

Waste Management in Japan

Editor: **H. ITOH**, *University of Nagoya, Japan*

This book contains contributions first presented in the special session Advanced Waste Treatment and Management in Japan at the Second International Conference on Waste Management and the Environment. Subjects discussed include the novel utilization of wasted materials for glass-ceramics or pollutant absorbers, hazardous waste detoxification and extraction techniques, the recycling of organic or agricultural wastes, and advanced incineration technology for thermal recycling.
The papers featured will help the international waste management community gain an appreciation of current issues in Japan together with their technical solutions.
ISBN: 1-84564-000-4   2004   192pp
£90.00/US$144.00/€135.00

WIT eLibrary

Home of the Transactions of the Wessex Institute, the WIT electronic-library provides the international scientific community with immediate and permanent access to individual papers presented at WIT conferences. Visitors to the WIT eLibrary can freely browse and search abstracts of all papers in the collection before progressing to download their full text.

Visit the WIT eLibrary at:
http://www.witpress.com

Water Pollution VII

Modelling, Measuring and Prediction

Editors: **C.A. BREBBIA**, *Wessex Institute of Technology, UK, and* **D. ALMORZA** *and*
D. SALES, *University of Cadiz, Spain*

This book features most of the papers presented at the Seventh International Conference on this subject. Almost 50 contributions providing some of the latest results are divided under headings such as: Experimental and Laboratory Work; and Agricultural Pollution.
Series: Progress in Water Resources, Vol 9
ISBN: 1-85312-976-3   2003   528pp
£158.00/US$249.00/€237.00

Risk Analysis IV

Editor: **C.A. BREBBIA**, *Wessex Institute of Technology, UK*

This volume contains over 70 papers from the fourth in the popular international conference series on this subject. Topics covered include: Seismic Risk; Landslides and Slope Movements; Floods and Droughts; Man-Made Risk; Estimation of Risk; Risk Assessment and Management; Risk Mitigation; and Hazard Prevention.
Contributions from three special sessions highlighting the work of renowned international experts are also featured. These deal with Geomorphic Hazard and Risk, Seismic Risk Analysis in Mediterranean Cities, and Landslides from Hazard to Risk Prevention.
Series: Management Information Systems, Vol 9
ISBN: 1-85312-736-1   2004   832pp
£291.00/US$465.00/€436.50